Respiratory
Pharmacology and
Pharmacotherapy

Series Editors:

Dr. David Raeburn
Discovery Biology
Rhône-Poulenc Rorer Ltd
Dagenham Research Centre
Dagenham
Essex RM10 7XS
England

Dr. Mark A. Giembycz
Department of Thoracic Medicine
National Heart and Lung Institute
Imperial College of Science, Technology and Medicine
London SW3 6LY
England

Nitric Oxide in Pulmonary Processes: Role in Physiology and Pathophysiology of Lung Disease

Edited by
M. G. Belvisi
J. A. Mitchell

Springer Basel AG

Editors:

Dr. Maria G. Belvisi
Pharmacology Department
Rhône-Poulenc Rorer
Research & Development
Rainham Road South
Dagenham, Essex RM 10 7XS
UK

Dr. Jane A. Mitchell
Unit of Critical Care Medicine
Imperial College Medical School
Royal Brompton Hospital
Sidney Street
London SW3 6NP
UK

Library of Congress Cataloging-in-Publication Data

Nitric oxide in pulmonary processes : role in physiology and
    pathophysiology of lung disease / edited by M. G. Belvisi, J. A. Mitchell.
        p.   cm. – (Respiratory pharmacology and pharmacotherapy)
    Includes index.
        ISBN 978-3-0348-9582-8   ISBN 978-3-0348-8474-7 (eBook)
    DOI 10.1007/978-3-0348-8474-7
    1. Lungs – Physilogy.   2. Nitric oxide – Physiological effect.
    3. Lungs – Pathophysiology.   4. Nitric oxide – Pathophysiology.
    I. Belvisi, M. G. (Maria G.) II. Series.
        [DNLM: 1. Lung – physiology.   2. Nitric Oxide – physiology.   3. Lung
    Diseases – drug therapy.   4. Lung Diseases – physiopathology.
    5. Nitric Oxide – therapeutic use.   WF 600 N7315 1999]
    QP121.N575   2000
    612.2 – dc21
DNLM/DLC
for Library of Congress

Die Deutsche Bibliothek – CIP-Einheitsaufnahme

Nitric oxide in pulmonary processes : role in physiology and
pathophysiology of lung disease / ed. by M. G. Belvisi ; J. A.
Mitchell. – Basel ; Boston ; Berlin : Birkhäuser, 2000
        (Respiratory pharmacology and pharmacotherapy)

    ISBN 978-3-0348-9582-8

© 2000 Springer Basel AG
Originally published by Birkhäuser Verlag in 2000
Softcover reprint of the hardcover 1st edition 2000
Printed on acid-free paper produced from cholorine-free pulp. TCF ∞
Cover design: Markus Etterich

ISBN 978-3-0348-9582-8

9 8 7 6 5 4 3 2 1

Contents

List of Contributors VII

Foreword IX

Introduction to Nitric Oxide Biology

1. Nitric Oxide Synthesis and Actions
   David Bishop-Bailey and Jane A. Mitchell 3

2. Reactive Oxygen and Reactive Nitrogen Species in the Lung
   Gregroy J. Quinlan and Nicholas J. Lamb 21

Role of Endogenous Nitric Oxide in the Lung

3. Non-Adrenergic Non-Cholinergic Neurotransmission
   in the Airways: Role of Nitric Oxide
   Maria G. Belvisi and Alan Gibson 41

4. Localisation of Nitric Oxide Synthases in the Lung
   Axel Fischer 71

5. Role of Nitric Oxide in the Regulation of Pulmonary Vascular
   Tone
   Shu Fang Liu and Timothy W. Evans 89

6. Nitric Oxide and Bronchial Hyperresponsiveness
   Frans P. Nijkamp and Gert Folkerts 111

7. Bronchodilator Actions of Nitric Oxide and Related Compounds
   Sanjay Mehta and Jeffrey M. Drazen 127

8. Role of Nitric Oxide in Airway Inflammation
   El-Bdaoui Haddad 151

**Therapeutic Potential of Inhalded Nitric Oxide and Nitric Oxide
Synthase Inhibitors in Lung Disease**

9. Nitric Oxide in Exhaled Air: Relevance in Inflammatory
   Lung Disease
   Peter J. Barnes and Sergei A. Kharitonov 167

10. Luminal Nitric Oxide in the Upper Airways: Implications
    for Local and Distal Sites of Action
    Kjell Alving, Jon O.N. Lundberg, Johan Rinder
    and Eddie Weitzberg. 185

11. Inhaled Nitric Oxide as a Therapy for Diseases
    of the Pulmonary Vasculature
    Helen M. Marriott and Timothy W. Higenbottam 201

12. Combinded Use of Nitric Oxide and Nitric Oxide Synthase
    Inhibitors as a Possible Therapeutic Approach
    Christoph Thiemermann 209

Index 227

List of Contributors

Kjell Alving, Department of Physiology and Pharmacology, Karolinska Institute, S-171 77 Stockholm, Sweden; e-mail: kjell.alving@fyfa.ki.se

Peter J. Barnes, Department of Thoracic Medicine, National Heart and Lung Institute, Imperial College School of Medicine, Dovehouse Street, London SW3 6LY, UK; e-mail: p.f.barnes@ic.ac.uk

Maria G. Belvisi, Pharmacology Department, Rhône-Poulenc Rorer Research & Development, Rainham Road South, Dagenham, Essex RM 10 7XS, UK; e-mail: Maria.Belvisi@rp-rorer.co.uk

David Bishop-Bailey, Department of Physiology, University of Connecticut Health Center, 263 Farmington Avenue, Farmington, CT 06030, USA; e-mail: Bishop@sun.uchc.edu

Jeffrey M. Drazen, Pulmonary and Critical Care Division, Brigham and Women's Hospital, Harvard Medical School, 75 Francis Street, Boston, MA 02115, USA

Timothy W. Evans, Unit of Critical Care, Royal Brompton Hospital, National Heart and Lung Institute at Imperial College, Sydney Street, London SW3 6NP, UK; e-mail: t.evans@rbh.nthames.nhs.uk

Axel Fischer, Department of Anatomy and Cell Biology, Justus-Liebig-University, Aulweg 123, D-35385 Giessen, Germany; e-mail: axel.fischer@anatomie.med.uni-giessen.de

Gert Folkerts, Department of Pharmacology and Pathophysiology, Faculty of Pharmacy, University of Utrecht, NL-3508 TB Utrecht, The Netherlands; e-mail: G.Folkerts@pharm.uu.nl

Alan Gibson, Pharmacology Group, Biomedical Sciences Division, King's College London, Manresa Road, Chelsea, London SW3 6LX, UK

El-Bdaoui Haddad, Pharmacology Department, Rhône-Poulenc Rorer Research & Development, Rainham Road South, Dagenham, Essex RM 10 7XS, UK; e-mail: el-bdaoui.haddad@rp-rorer.co.uk

Timothy W. Higenbottam, Section of Respiratory Medicine, Clinical Sciences Division (CSUHT), University of Sheffield, Floor F, The Medical School, Beech Hill Road, Sheffield S10 2RX, UK; e-mail T.Higenbottam@shef.ac.uk

Sergei A. Kharitonov, Department of Thoracic Medicine, National Heart and Lung Institute, Imperial College School of Medicine, Dovehouse Street, London SW3 6LY, UK; e-mail: s.kharitonov@ic.ac.uk

Nicholas J. Lamb, Unit of Critical Care, Royal Brompton Hospital, National Heart and Lung Institute at Imperial College, Sydney Street, London SW3 6NP, UK; e-mail: n.lamb@ic.ac.uk

Shu Fang Liu, Long Island Jewish Medical Center, Albert Einstein College of Medicine, 270-5 76th Avenue, New Hyde Park, NY 11040, USA; e-mail: sliu@lij.edu

Jon O.N. Lundberg, Department of Physiology and Pharmacology, Karolinska Institute, S-17177 Stockholm, Sweden; e-mail: jon.lundberg@fyfa.ki.se

Helen M. Marriott, Section of Respiratory Medicine, Clinical Sciences Division (CSUHT), University of Sheffield, Floor F, The Medical School, Beech Hill Road, Sheffield S10 2RX, UK; e-mail: H.M.Marriott@shef.ac.uk

Sanjay Mehta, Pulmonary Division, Departments of Medicine and Pharmacology/Toxicology, London Health Sciences Center, 375, South St., University of Western Ontario, London, Ontario, Canada NGA 4G5; e-mail: sanjay.mehta@lhsc.on.ca

Jane A. Mitchell, Unit of Critical Care, Royal Brompton Hospital, National Heart and Lung Institute at Imperial College, Sydney Street, London SW3 6NP, UK

Frans P. Nijkamp, Department of Pharmacology and Pathophysiology, Faculty of Pharmacy, University of Utrecht, NL-3508 TB Utrecht, The Netherlands; e-mail: F.P.Nijkamp@pharm.uu.nl

Gregory J. Quinlan, Unit of Critical Care Medicine, Royal Brompton Hospital, National Heart and Lung Institute at Imperial College, Sydney Street, London SW3 6NP, UK; e-mail: g.quinlan@rbh.nthames.nhs.uk

Johan Rinder, Department of Surgical Sciences, Karolinska Hospital, S-171 76 Stockholm, Sweden

Christoph Thiemermann, The William Harvey Research Institute, The Medical College of St. Bartholomew's Hospital, Charterhouse Square, London EC1M 6BQ, UK

Eddie Weitzberg, Department of Surgical Sciences, Karolinska Hospital, S-171 76 Stockholm, Sweden; e-mail: eddie.weitzberg@neuro.ks.se

Foreword

It is now more than two decades since Ferid Murad and co-workers showed that nitric oxide (NO) could activate soluble guanylyl cyclase and raise intracellular levels of cyclic guanosine monophosphate (cGMP). We now know that the cGMP pathway is the effector mechanism for the great majority of the actions of NO. Several years later the seminal report by Furchgott and Zawadzki showed that endothelial cells release a relaxing factor endothelial-derived relaxing factor (EDRF) when stimulated with agonists. It is now clear, after reports by Furchgott, Ignarro and Moncada and their co-workers, that EDRF is the gas NO, formed from the amino acid L-arginine. Since the early 1980s interest in NO and its pathways of synthesis and action has increased enormously as the importance of the endogenous release of this simple gas has become apparent. Moreover, in 1998 the work of Murad, Ignarro and Furchgott on NO in the cardiovascular system was acknowledged by the Nobel Committee.

NO has many roles in the human body. It is a very important vasodilator, acting as an endogenous "breaking mechanism" to sympathetic tone. It is also involved in the control of smooth muscle function in other structures of the body such as in the gastrointestinal and urogenital tracts. For example, we have all listened with interest at the success of the new antiimpotence drug, Viagra, which works by inhibiting the breakdown of cGMP and thereby increasing the effectiveness of NO. In addition, NO formed by immune cells kills invading pathogens and tumour cells. However, nowhere is the presence of NO felt more strongly than in the lung, where blood vessels, airways and resident as well as invading white blood cells release and respond to it. For this reason the following chapters are dedicated to the most important aspects of how NO regulates the physiology and pathophysiology of the lung. In this setting, the biochemistry and pharmacology of the different isoforms of nitric oxide synthase (NOS) are discussed as well as synthetic nitro (NO) mimetics. Where possible, attention has been paid to discussing the relevance of the NO pathway in human tissues and in human disease states which specifically affect the lung, such as asthma, chronic obstructive pulmonary disease, pulmonary hypertension and adult respiratory distress syndrome.

We hope that this book will be of interest to scientists and clinicians with interests either in the general role of NO in the human body or more specifically in the multitude of structures that constitute the lung.

Jane A. Mitchell and Maria G. Belvisi

Introduction to Nitric Oxide Biology

Nitric Oxide in Pulmonary Processes:
Role in Physiology and Pathophysiology of Lung Disease
ed. by M. G. Belvisi and J. A. Mitchell
© 2000 Birkhäuser Verlag Basel/Switzerland

CHAPTER 1
Nitric Oxide Synthesis and Actions

David Bishop-Bailey[1] and Jane A. Mitchell[2]

[1] *Department of Physiology, University of Connecticut Health Center, Farmington, CT 06030, USA*
[2] *Unit of Critical Care Medicine, Imperial College Medical School at the Royal Brompton Hospital, Sydney Street, London SW3 6NP, UK*

1   Introduction
2   Nitric Oxide Synthesis by Different Cell Types
3   Release of NO by Nerves: Neuronal (nNOS) NOS
3.1 Regulation of nNOS Expression
4   Release of NO by Endothelial Cells: Endothelial (eNOS) NOS
4.1 Regulation of eNOS Expression
5   Release of NO by Cells Induced to Express NOS: Inducible (iNOS) NOS
5.1 Regulation of iNOS Expression
6   Classification of NOS Isoforms
7   Substrate and Substrate Analogue (i.e. Inhibitors) Interactions with Different NOS isoforms
8   Effector Mechanisms Utilised by NO
8.1 Activation of Guanylyl Cyclase
8.2 Interactions of NO with Thiols
8.3 Mutagenesis of DNA
8.4 Interactions between Superoxide Anions and NO: Formation of Peroxynitrite
8.5 Direct Toxicity
8.6 Interactions with Enzymes
9   Concluding Remarks
10   References

1. Introduction

Nitric oxide (NO) is the ubiquitous activator of soluble guanylyl cyclase resulting in smooth muscle relaxation. In addition, NO can activate/inhibit a number of other proteins that influence cellular responses. Within a physiological setting, NO release by endothelial cells or nerves contributes to homeostatic processes in every organ system in the body. NO is also released as a primary defence mechanism by immune cells. However, when NO production becomes excessive, its release can contribute to the processes of inflammation and/or cardiovascular dysfunction.

The ability of NO to perform its different functions in the body is largely made possible by the presence of multiple isoforms of the enzyme NO synthase (NOS) which can be induced, upregulated or suppressed depending upon requirement. This chapter will discuss the relevance of the different isoforms of NOS in the regulation of physiological and pathophysiological events.

Constitutive forms   inducible form

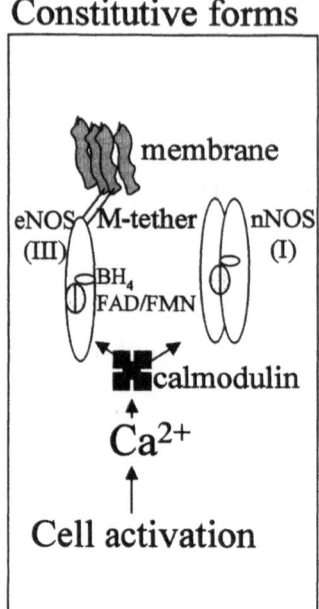 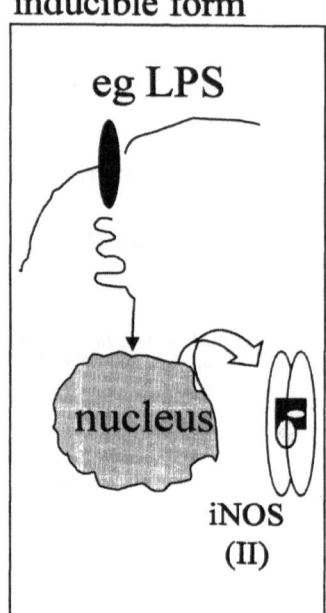

Figure 1. Cellular location of eNOS, nNOS and iNOS. eNOS (type III) is a membrane bound protein due to a myristylation tether (M-tether). eNOS and nNOS contain FAD, FMN and BH_4 tightly bound to the enzyme. When cells are activated intracellular calcium is increased which binds to calmodulin and activates it. The calcium/calmodulin complex then binds to both eNOS and nNOS resulting in activation. In order for iNOS to be present in cells, they first need to be stimulated with an inducing agent, such as lipopolysaccharide (LPS). Transduction and transcription factors are activated resulting in the synthesis of new iNOS protein. iNOS protein has FAD, FMN, BH_4 and calcium activated calcium tightly bound to the mature enzyme and therefore does not require additional cellular stimulation to produce NO.

2. Nitric Oxide Synthesis by Different Cell Types

The first examples of the actions of endogenously released NO in mammals were observed in isolated blood vessels. In these studies, activation of the endothelial layer resulted in relaxation of the underlying smooth muscle and an unknown factor, endothelial-derived relaxing factor (EDRF) was identified [1]. The identity of EDRF was not established until 1987 when Palmer and colleagues showed that it was indistinguishable from NO [2]. Around this time it was also found that NO was a neurotransmitter [3] used by the inhibitory non-adrenergic non-cholineric (iNANC) nerves [4] and in the central nervous system [5] and that it was an intermediate in the formation of nitrite and nitrate by activated macrophages [6]. The fact that these three cellular sources of NO (i.e. endothelial cells, neurons and inflammatory cells; see Fig. 1) had been identified was to influence the progress and direction of future biochemical studies of the enzymes that produce it.

3. Release of NO by Nerves: Neuronal (nNOS) NOS

Despite endothelial cells being the first location identified for NO production, a neuronal source was initially used for characterisation and purification of NOS. In 1990, just one year after NO had been identified as a mediator release by rat cerebral tissue. Bredt and Snyder had purified NOS from this tissue [7]. This first NOS isoform was called neuronal NOS (nNOS) because of its cellular origin. nNOS is a homodimer with sub-units of approximately 150 kDa. It is a soluble protein that requires nicotinamide dinucleotide phosphate (NADPH), calcium, calmodulin [7, 8] as well as tetrahydrobiopterin (BH$_4$) [9] for full activity. These characteristics were utilised in a number of variations on the original purification scheme which included columns packed with 2'5' ADP sepharose (which binds NADPH requiring proteins) and affinity columns for calmodulin.

For nNOS, NADPH serves as an electron donor whilst calcium activated calmodulin binds to the relevant site on the enzyme producing a conformational change consistent with activation. The nature of the requirement of nNOS for BH$_4$ is less clear although it is thought that it may act as a redox reagent, like NADPH [9] and/or to stabilise the NOS protein [10].

Antibodies raised by Bredt and Snyder to purified nNOS showed immuno-histochemically localisation in rat brain in discrete neuronal populations, mainly in the cerebellum and the olfactory bulb; areas associated with roles in hormone release and visualisation, respectively. In these neuronal areas, a co-localisation with NADPH diaphorase staining was observed [11]. Although the functional relevance of diaphroase is unclear, all the NOS isoforms purified to date possess NADPH-dependent diaphorase activity [11–13].

Neuronal cDNA for nNOS was cloned and expressed in human kidney 293 cells [14]. The cDNA coded a protein that had structural homology with cytochrome P450 reductase with recognition sites for L-arginine, NADPH, flavin adenine dinucleotide (FAD), flavin nucleotides, calmodulin and phosphorylation. In most cases FAD and flavin mononucleotide (FMN) are so tightly bound to NOS that they are purified along with the protein and so are not required as additional factors. nNOS activity has also been shown to be present in peripheral iNANC neurons purified from the rat anococcygeus [15], and the bovine retractor penis muscle [16]. NO release by iNANC nerves is particularly important in human airways where it serves as a bronchodilator. The role of NO released in the airway is discussed in detail elsewhere in the relevant chapters of this book.

3.1. Regulation of nNOS Expression

Although nNOS is a constitutive form of the enzyme, its activity can by modulated by a number of different stimuli [17]. nNOS is upregulated at the mRNA or protein level by stimuli including heat, electrical activation and light [18–20]. A reduction in the expression of nNOS is associated with mediators of sepsis including endotoxin and cytokines [17]. nNOS may also be increased as a response to injury after ischemia [21]. Indeed, several *in vivo* studies illustrate a time-dependent increase in nNOS mRNA after hypoxia [22–24]. Increased levels of enzyme in these models may be a result of specific hypoxia-induced factors acting on designated response elements in the nNOS gene, as occurs for other similarly regulated response proteins [25]. In support of this, sequence consensus for the binding of hypoxia inducible factor-1 has been described on the nNOS gene.

In addition to stress, nNOS can be modulated by a number of different chemical agents. Inhibition of glutamatergic transmission increases nNOS expression in cerebral nerves [26]. By contrast, increasing endogenous levels of acetylcholine (using a cholinesterase inhibitor) increases nNOS levels in the hippocampus [27]. Moreover, nNOS expression is increased by some sex hormones including estradiol and testosterone [28, 29] and reduced by corticosterone [30].

4. Release of NO by Endothelial Cells: Endothelial (eNOS) NOS

Endothelial cells from all locations of the circulation express a distinct iso-form of NOS named eNOS. eNOS was initially thought to be, like nNOS, a soluble protein [31, 32]. However, subsequent studies clearly showed that the majority of eNOS resides in the particulate fractions of cells [33, 34]. The purified particulate eNOS was however, found to have a number of similarities to nNOS. For instance eNOS requires calcium, calmodulin, NADPH [35] and BH_4 [36] for full activity. It is also similar in size to nNOS with a denatured molecular mass of approximately 135 kDa [35]. Nevertheless, eNOS and nNOS are the products of separate genes [37]. Bovine endothelial cDNA [37] coded a 4.8 kb transcript which gives rise to a protein with an approximate Mr of 135 kDa. The amino acid sequence predicted the same regulatory sites and NADPH-dependent diaphorase activity as previously published for the nNOS. Similar results have been published using human umbilical vein endothelial cell cDNA [38], with a predicted Mr of 144 kDa. eNOS cDNA, unlike nNOS cDNA, encodes for a N-myristylation site [39], which does not influence catalytic activity but results in the tethering of this isoform to the membrane fraction [39].

4.1. Regulation of eNOS Expression

The mechanisms involved in the regulation of eNOS are still being investigated. However, physical forces of shear and strain increase its expression in endothelial cells *in vitro* and *in vivo* [40–42]. In addition a putative shear stress response element has been described in the promoter region of both human and bovine eNOS gene [43, 44]. Hypoxia upregulates eNOS expression in pulmonary endothelial cells [45] and some reports, but not others, have shown a similar phenomenon in endothelium from systemic vessels [17].

Some growth factors increase eNOS expression in endothelial cells. For example transforming growth factor (TGF-β) increase eNOS mRNA and protein as a result of enhanced promoter activity [46]. There is some controversy surrounding the changes in eNOS expression in proliferating cells. For instance one study has shown that eNOS mRNA and protein are increased in proliferating versus resting cells. This increased expression of enzyme is thought to be a result of increased mRNA stability [47]. By contrast, another group found that eNOS mRNA was actually less stable resulting in lower levels of enzyme in proliferating cells compared to resting cells [48]. These conflicting observations may reflect the complexity of responses produced by NO in different cells and also the variability in responses of cultures at different passages in different laboratories.

There are now a number of studies reporting clear effects of different cytokines on the expression of eNOS [17]. For example, tumor necrosis factor α (TNF-α) can down-regulate eNOS [17] by destabilising mRNA. Whilst a combination of interferon (IFN) and endotoxin can up-regulate eNOS expression in bovine aortic endothelial cells [49]. This is not however, a consistent observation. In a number of studies endotoxin administration *in vivo* results in the down-regulation of eNOS [50], an effect that may be attributed to increases in endogenous levels of TNF.

As is the case for nNOS, sex hormones have been shown to increase levels of eNOS. Indeed, pregnancy and estradiol, but not progesterone or testosterone, increase eNOS mRNA, protein and activity [51, 52]. Similar observations have been made *in vitro* using cultured immortalised endothelial cells. Here estrogen increased eNOS mRNA and activity by increasing the promoter activity via an estrogen responsive element [53].

5. Release of NO by Cells Induced to Express NOS: Inducible (iNOS) NOS

During the 1980s, a number of experiments involving the measurement of nitrite/nitrate excretion by humans and laboratory animals *in vivo* and by macrophage cell lines *in vitro* provided a clear link between infection and NO formation [54, 55]. For instance, lipopolysaccharide (LPS) induces the synthesis of nitrates/nitrites by macrophages which was found to be dependent on the presence of L-arginine, and L-citrulline was formed as a biproduct [56]. Similarly, the cytotoxic ability of LPS-activated macrophages to inhibit mitochondrial respiration, metabolism and DNA synthesis in tumour cells was found to be L-arginine dependent, and associated with the formation of citrulline and nitrite [57]. Moreover analogues of L-arginine where guanidino nitrogen groups had been substituted were found to inhibit both nitrite formation, and the cytotoxic activities of macrophages [57]. It is now clear that inflammatory and infective agents 'induce' cells to express a distinct form of NOS, inducible NOS (iNOS), and that NO is the active intermediate in nitrite/nitrate production by macrophages.

The induction of iNOS has now been demonstrated in most cell types *in vitro* [58–60] and in all organs of the rat *in vivo* [61]. However, there has been considerable controversy surrounding the relative ease of induction of iNOS in rat and murine tissues compared to human. Nevertheless there are a number of studies using different cell types, which clearly demonstrate that active iNOS is expressed in human tissues [58–60, 62].

iNOS, unlike its constitutive counterparts, can be regulated by anti-inflammatory steroids such as dexamethasone [63] and is not dependent on free calcium or calmodulin [64]. The production of NO, therefore only occurs after a lag phase, due to the necessary induction of iNOS protein and results in the release of relatively large amounts of NO.

iNOS was purified first from the cytosol of the mouse macrophage cell line RAW 264.7, activated with LPS and IFN-γ [65], and rat peritoneal macrophages activated with LPS. The protein found had an Mr of approximately 130 kDa. The active iNOS appeared as a dimer (approximate Mr 250 kDa), requiring NADPH, BH$_4$, FAD and FMN, but not exogenous calcium or calmodulin for full activity [65]. Macrophage cDNA was cloned and expressed from LPS and IFN-γ-treated RAW 264.7 macrophages [66]. The sequenced cDNA codes a protein similar to cNOS isoforms, with a predicted Mr of 130 kDa, and binding sites for FAD, FMN, NADPH and interestingly calmodulin [66]. Similar results were obtained with cDNA from IFN-γ-stimulated smooth muscle cells [67]. Further studies demonstrated that the iNOS contains activated calmodulin which is extremely tightly bound [68], thereby explaining the lack of requirement for exogenous calcium for this isoform.

5.1. Regulation of iNOS Expression

Unlike studies on nNOS and eNOS expression, which display some level of controversy, there is a strong consensus of opinion that iNOS is induced by proinflammatory cytokines and/or endotoxin. Specifically, interleukin-1β, TNF-α and IFN-γ alone or in combination induce iNOS in a wide range of cell types [58–60]. Moreover, growth factors such as platelet-derived growth factor inhibit the induction of iNOS [59]. The large and increasing number of proinflammatory agents demonstrated to induce iNOS and the pathways involved in its induction are beyond the scope of this chapter and are fully discussed in detail elsewhere [58–60].

6. Classification of NOS Isoforms

After the different forms of NOS had been purified, antibodies were raised that recognised nNOS, eNOS or iNOS. Studies using these antibodies revealed that NOS isoforms were expressed in other cell types. For instance nNOS is present in epithelial as well as nerves of the airway and gut [17]. In addition to endothelial cells eNOS is present in bone cells [17]. Moreover, iNOS is expressed constitutively in certain cells including those of the macula densor [58]. For these reasons the historical classification of eNOS, nNOS and iNOS has been modified to represent the order of purification of the enzyme. Thus, nNOS becomes NOS1, iNOS beomes NOS2 and eNOS becomes NOS3. However, for the purposes of this chapter the original classification will continue to be used.

7. Substrate and Substrate Analogue (i. e. Inhibitors) Interactions with Different NOS Isoforms

In each case the substrate for NO formation by different NOS enzymes is L-arginine (see Fig. 2). The K_m for L-arginine differs marginally between enzymes from $1-5$ µM. The exact way in which NO and L-citrulline are formed from L-arginine is not fully understood, though a proposed mechanism has been suggested [69, 70]. The initial step in NO biosynthesis is the conversion of L-arginine to the intermediate N^G-hydroxy-L-arginine [69] by substitution of oxygen for one of the guanidino nitrogens. In addition, endogenous N^G-hydroxy-L-arginine itself is a substrate for the enzyme [71]. Less is known of the conversion of N^G-hydroxy-L-arginine to L-citrulline and NO, apart from a requirement of NADPH. Inhibition of this step by carbon monoxide [70] though, suggests a role for the iron centre

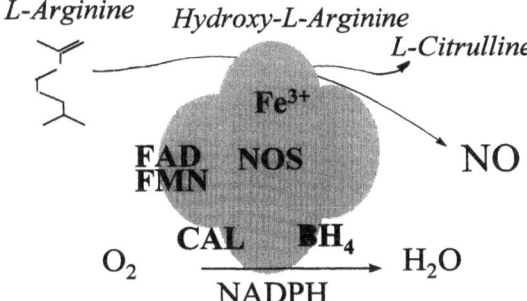

Figure 2. Formation of NO from L-arginine. All NOS isoforms are FAO, FMN containing heme (Fe^{3+}) proteins, which require activated calmodulin, NAOPH, and BH_4 for full catalytic activity. Although the full process by which L-Arginine is converted to NO and L-citrulline is not known, the initial catalytic step is the conversion of L-Arginine to N^G-hydroxy-L-arginine by substitution of oxygen for one of its guanidino nitrogens.

Table 1

Substrate related inhibitors	
Non-selective	L-NMMA, Asymetric-dimethy-L-arginine, N-iminoethyl-L-ornithine, N-amino-L-Arg, N-nitro-L-Arg, N-nitro-L-Arg methyl ester (L-NAME)
iNOS selectivity	Aminoguanidine, Isothioureas, 1400 W
nNOS selectivity	N-nitro-L-Arg-p-nitroanaline, 7-nitro indazole (and analogues)

Others	
Flavoprotein binders	Diphenylene iodonium, Iodonium diphenyl, Di-2-thienyl iodonium
Calmodulin binders	Calcineurin, Trifluroperazine, N-(4-aminobuty)-5-chloro-2-naphthalensulfonamide, N-(6-aminohexyl)-1-naphthalen-sulfonamide
Heam binder	Carbon monoxide, NO
Depleter of BH$_4$	2,4-Diamino-6-hydroxypyrimidine
Inhibitors of iNOS Induction	Corticosteriods, TGF-β-1/2/3, Interleukin (IL)-4, IL-10, Prostaglandin E$_2$/Iloprost
Inhibitor of NADPH Consumption	Imidazole, Phenylimidazole
Binding NO	Haemo-proteins, Oxidised lipoproteins

(Fe^{3+}) of the enzyme. The formation of NO from L-arginine requires a five electron oxidation, and molecular oxygen is incorporated into both L-citrulline and NO, indicating NOS as a dioxygenase enzyme [72].

Analogues of L-arginine where groups are substituted on to one or more of the guanidino nitrogens, have generally proved to be inhibitors of NOS. Moreover, different analogues of L-arginine have varying potencies as inhibitors of eNOS and nNOS versus iNOS. This phenomenon was first described with N^{G}monomethyl-L-arginine (L-NMMA) versus N^{G}nitro-L-arginine methylester (L-NAME). Indeed, L-NAME is a more potent inhibitor than L-NMMA of the constitutive forms of NOS (eNOS and nNOS). By contrast L-NMMA is either more potent than L-NAME or of similar potency to L-NAME as an inhibitor of iNOS. There are now a number of 'selective' inhibitors for different forms of NOS (see Tab. 1) [73–76).

8. Effector Mechanisms Utilised by NO

8.1. Activation of Guanylyl Cyclase

Organic nitrates such as amyl nitrate or glycerol trinitrate, have been used clinically for the treatment of angina pectoris for over 100 years. The effects commonly seen with organic nitrate treatment are flushing, tachycardia and

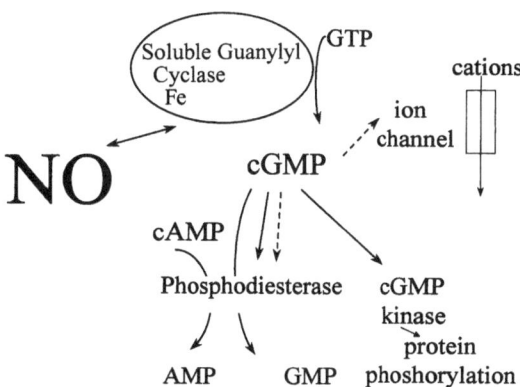

Figure 3. Activation of soluble guanylyl cyclase by NO. NO diffuses through and between cells. Once in the cytoplasm, NO activates soluble guanylyl cyclase via modification of the heam centre. GTP is then converted to cGMP which can then go on to modulate a number of downstream targets including G kinase (cGMP kinase) or ion channels. The intracellular levels of cGMP are tightly regulated by phosphodiesterase enzymes which metabolise it to GMP. Solid line indicates positive effects, while dashed line indicates negative effects.

a fall in blood pressure. All organic nitrates relax vascular and non-vascular smooth muscle via the release of NO and activation of soluble guanylyl cyclase [77] causing an increase in intracellular cGMP (see Fig. 3).

NO reversibly binds to heam in soluble guanylyl cyclase to form nitrosyl complexes, which activate the enzyme to cause cGMP production. It is now clear that NO formed endogenously by NOS produces many of its effects by activation of guanylyl cyclase. In many cases, cGMP mediates the effects of NO via activation of cytosolic G kinases [78]. Much of the evidence linking cGMP-mediated events to G kinase has come from the use of kinase inhibitors, such as cGMP analogues. However, these analogues are only selective for G kinase and have generally been used along-side selective/specifc inhibitors of other kinases (e.g. protein kinases A or C) to more conclusively demonstrate the involvement of G kinase in a particular response.

One effect of G kinase activation is to reduce inositol triphosphate (IP$_3$) generation, which consequently results in inhibition of inositol phosphate accumulation. Indeed, NO has been shown to reduce inositol phosphate generation in a number of preparations including blood vessels and platelets [79, 80]. However, the intermediate steps between G kinase activation and inositol phosphate inhibition are not clear. It has been suggested that G kinase activation can result in phosphorylation and inhibition of G proteins [81–83]. Alternatively G kinase may modulate the activity of some forms of phospholipase C [84, 85]. It is not clear whether the putative actions of G kinase on G proteins or phospholipase enzymes are direct or indirect via intermediate candidates, such as the actin-binding protein VASP, whose phosphorylation correlates well with phospholipase C activity in plateletes

[86]. NO can also exert its inhibitory effects on calcium release via a G kinase-mediated phosphorylation of the IP$_3$ receptor. G kinase-mediated phosphorylation of IP$_3$ receptors has been demonstrated in smooth muscle and platelets [87–89] but not in all cells.

Recently a role for NO and G kinase in modulating calcium release from ryanodine sensitive stores has been established. Here, NO mediates the formation of cADP ribose (a metabolite of NAD$^+$), which directly affects ryanodine-sensitive calcium stores. More recently, it has been shown that NO can also directly activate ryanodine-sensitive calcium stores in skeletal (type 1) and cardiac (type 2) tissue by nitrosolating regulatory thiols [90].

Release/sequestration from/to intracellular stores and entrance from the extracellular environment manage intracellular calcium levels. In addition to the effects of G kinase on movements from intracellular stores, there is also evidence to suggest that NO can modulate calcium exchange with the extracellular environment. For instance NO has a dual action on store operated calcium channels. At low levels of NO and cGMP store-operated calcium channels are activated, whilst at high concentrations these channels are inhibited [91]. NO can also affect the functioning of second messenger-operated calcium channels, particularly those linked to muscarinic receptors [92–94]. In addition NO, via G kinase activation, has been shown to activate second messenger operated calcium channels likened to growth factor receptors [95, 96].

It should be remembered that there are some cells in which calcium homeostasis is relatively unaltered by NO [78], an effect, which may reflect the lack of G kinase-mediated pathways in those cells.

8.2. Interactions of NO with Thiols

NO signalling is achieved through both cGMP-dependent (as discussed above) and cGMP-independent mechanisms (see Fig. 4). An important example of cGMP-independent actions of NO are those achieved by nitrosylation of thiol groups leading to modification of protein function [97]. When NO combines with thiol groups, a stable bioactive NO-like moiety can be formed. Such molecules include S-nitroso-N-acetylpenicillamine (SNAP), S-nitrosoglutathione and S-nitrosocysteine. These modified molecules have been suggested to have similar biological actions as EDRF and NO on smooth muscle preparations [98]. However, further studies using traditional bioassay techniques have concluded that this is not the case. A number of other molecules can be polynitrosylated by NO from iNOS induced in murine macrophages *in vitro*, or in the tracheal secretions of humans being treated with inhaled NO therapy [97, 99, 100]. The various ways in which nitrosylation and polynitrosylation can modify protein structure and function are discussed in detail elsewhere [97, 99, 100].

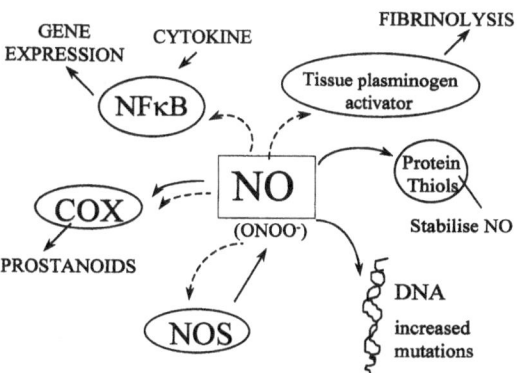

Figure 4. Effects of NO on cellular components. In addition to activation of soluble guanylyl cyclase, NO (either directly, or as peroxynitrite; ONOO⁻) can modulate a number of other proteins resulting in alterations in cellular function, some of these are shown in this figure.

8.3. Mutagenesis of DNA

NO can cause profound effects on living cells by directly modifying nuclear components. Non-inherited genetic diseases and cancers involve the spontaneous mutation of DNA. Interactions of NO with isolated DNA, RNA and nucleotides or nuclear components in intact human cells, causes deamination leading to an increased number of mutations [100]. The mechanism by which this occurs is not completely understood but is thought to involve nitrosylation of nucleotide residues [97, 99].

8.4. Interactions between Superoxide Anions and NO: Formation of Peroxynitrite

The combination of NO with superoxide anions leads to the detoxification of both, but a hydroxyl radical (a potent oxidant) may be formed as a biproduct of the reaction [101]. Superoxide anions can also combine with NO to form peroxynitrite, a potent oxidant which can contribute to many of the damaging effects of NO, leaving nitrotyrosylated proteins as a marker [102]. The relative effects of NO can therefore change depending on the availability of superoxide, which itself is removed by isoforms of superoxide dismutase (SOD) [103]. Thus the level of SOD activity present in tissues is a very important component in the overall effect of NOS activation.

It has recently been suggested that NOS activity alone can result in the generation of peroxynitrite. This is most likely to occur at low arginine concentrations, when NOS is capable of producing superoxide anions along with NO [104]. The interactions between NO, superoxide and peroxynitrite are discussed in detail in chapter 2 in this book.

8.5. Direct Toxicity

Large amounts of NO from iNOS have anti-bacterial, anti-fungal, and anti-viral properties. It is now thought that peroxynitrite, rather than NO itself, is responsible for some of the cytotoxic effects associated with immune cells expressing iNOS. Although the mechanisms involved in NO-mediated cell/pathogen killing are not completely understood, NO has number of actions which contribute to this property. Binding of NO (or peroxynitrite [106]) to the Fe-S group of aconitase, an important enzyme in the tricar-boxylic acid – respiration cycle, inactivates this enzyme [105]. Aconitase is also an important iron-regulatory protein. These proteins bind to the iron response elements of RNA, encoding a number of proteins involved in iron homeostasis. Indeed, NO inhibition of aconitase in hepatoma cells, increased its binding to the iron response element and subsequent suppression of ferratin synthesis [105].

In addition to effects on aconitase activity, NO or peroxynitrite can mediate cellular toxicity by (i) inhibiting ribonucleotide reductase, an important rate-limiting enzyme in DNA synthesis, (ii) inhibition of mitochondrial electron transport or (iii) damage to DNA. The latter mechanism is thought to involve the activation of poly adenosine diphosphate ribose synthase (PARS) [106]. Once activated PARS initiates continual cyclical DNA damage resulting in cellular depletion of adenosine triphosphate (ATP) and NAD^+ and ultimately cell death [106].

8.6. Interactions with Enzymes

There is now an increasing list of enzymes, which are activated or inhibited by NO. Indeed, NOS itself can be modulated by NO. NO can inhibit NOS activity directly or as a result of inhibition of the induction of iNOS [107]. In addition NO can stimulate or inhibit cyclooxygenase (COX) [107]. NO can activate COX by providing either hydroperoxide substrate by formation of peroxynitrite [108], or free radical initiator substrate support. The inhibition effects of NO on COX may, however, be through nitrotyro sylation or interaction with the haem centre [107]. Alternatively, NO can inhibit the induction of COX protein [109], though the mechanism by which this occurs is unknown. As previously mentioned, NO activates cGMP dependent kinase, directly interacts with nucleotides, effects iron homeostasis, and may also through nitrotyrosylation inhibit the binding of nuclear factor κB to DNA [99].

9. Concluding Remarks

The synthesis of NO by mammalian cells was once thought to be impossible. However, it is now clear that this simple gas can regulate processes in all bodily organs. Its primary targets seem to be vascular smooth muscle and circulating blood elements in the cardiovascular system, smooth muscle in the airways and the gastrointestinal tract, the central nervous system and invading pathogens or cancer cells. The functions of NO are partially achieved by a highly developed mechanism for the regulation of its release. Thus, small quanta of NO are formed by calcium activation of the constitutive forms eNOS and nNOS, whilst large cytotoxic amounts of NO are formed by the calcium-independent iNOS. A further layer of regulation is provided for by the different transduction mechanisms utilised by NO in different cells. The most important effector pathway for NO is activation of the soluble form of guanylyl cyclase.

We now seem to have a wealth of information relating to NO biology in health. However, we are only just beginning to understand how dysfunctions in the L-arginine – NO – cGMP pathway contribute to diseases in humans. A better understanding of the physiological and pathophysiological functions of NO in such diseases will undoubtedly lead to new therapies.

10. References

1 Furchgott R, Zawadzki JV (1980) The obligatory role of endothelial cells in relaxation of arterial smooth muscle by acetylcholine. *Nature* 288: 373–376

2 Palmer RJM, Ferrigo AG, Moncada S (1987) Vascular endothelial cells synthesise nitric oxide from L-arginine. *Nature* 325: 664–666

3 Garthwaite J (1991) Glutamate, nitric oxide and cell-cell signalling in the nervous system. *TINS* 14: 61–67

4 Gillespie JS (1972) The rat anococcygeus muscle and it response to nerve stimulation and to some drugs. *Br J Pharmacol* 45: 404–416

5 Garthwaite J, Charles SL, Chess-Williams R (1988) Endothelium-derived relaxing factor release on activation of NMDA receptors suggest a role as intercellular messenger in the brain. *Nature* 336: 385–388

6 Hibbs JB, Taintor RR, Vavrin Z, Rachlin EM (1988) Nitric oxide: A cytotoxic activated macrophage effector molecule. *Biochem Biophys Res Comm* 157: 87–94

7 Bredt D, Snyder S (1990) Isolation of nitric oxide synthase, a calmodulin-requiring enzyme. *Proc Natl Acad Sci* 86: 682–685

8 Schmidt HHHW, Pollock JS, Nakane M, Gorsky LD, Förstermann U, Murad F (1991) Purification of a soluble isoform of guanylyl cyclase-activating factor synthase. *Proc Natl Acad Sci* 88: 865–869

9 Mayer B, John M, Bohme E (1990) Purification of a calcium/calmodulin-dependent nitric oxide synthase from porcine cerebellum. Co-factor role of tetrahydrobiopterin. *FEBS Lett* 277: 215–219

10 Giovanelli J, Campos KL, Kaufman S (1991) Tetrahydrobiopterin, a cofactor for rat cerebella nitric oxide synthase, does not function as a reactant in the oxygenation of arginine. *Proc Natl Acad Sci* 88: 7091–7095

11 Hope BT, Michael GJ, Knigge KM, Vincent SR (1991) Neuronal NADPH diaphorase is a nitric oxide synthase. *Proc Natl Acad Sci* 88: 2811–2814

12 Mitchell JA, Kohlhass KL, Matsumoto T, Förstermann U, Warner TD, Murad F (1992) Induction of NADPH dependent diaphorase and NO synthase activity occurs simultaneously in aortic smooth muscle and cultured macrophages. *Mol Pharmacol* 41: 1163–1168

13 Lamas S, Marsden PA, Li GK, Tempst P, Michel T (1992) Endothelial nitric oxide synthase: molecular cloning and characterisation of a distinct constitutive enzyme. *Proc Natl Acad Sci* 89: 6348–6352

14 Bredt DS, Hwang PM, Glatt CE, Lowenstein C, Reed RR, Snyder SH (1991) Cloned and expressed nitric oxide synthase structurally resembles cytochrome P-450 reductase. *Nature* 351: 714–718

15 Mitchell JA, Sheng H, Föstermann U, Murad F (1991) Characterisation of nitric oxide synthase in non-adrenergic-non-cholinergic nerve containing rat anococcygeus. *Br J Pharmacol* 104: 289–291

16 Sheng H, Schmidt H, Nakane M, Mitchell JA, Pollock JS, Förstermann U, Murad F (1991) Characterisation and localisation of nitric oxide synthase in non-adrenergic non-cholinergic nerves from bovine retractor penis muscles. *Br J Pharmacol* 106: 768–773

17 Forsterman U, Boissel JP, Kleinert H (1998) Expressional control of the 'constitutive' isoforms of nitric oxide synthase (NOSI and NOSII). *FASEB J* 12: 773–790

18 Sharma HS, Westman J, Alm P, Sjoquist PO, Cervos J, Nyberg F (1997) Involvement of nitric oxide in the pathophysiology of acute heat stress in the rat. Influence of a new anti-oxidant compound H-290/51. *Ann N Y Acad Sci* 813: 581–590

19 Reiser PJ, Kline WO, Vaghy PL (1997) Induction of neuronal type nitric oxide synthase in skeletal muscle by chronic electrical stimulation *in vivo*. *J Appl Physiol* 82: 1250–1255

20 Goldstein J, LopezGostra JJ, Saavedra JP (1997) Changes in NADPH diaphorase activity and neuronal nitric oxide synthase in rat retina following constant illumination. *Neurosci Lett* 231: 45–48

21 Zhang ZG, Chopp M, Gautam S, Zaloga C, Schmidt HHHW, Pollock JS, Förstermann U (1994) Up-regulation of neuronal nitric oxide synthase mRNA and selective sparing of nitric oxide synthase-containing neurones after focal cerebral ischaemia in rat. *Brain Res* 654: 85–95

22 Shaul PW, North AJ, Brannon TS, Ujie K, Wells IB, Nisen PA, Lowenstein CJ, Snyder SH, Star RA (1995) Prolonged *in vivo* hypoxia enhances nitric oxide synthase type I and type III gene expression in adult rat lung. *Am J Resp Cell Mol Biol* 13: 167–174

23 Prabhakar NR, Rao S, Premknmar D, Pieramiei SP, Kumar GK, Kalaria RK (1996) Regulation of neuronal nitric oxide synthase gene expression by hypoxia. Role of nitric oxide in respiratory adaption to low pO_2. *Adv Exp Med Biol* 410: 345–348

24 Guo Y, Ward MB, Beasjours S, Mori M, Hussain SNA (1997) Regulation of cerebellar nitric oxide production in response to prolonged *in vivo* hypoxia. *J Neurosci Res* 49: 89–97

25 Kvieukova I, Wenger KH, Marti HH, Gassmann M (1995) The transcription factor ATP-1 and GREB-1 bind constitutively to the hypoxia-inducible factor-1 (HOF-1) DNA recognition site. *Nucleic Acids Res* 23: 4542–4550

26 Baader SL, Schilling K (1996) Glutamate receptors mediate dynamic regulation of nitric oxide synthase expression in cerebellar granule cells. *J Neurosci* 16: 1440–1449

27 Bagetta G, Corasania MT, Mehao G, Paoletti AM, Finazzi A, Nistico G (1993) Lithium increases the expression of nitric oxide synthase mRNA in the hippocampus of rat. *Biochem Biophys Res Comm* 197: 1132–1139

28 Luckman SM, Huckett L, Bicknell RJ, Voisin DL, Herbison AE (1997) Up-regulation of nitric oxide synthase messenger RNA in an integrated forebrain circuit involved in oxytocin secretion. *Neuroscience* 77: 37–48

29 Reily CM, Zamorano P, Stopper VS, Mills TM (1997) Androgenic regulation of NO availability in rat penile erection. *J Androl* 18: 110–115

30 Weber CM, Eke BC, Mains MD (1994) Corticosterone regulates heme oxygenase-2 and NO synthse transcription and protein expression in rat brain. *J Neurochem* 63: 953–962

31 Palmer RJM, Moncada S (1989) A novel citrulline-forming enzyme implicated in the formation of nitric oxide by vascular endothelial cells. *Biochem Biophys Res Comm* 158: 524–526

32 Mulsch A, Bassenge E, Busse R (1989) Nitric oxide synthase in endothelial cells: evidence for a calcium-dependent mechanism. *Naunyn Schmiedeberg's Arch Pharmacol* 340: 767–770

33 Förstermann U, Pollock JS, Schmidt HHHW, Heller M, Murad F (1991) Calmodulin-dependent endothelium-derived relaxing factor/nitric oxide synthase activity is present in the particulate and soluble fractions of bovine aortic endothelial cells. *Proc Natl Acad Sci* 88: 1788–1792

34 Mitchell JA, Förstermann U, Warner TD, Pollock JS, Schmidt HHHW, Heller M, Murad F (1991) Endothelial cells have a particulate enzyme system responsible for EDRF formation: measurement by vascular relaxation. *Biochem Biophys Res Comm* 176: 1417–1423

35 Pollock JS, Förstermann U, Mitchell JA, Warner TD, Schmidt HHHW, Nakane M, Murad F (1991) Purification and Characterisation of EDRF synthase. *Proc Natl Acad Sci* 88: 10480–10485

36 Pollock JS, Werner F, Mitchell JA, Förstermann U (1993) Characterisation of EDRF/NO synthase as a FAD/FMN containing flavoprotein. *Endothelium* 1: 147–152

37 Sessa WC, Harrison JK, Barber CM, Zeng D, Durieux ME, Anglo DD, Lynch KR, Peach MJ (1992) Molecular cloning and expression of a cDNA encoding endothelial cell nitric oxide synthase. *J Biol Chem* 267: 15274–15276

38 Janssens SP, Shimouchi A, Quertermous T, Bloch CD, Bloch KD (1992) Cloning and expression of a cDNA encoding human endothelium-derived relaxing factor/nitric oxide synthase. *J Biol Chem* 194: 420–424

39 Sessa WC, Barber CM, Lynch KR (1993) Mutation of N-myristolation site converts endothelial cells nitric oxide synthase from a membrane to a cytosolic protein. *Circ Res* 72: 921–924

40 Nishida K, Harrison DG, Navas JP, Fisher AA, Docker SP, Uematsu M, Nerem RM, Alexander RW, Muphy TJ (1992) Molecular cloning and characterisation of the constitutive bovine aortic endothelial cell synthase. *J Clin Invest* 90: 2092–2096

41 Sessa WC, Pritchard K, Seyedi N, Wang J, Hints TH (1994) Chronic exercise in dogs increases coronary vascular nitric oxide production and endothelial nitric oxide synthase gene expression. *Circ Res* 74: 349–353

42 Xino Z, Zhang Z, Dramond SL (1997) Shear stress induction of the endothelial nitric oxide synthase gene is calcium-dependent but not calcium activated. *J Cell Physiol* 17: 205–211

43 Marsden PA, Heng HH, Scherer SW, Stewart RJ, Hall AV, Shi XM, Tsui LC (1993) Structure and chromosomal localisation of the human constitutive endothelial nitric oxide synthase. *J Biol Chem* 268: 17478–17488

44 Venema TG, Nishida K, Alexander RW, Harrision DG, Murphy TJ (1994) Organization of the bovine gene encoding the endothelial nitric oxide synthase. *Biochem Biophys Res Comm* 1218: 413–420

45 Ziesche R, Perkov V, Williams J, Zakeri SM, Mosgoller W, Knofler M, Block LH (1996) Lipopolysaccharide and interleukin 1 augment the effects of hypoxia and inflammation in human pulmonary arterial tissue. *Proc Natl Acad Sci* 93: 12478–12483

46 Inoue N, Venema RC, Sayegh HS, Ohara Y, Murphy TJ, Harrision DC (1995) Molecular regulation of the bovine endothelial cell nitric oxide synthase by transforming growth factor beta. *Arterioscler Thromb Vasc Biol* 15: 1255–1261

47 Arnal JR, Yamin J, Dockery S, Harrision DG (1994) Regulation of endothelial nitric oxide synthase mRNA protein and activity during cell growth. *Am J Physiol* 36: C1381–C1388

48 Flower MA, Wang Y, Stewart RJ, Patel M, Marsden PA (1995) Reciprocal regulation of endothelin-1 and endothelial constitutive NOS in proliferating endothelial cells. *Am J Physiol* 269: 111988–111997

49 Bucher M, Itter KP, Zimmermann M, Wolf K, Hobbhahn J, Kurtz A (1997) Nitric oxide synthase isoform III gene expression in rat liver is up-regulated by lipopolysaccharide and lipoteichoic acid. *FEBS* 412: 511–514

50 Liu SF, Adcock IM, Old RW, Barnes PJ, Evans TW (1996) Differential regulation of the constitutive and inducible nitric oxide synthase mRNA by lipopolysaccharide treatment *in vivo* in the rat. *Crit Care Med* 24: 1219–1225

51 Weiner CP, Lizasoain I, Baylis SA, Knowles RG, Charles IG, Moncada S (1994) Induction of calcium-dependent nitric oxide synthase by sex hormones. *Proc Natl Acad Sci* 91: 5212–5216

52 Guetz RM, Morano I, Calovini T, Studer R, Holts J (1994) Increased expression of endothelial constitutive nitric oxide synthase during pregnancy. *Biochem Biophys Res Comm* 205: 905–910

53 Kleinert H, Wallerath T, Euchenhofer Ce, Biedert I, Li H, Förstermann U (1998) Estrogens increase transcription of the human endothelial NO synthase gene: analysis of the transcription factors involved. *Hypertension* 31: 582–588

54 Green LC, Ruiz de Luzuriaga K, Wagner DA, Rand W, Istfan N, Young RV, Tannenbaum SR (1981) Nitrate biosynthesis in man. *Proc Natl Acad Sci* 78: 7764–7768

55 Stuehr DJ, Marletta MA (1987) Synthesis of nitrite and nitrate in murine macrophage cell lines. *Cancer Res* 47: 5590–5594

56 Iyengar R, Stuehr DJ, Marletta MA (1978) Macrophage synthesis of nitrite, nitrate and N-nitrosamines: precursors and role of the respiratory burst. *Proc Natl Acad Sci* 84: 6369–6373

57 Hibbs JB, Taintor RR, Vavrin Z, Rachlin EM (1988) Nitric oxide: A cytotoxic activated macrophage effector molecule. *Biochem Biophys Res Comm* 157: 87–94

58 Cohen J, Evans TJ, Spink J (1998) Cytokine regulation of inducible nitric oxide synthase in vascular smooth muscle cells. *Proc Clin Biol Res* 397: 169–177

59 Wong JM, Billiar TR (1995) Regulation of inducible nitric oxide synthase during sepsis and acute inflammation. *Adv Pharmacol* 34: 155–170

60 Nathan C (1997) Inducible nitric oxide synthase: What difference does it make? *J Clin Invest* 100: 2417–2423

61 Mitchell JA, Kohlhass KL, Sorrentino R, Murad F, Warner TD, Vane JR (1993) Induction of calcium-independent NO synthase in rat mesentery: possible role in the hypotension associated with sepsis. *Br J Pharmacol* 109: 265–300

62 Chester AH, Borland JAA, Buttery LDK, Mitchell JA, Cunningham DA, Hafizi S, Hoare GS, Springall DR, Polack JM, Yacoub MH (1998) Induction of nitric oxide synthase in human vascular smooth muscle: interactions between proinflammatory cytokines. *Cardio-vasc Res* 38: 814–821

63 Radomski MW, Palmer RMJ, Moncada S (1990) Glucocorticoids inhibit the expression of an inducible, but not the constitutive, nitric oxide synthase in vascular endothelial cells. *Proc Natl Acad Sci* 87: 10043–10047

64 Busse R, Mulsch A (1990) Induction of nitric oxide synthase by cytokines in vascular smooth muscle cells. *FEBS Lett* 275: 87–90

65 Stuehr DJ, Cho HJ, Kwon NS, Weise M, Nathan C (1991) Purification and characterisation of the cytokine induced macrophage nitric oxide synthase: A FAD and FMN-containing flavoprotein. *Proc Natl Acad Sci* 88: 7773–7777

66 Lowenstein CJ, Glatt CS, Bredt DS, Snyder S (1992) Cloned and expressed macrophage nitric oxide synthase contrast with the brain enzyme. *Proc Natl Acad Sci* 89: 6711–6715

67 Nunokawa Y, Nobuhiro I, Tanaka S (1993) Clonong of inducible nitric oxide synthase in rat vascular smooth muscle cells. *Biochem Biophys Res Comm* 191: 89–94

68 Cho HJ, Xie QW, Calaycay J, Mumford RA, Swiderek KM, Lee TM, Nathan C (1992) Calmodulin is a tightly bound subunit of calcium-calmodulin independent nitric oxide synthase. *J Exp Med* 176: 599–604

69 Marletta MA (1993) Nitric oxide synthase structure and mechanism. *J Biol Chem* 268: 12231–12331

70 Ignarro LJ (1990) Biochemistry and metabolism of endothelium derived nitric oxide. *Ann Rev Pharmacol Toxicol* 30: 535–560

71 Mitchell JA, Pollock JS, Nakane M, Warner TD, Kerwin JF, Murad F (1992) NG-hydroxy-L-arginine as a substrate for constitutive nitric oxide synthase purified from endothelial cells and brain: comparison with L-arginine. In: S Moncada, A Higgs (eds) *Biology of Nitric oxide*. Portland Press, 66–68

72 Leone AM, Palmer RMJ, Knowles RG, Francis PL, Ashton DS, Moncada S (1991) Constitutive and inducible nitric oxide synthase incorporate molecular oxygen into both nitric oxide and citrulline. *J Biol Chem* 266:23790–23795

73 Nathan CF, Hibbs JB (1991) Role of nitric oxide synthesis in macrophage antimicrobial activity. *Curr Opin Immunol* 3: 65–70

74 Southern GJ, Szabo C, Thiemermann C (1995) Isothioureas: potent inhibitors of nitric oxide synthase with variable isoform selectivity. *Br J Pharmacol* 114: 510–516

75 Moore PK, Wallace P, Gaffen Z, Hart SL, Babbedge RC (1993) Characterisation of the novel nitric oxide synthase inhibitor 7-nitro indazole and related indazoles: antinociceptive and cardiovascular effects. *Br J Pharmacol* 110: 219–224

76 Vallance P, Leone A, Calver A, Collier J, Moncada S (1992) Endogneous dimethylarginine as an inhibitor of nitric oxide synthesis. *J Cardiovasc Pharmacol* 20: S60–S62

77 Murad F, Mittal CK, Arnold WP, Katsuki S, Kimura H (1978) Guanylate cyclase: activation by azide, nitrocompounds, nitric oxide and hydroxyl radicals and inhibition by haemoglobin and myoglobin. *Adv Cyclic Nucleotide Res* 9: 145–158

78 Clementi E (1998) Role of nitric oxide and its intracellular signalling pathways in the control of calcium homeostasis. *Biochem Pharmacol* 55: 713–718

79 Rapport RM (1986) Cyclic guanosine monophosphate inhibition of contraction may be mediated through inhibition of phosphatidylinositol hydrolysis in rat aorta. *Circ Res* 58: 407–410

80 Nakashima S, Tohmatsu T, Hattori H, Okano Y, Nozawa Y (1986) Inhibitory action of cyclic GMP on secretion, polyphosphoinositide hydrolysis and calcium mobilization in thrombin-stimulated human platelets. *Biochem Biophys Res Comm* 135: 1099–1104

81 Hirata M, Kohse KP, Chang CH, Ikebe T, Murad F (1990) Mechanism of cyclic GMP inhibition of inositol phosphate formation in rat aorta segments and culture bovine aortic endothelial cells. *J Biol Chem* 265: 1268–1273

82 Light DB, Corbin JD, Stanton BA (1990) Dual ion-channel regulation by cyclic GMP-dependent protein kinase. *Nature* 344: 336–339

83 Nguyen BL, Saitoh M, Ware A (1991) Interaction of nitric oxide and cGMP with signal transduction in activated platelets. *Am J Physiol* 261: H1043–H1052

84 Clementi E, Sciorati C, Riccio M, Miloso M, Meldolesi H, Nistico G (1995) Nitric oxide action of growth factor-elicited signals. *J Biol Chem* 270: 22277–22282

85 Clementi E, Vecchio I, Sciorati C, Nistic G (1995) Nitric oxide modulation of agonist-evoked intracellular calcium release in neurosecretory PC-12 cells. Inhibition of phospholipase C activity via cyclic GMP-dependent protein kinase I. *Mol Pharmacol* 47: 517–524

86 Halbrugge M, Friederich C, Eigenthaler M, Schanzenbacher P, Walker U (1990) Stoichiometric and reversible phosphoarylation of a 56-kDa protein in human platelets in response to cGMP and cAMP-elevating vasodilators. *J Biol Chem* 265: 3088–3093

87 Komalavilas P, Lincoln TM (1996) Phosphorylation of the inositol 1,4,5-triphosphate receptor. *J Biol Chem* 271: 21933–21938

88 Komlavilas P, Lincoln TM (1994) Phosphorylation of the inositol 1,4,5-triphosphate receptor by cyclic GMP-dependent protein kinase. *J Biol Chem* 269: 8701–8707

89 Cavallini L, Coassin M, Borean A, Alexandre A (1996) Prostacyclin and sodium nitroprusside inhibit the activity of the platelet inositol 1,4,5-triphosphate receptor and promote its phosphorylation. *J Biol Chem* 271: 5545–5551

90 Stoyanovsky D, Murphy T, Anno PR, Kim YM, Salama G (1997) Nitric oxide activates skeletal and cardiac ryanodine receptors. *Cell Calcium* 21: 19–29

91 Xu X, Star RA, Tortorici G, Muallem S (1994) Depletion of intracellular calcium stores activates nitric oxide synthase to generate cGMP and regulate calcium influx. *J Biol Chem* 269: 12643–12653

92 Pandol SJ, Schoeffield-Payne MS (1990) Cyclic GMP mediates the agonist stimulated increas in plasma membrane calcium entry in the pancreatic acinar cell. *J Biol Chem* 265: 12846–12855

93 Matches C, Thompson SH (1996) The relationship between depletion of intracellular calcium stores and activation of calcium current by muscarinic receptors in neuroblastoma cells. *J Neuroci* 6: 1702–1709

94 Liu PS, Shaw YH (1997) Arginine-modulated receptor activated calcium influx via a NO/cyclic GMP pathway in human SK-N-SH neuroblastoma cells. *J Neurochem* 68: 376–382

95 Clementi E, Sciorati C, Nistico G (1995) Growth factor-induced calcium responses are differentially modulated by nitric oxide via a cGMP-dependent pathway. *Mol Pharmacol* 84: 1068–1077

96 Pfeifer A, Nurnberg B, Kamm S, Uhde M, Schult G, Ruth P, Hofmann F (1995) Cyclic GMP-dependent protein kinase blocks pertussis toxin-sensitive hormone receptor signalling pathways in Chinese hamster ovary cells. *J Biol Chem* 270: 9052–9059

97 Brune B, Mohr S, Messmer UK (1996) Protein thiol modification and apopototic cell death as cGMP-independent nitric oxide signalling pathways. *Rev Physiol Biochem Pharmacol* 127: 1–30

98 Myers PR, Minor RL, Guerra R, Bates JN, Harrision DG (1990) Vasorelaxant properties of the endothelium-derived relaxing factor more closely resembles S-nitrosocysteine than nitric oxide. *Nature* 345: 161–163

99 Upchurch GR, Welch GN, Loscalzo J (1996) The vascular biology of S-nitrosothiols, nitrosated derivatives of thiols. *Vasc Med* 1: 25–33

100 Butler AR, Rhodes P (1997) Chemistry, analysis and biological roles of S-nitrosothiols. *Anal Biochem* 249: 1–9

101 Beckman JS, Beckman TW, Chen J, Marshall PA, Freeman BA (1990) Apparent hydroxyl radical production by peroxynitrite: implications for endothelial injury from nitric oxide and superoxide. *Proc Natl Acad Sci* 87: 1620–1624
102 Beckman JS, Koppenol WH (1996) Nitric oxide, superoxide and peroxynitrite: the good the bad and the ugly. *Am J Physiol* 271: C1424–C1437
103 Chabot F, Mitchell JA, Gutteridge JMC, Evans TW (1998) Reactive oxygen species and acute lung injury. *Eur Resp J* 11: 754–757
104 Pryor WA, Squadrito GL (1995) The chemistry of peroxynitrite: a product form the reaction of nitric oxide with superoxide. *Am J Physiol* 268: L699–722
105 Hibbs JB, Taintor RR, Vavrin Z, Granger DL, Drapier JC, Amber IJ, Lancaster JR (1990) Synthesis of nitric oxide form terminal guanidino nitrogen atom of L-arginine: a molecular mechanism regulating cellular proliferation that targets intracellular iron. Nitric oxide from L-arginine: A bioregulatory system. 189–223
106 Szabo C (1998) Role of poly(ADP-ribose)synthase in inflammation. *Eur J Pharmacol* 350: 1–19
107 Mitchell JA, Larkin S, Williams TJ (1995) Cyclooxygenase-2: regulation and relevance in inflammation. *Biochem Pharmacol* 50: 1535–1542
108 Landino LM, Crews BC, Timmons MD, Morrow JD, Marnett LJ (1996) Peroxynitrite, the coupling product of nitric oxide and superoxide, activates prostaglandin biosynthesis. *Proc Natl Acad Sci* 93: 15069–15074
109 Swierkosz TA, Mitchell JA, Warner TD, Botting RM, Vane JR (1995) Co-induction of nitric oxide synthase and cyclo-oxygenase; interactions between nitric oxide and prostanoids. *Br J Pharmacol* 114: 1335–1342

Nitric Oxide in Pulmonary Processes:
Role in Physiology and Pathophysiology of Lung Disease
ed. by M. G. Belvisi and J. A. Mitchell
© 2000 Birkhäuser Verlag Basel/Switzerland

CHAPTER 2
Reactive Oxygen and Reactive Nitrogen Species in the Lung

Gregory J. Quinlan and Nicholas J. Lamb

Unit of Critical Care, Royal Brompton Hospital, National Heart and Lung Institute at Imperial College, Sydney Street, London SW3 6NP, UK

1   Introduction
1.1 Definitions
2   Reactive Oxygen Species (ROS)
2.1 Organic Oxygen Radicals
2.2 Reactive Nitrogen Species (RNS)
2.3 Summary
3   ROS and RNS and Their Role in Lung Injury
3.1 Acute Respiratory Distress Syndrome (ARDS)
3.2 Hyperoxia
3.3 Ischaemia Reperfusion Injury
3.4 Inflammatory Cells
3.5 Antioxidants
3.6 Other Lung Diseases
4   ROS and RNS as Second Messengers
5   Concluding Remarks
6   References

1. Introduction

Reactive oxygen species (ROS) and reactive nitrogen species (RNS) have been implicated as contributing to the pathogenesis of a broad spectrum of diseases [1, 2]. Historically, oxygen free radicals were primarily considered to be aggressive species, indeed the superoxide ($O_2^{\cdot-}$) theory of oxygen toxicity is based on this hypothesis, (reviewed in 3). There is circumstantial evidence to support this view, some of which will be reviewed elsewhere in this chapter. However, other roles for free radicals – or more appropriately ROS and RNS – have recently emerged, most notably as signal or second messenger molecules. It seems therefore that these species can have differing effects which are dependent on their levels of production and on antioxidant defences. This chapter will mainly be concerned with the deleterious consequences associated with these reactive species, particularly in the lung, with special reference to acute lung injury (ALI) and acute respiratory distress syndrome (ARDS).

1.1. Definitions

A biological definition of a free radical is "any chemical species capable of independent existence that contains one or more unpaired electrons" [4]. Classically, free radicals are thought of as highly reactive species, but this is often not the case. Ground state molecular oxygen and nitric oxide (NO) have unpaired electrons, and therefore are free radicals, although neither are particularly reactive species. However, other related reactive oxidants like ozone and peroxynitrite (ONOO⁻), or species such as hydrogen peroxide (H_2O_2), with the potential to form reactive species, are not free radicals. For this reason, the terms reactive oxygen species (ROS) for oxygen containing species, and reactive nitrogen species (RNS) for nitrogen containing species, have been introduced to allow free radicals and other related species to be included within common definitions.

2. Reactive Oxygen Species (ROS)

Oxygen is an essential requirement for aerobic life forms, as the terminal electron acceptor at the end of the respiratory chain. During aerobic metabolism carbohydrate is oxidised whilst oxygen is reduced by the sequential addition of four electrons, leading to the formation of water. Various ROS are produced as intermediates during this process (equations 1–4):

$$O_2 + e^- + H^+ \rightarrow HO_2^{\cdot} \text{ (hydroperoxyl radical)} \tag{1}$$
$$HO_2^{\cdot} \rightarrow H^+ + O_2^{\cdot-}$$

$$O_2^{\cdot-} + 2\,H^+ + e^- \rightarrow H_2O_2 \tag{2}$$

$$H_2O_2 + e^- \rightarrow OH^- + {\cdot}OH \text{ (hydroxyl radical)} \tag{3}$$

$${\cdot}OH + e^- + H^+ \rightarrow H_2O \text{ (water)} \tag{4}$$

$O_2^{\cdot-}$ although a free radical anion, is a weak oxidising agent, capable of oxidising thiols and ascorbic acid. It is, however, a much stronger reducing agent, capable of reducing several iron complexes. At physiological pH it is unstable and rapidly dismutates to H_2O_2, a process which is accelerated by the antioxidant enzyme superoxide dismutase (SOD).

H_2O_2 is an uncharged molecule, readily soluble in water, with the ability to enter and leave cells easily. It is not a very reactive species, but can ultimately lead to the formation of the most aggressive oxygen free radical known, the hydroxyl (˙OH) radical. H_2O_2 levels are regulated *in vivo* by glutathione peroxidase, and catalase antioxidant enzymes.

The ˙OH radical can be formed via the iron (Fenton reaction) or copper catalysed decomposition of H_2O_2. This reaction emphasises the importance of redox active transition metal ions in free radical chemistry and oxygen toxicity. The ·OH radical is an extremely reactive oxidant that attacks most biological molecules at almost diffusion-controlled rates. This extreme reactivity, however, limits its ability to cause damage at any distance from its site of formation, although it can initiate radical chain reactions such as lipid peroxidation [4]. Recently iron-independent mechanisms for *in vivo* ·OH production have been proposed, either via the decomposition of peroxynitrous acid [5] or from the reaction of $O_2^{\cdot-}$ with hypochlorous acid (a neutrophil derived oxidant) [6]. Both mechanisms are, however, still open to debate [7, 8].

Ozone is a powerful oxidant and toxic pollutant which has been implicated in various respiratory disorders including asthma [9]. It is capable of causing oxidative damage to biomolecules such as DNA, lipids, and carbohydrates [10, 11].

Ground state molecular oxygen (O_2) is classified as a free radical as it contains two unpaired electrons with parallel spins. This spin restriction limits its reactivity. It can, however, react by accepting electrons one at a time, in reactions involving transition metal ions such as iron and copper. More reactive forms of oxygen can also be formed, as a result of energy input into ground state oxygen, and are known collectively as singlet oxygen. Two forms exist, ($^1\Sigma g^+O_2$) is the most reactive, and is a free radical containing two unpaired electrons with opposite spins. It rapidly decays to the ($^1\Delta gO_2$) form, which is not a free radical as both electrons now occupy the same orbital. Singlet oxygen can also be formed from the interaction of H_2O_2 with the hypochlorite ion, a reaction that may be of biological significance. Its formation *in vivo* is most often associated with photosensitization reactions.

Hypochlorous acid is a potent bleaching agent, produced by the lysosomal enzyme, myeloperoxidase, of activated neutrophils. Its key function is as a microbial killing agent. Production of this powerful oxidant can, however, also have detrimental effects. It readily oxidises or chlorinates many biological molecules including thiols, amines and nucleotides [12], and causes intramolecular crosslinking of proteins [13]. Hypochlorous acid can interact with other ROS or decompose to form other damaging oxidants including the ·OH radical (either independently [6] or via iron catalysis [8]). Recently hypochlorous acid has been shown to form a potent chlorinating and nitrating species on interaction with nitrite [13, 14].

2.1. Organic Oxygen Radicals

Lipid peroxides can be formed in biological systems by a variety of mechanisms. Purposeful enzyme catalysed lipid peroxidation occurs in both animal and plant tissues to produce bioactive substances collectively known as eicosanoids. Various ROS are also capable of initiating lipid peroxidation that can lead to deleterious consequences. Singlet oxygen is capable of reacting directly with carbon-carbon double bonds to produce lipid hydroperoxides [16]. Other non-radical oxidants such as ozone, $ONOO^-$, and hypochorite have also been implicated in lipid peroxidation processes [17–19]. The $^.OH$ radical, if formed locally reacts with unsaturated fatty acids resulting in the formation of peroxy radicals capable of initiating further peroxidation. Stable lipid peroxides can also be formed, these are not free radicals, but in the presence of iron or copper ion catalysts form alkoxyl or peroxyl radicals, which are also able to propagate the peroxidation process.

2.2. Reactive Nitrogen Species (RNS)

NO, contrary to popular belief is not a particularly reactive molecule, except under certain circumstances (reactions with other free radicals). It is an environmental pollutant and is also found in cigarette smoke. NO is produced *in vivo* both constitutively and inducibly via the NO synthase (NOS) enzyme systems. Its biological functions are indistinguishable from those of endothelial-derived relaxing factor (EDRF) and may also function as an antioxidant by inhibiting the ROS producing enzyme xanthine oxidase [20], by scavenging O_2^- [21], and by acting as a chain breaking antioxidant.

Nitrogen dioxide (NO_2) is a free radical gas, a pollutant, and a constituent of cigarette smoke. It is a powerful oxidant and may therefore be of some significance to respiratory diseases such as asthma [22]. NO_2 can be formed by reaction of nitrogen with molecular oxygen. However, this reaction is thought to be of little physiological relevance, as it is out competed by $ONOO^-$ formation [23].

$ONOO^-$ is not a free radical; it is however, a powerful oxidant, formed from the reaction of O_2^- with NO (reviewed in [23]), and possibly by NOS enzymes directly [24]. As an oxidant, $ONOO^-$ can damage lipids, DNA, and proteins [25–27]. It is also a nitrating and nitrosating species, able to nitrate tyrosine and tryptophan residues [28, 29], and nitrosate thiol groups to form nitrosothiols [30, 31]. It has been suggested that the major deleterious effect associated with its formation *in vivo*, is not as an oxidant but rather as a nitrating agent of proteins, the modification of which can result in a loss of function. High and low molecular mass nitrosothiols may act as an *in vivo* sink for NO, indicating a positive role for $ONOO^-$ formation *in vivo*. Indeed, reports have shown the ability of $ONOO^-$ to induce vasorelaxation, some via thiol dependent release of NO [32]. Other reports suggest further beneficial effects may be associated with the scavenging of O_2^-, as NO has been shown to protect against this type of ROS-mediated lung injury [33, 34]. Additionally, physiologically relevant doses of $ONOO^-$ have been found to be cardioprotective in a cat model of myocardial ischaemia and reperfusion [35].

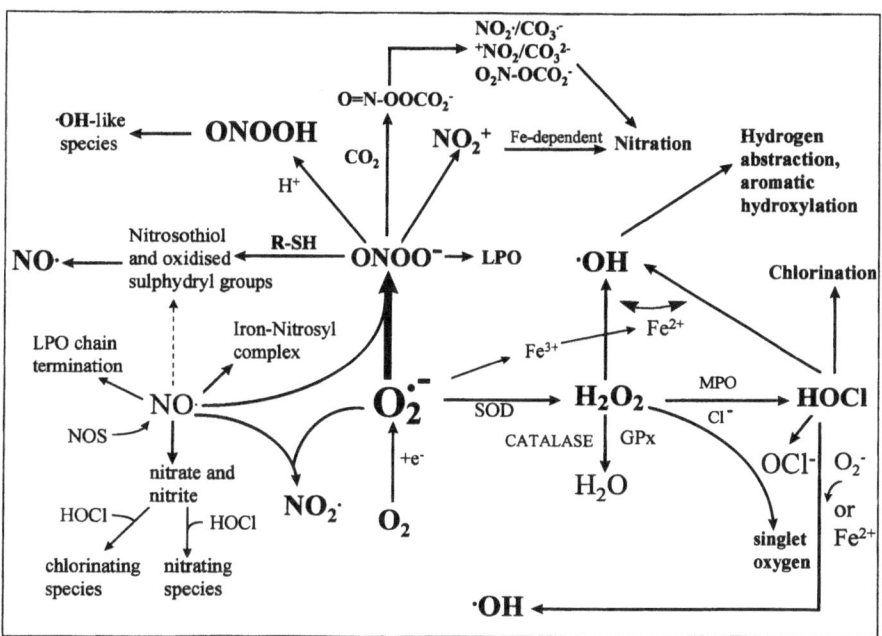

Figure 1. The interactions which may lead to the production of ROS and RNS *in vivo* are depicted. (LPO) lipid peroxidation, (GPx) glutathione peroxidase, (SOD) superoxide dismutase.

2.3. Summary

It is clear then that numerous ROS and RNS can be produced *in vivo*, and that there is a complex interrelationship between these species, which is further influenced by transition metal ion catalysts and antioxidants (see Fig. 1).

3. ROS and RNS and Their Role in Lung Injury

3.1. Acute Respiratory Distress Syndrome (ARDS)

ARDS is an acute form of inflammatory lung injury, precipitated by a variety of predisposing causes, many not directly related to the lung. It is characterised by non-cardiogenic pulmonary oedema and carries with it a high instance of mortality (for reviews see [36, 37]). ROS and RNS have been implicated as contributory factors to the onset and progression of ARDS, such species arise as a result of various processes (see Fig. 2).

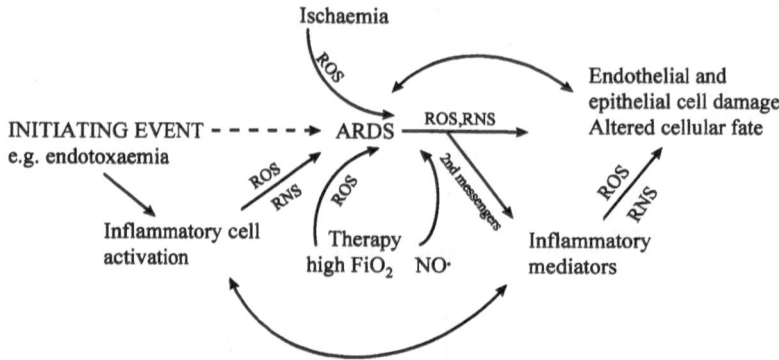

Figure 2. Possible sources of ROS and RNS in ARDS are illustrated.

3.2. Hyperoxia

It is now known that the deleterious effects of oxygen are attributable to the reactive nature of its reductive intermediates, this was first proposed as a theory by Gerschman and colleagues in 1954 [38]. ROS and RNS arise *in vivo* principally as a result of normal cellular metabolic processes. 1% of all oxygen consumed during aerobic respiration leaks from the respiratory chain of mitochondria as O_2^-, which is scavenged by endogenous anti-oxidants. However, exposure to normabaric concentrations of oxygen great-er than those found in normal air during hyperoxia, leads to increased leak-age of O_2^- from mitochondria and other organelles, with a consequent increase in H_2O_2 (for reviews see [39, 40]). The pathology of oxygen toxicity in the lungs of humans results in tissue damage and can lead to ALI [9]. Oxygen-induced lung damage leads to atelectasis, fibrin deposition, thickening and hyalinisation of alveolar membranes [41], and alterations in the composition and properties of surfactant [42]. Evidence for the involve-ment of oxidants in this form of lung injury is further strengthened by find-ings showing protection from oxygen toxicity after previous exposure to hyperoxia [43], endotoxin [44], or cytokines [45]. Protection results from the induction of lung antioxidant defences at the time of primary exposure. These defences include upregulation of antioxidant enzymes (SODs, cata-lase, glutathione peroxidases), iron-oxidising enzymes (caeruloplasmin) [46, 47], and protective peptides [48]. Recently, inhibitors of anion exchange and L-arginine have been shown to attenuate this form of lung injury, im-plicating the O_2^- anion and $ONOO^-$ in the injury process [49].

3.3. Ischaemia Reperfusion Injury

When tissues are deprived of oxygen (ischaemia) or oxygen tensions are reduced (hypoxia), biochemical changes result in cell damage and death. If oxygen is restored to tissues they can survive, but this is dependent on the length of time the tissue was deprived of oxygen and also on the type of tissue. However, studies have shown that on reoxygenation an additional cellular injury occurs which is mediated in part by the production of ROS and is known as ischaemia/reperfusion injury [50]. Several mechanisms for ROS production in ischaemia/reperfusion injury have been proposed but it is now thought that they may be formed as a result of changes to the mito-chondrial electron transport chain during ischaemia/hypoxia, which result in increased leakage of O_2^- when tissues are reperfused. The formation of eicosanoids relies on single electron transfer reactions, these biosynthetic processes are upregulated during ischaemia and may lead to ROS forma-tion (reviewed in [51]). Inflammatory cell activation and ROS release during the respiratory burst may also be involved in ischaemia/reperfusion injury, although some literature suggests that this is not a feature in the initial stages of injury [51]. Much research into ischaemia/reperfusion injury has concentrated on the enzyme xanthine oxidase (XOD) and its role in ROS production during ischaemia/reperfusion [50, 52, 53]. The enzyme exists in two isoforms, and is rate limiting in purine catabolism. The oxi-dase form of XOD is produced by limited proteolysis or oxidative modif-ication [54] as a result of neutrophil activation [55]. XOD catalyses the breakdown of purines to uric acid, coupled with the reduction of oxygen to O_2^- and H_2O_2. Appreciable conversion of the enzyme occurs during isch-aemia, and when oxygen is reintroduced, ROS are formed. Additionally, levels of substrates (hypoxanthine and xanthine) for the enzyme become elevated during the ischaemic period due to aberrant ATP metabolism [54], so increasing the prooxidant potential of XOD. Recently, substrate forma-tion rather than enzyme conversion has been shown to be of key importance in myocardial ischaemia/reperfusion injury [56]. A potential for XOD-mediated ROS production in patients with ARDS exists, as plasma and bronchoalveolar lavage fluid (BAL) hypoxanthine levels are found to be significantly elevated in non-surviving patients [57] and XOD is detectable in plasma from such patients [58]. Lung injury in the form of high per-meability pulmonary oedema is seen in animal studies where XOD and xanthine are instilled into the lungs of rabbits or rats [59, 60]. Further, lipo-polysaccharide (LPS)-induced pulmonary oedema in the mouse lung is associated with the induction of XOD activity [61].

The liver and the gut are particularly rich in XOD [62], which is present in relatively low amounts in the heart and lung [63], casting doubt on the role of XOD in ischaemia/reperfusion injury in these organs. However, recent evidence shows that XOD has a heparin-like binding site and is capable of binding to endothelial cells [64]. So raising the possibility that XOD may be released into the circulation, and may subsequently bind to the endothelium within organs where it is not normally found. Indeed, recent studies in animal models of gut and liver induced surgical ischaemia show lung injury attributable to the activity of XOD [65]. Further, XOD has now been demonstrated in animal [66], and human endothelial cells [67] where it contributes to lung injury through several mechanisms including oxidant formation [68]. XOD may contribute to ischaemia/reperfusion injury by promoting neutrophil sequestration in the lung by an O_2^--dependent mechanism [69] and by contributing to their adherence to cultured endothelial cells in the presence of xanthine [70]. It may also promote cytokine production and NF-κ B activation in lungs, as seen in a mouse models of haemorrhagic shock [71, 72].

3.4. *Inflammatory Cells*

Activated neutrophils and macrophages contain a membrane-bound nicotinamide dinucleotide phosphate (NADPH) oxidase enzyme, which produces O_2^- (the respiratory burst), and contributes to bacterial cell killing [73]. Recently, similar enzyme systems have been found in other cell types including lung fibroblasts [74]. Increased levels of O_2^- production have been demonstrated in animal models of ALI induced by oleic acid and endotoxemia [75, 76], and the NADPH oxidase inhibitor apocynin is known to attenuate sepsis induced lung injury in guinea-pigs [77]. Under normal physiological conditions O_2^- rapidly dismutates to H_2O_2 an effect which can also be seen during the respiratory burst of neutrophils [78]. H_2O_2 is detectable in breath condensates of patients with ARDS, at significantly elevated levels compared to ventilated non-ARDS control patients [79], and in patients with hypoxemic respiratory failure [80]. Additionally it can be detected in the urine of critically ill patients with sepsis and ARDS [81], (reviewed in [82]). The ·OH radical is formed from H_2O_2 in the presence of redox active iron, and recently this form of iron has been measured in human BAL fluid [83]. This may have implications for ROS mediated lung injury in acute inflammatory states such as ARDS and ALI. Indeed evidence for ·OH mediated damage to BAL fluid protein measured as non-enzyme formed tyrosine isomers (makers of ·OH formation), has been found in these patients [84]. The ·OH radical is also capable of initiating lipid peroxidation. Animal models of acute lung injury show increases in non-specific markers of lipid peroxidation, such as thiobarbituric reactive substances (TBARS) in lung tissue [85] and conjugated dienes in plasma [86], the levels of which are related to the degree of lung injury. In humans with ARDS, elevated plasma levels of TBARS have been found accompanied by decreased levels of unsaturated fatty acids and vitamin E [87]. Plasma TBARS levels have also been shown to correlate well with the Murray lung injury score in ARDS patients, although the mechanisms involved may not be entirely neutrophil dependent [88]. Mechanical ventilation may also contribute to plasma lipid peroxidation in such critically ill patients [89]. However, 4-hydroxy-2-nonenal (HNE) is a more reliable indicator of lipid peroxidation. It is a specific aldehydic n-6 fatty acid oxidation product, which has been demonstrated *in vivo* (reviewed in [90]). HNE can be cytotoxic, chemotactic, inhibit some enzymes and be produced by lung neutrophils in the rat [91]. Elevated levels of this bio-active aldehyde have been reported in the plasma of patients with ARDS [92]. HNE and other products of lipid peroxidation are markers of oxidative damage, but additionally may contribute to injurious processes in the lung. For instance, linoleic acid hydroperoxides which induce broncho- and vasoconstriction in isolated rat lungs [93], are toxic to endothelial cells [94], and lead to increased phospholipid oxidation [95]. The other oxidant produced by neutrophils is hypochlorous acid. Evidence to implicate this aggressive ROS in lung injury is strengthened by findings of subcellular matrix damage of the endothelium [96], and loss of lung surfactant surface tension function [97]. Recently, chlorinated tyrosine residues (markers of hypochlorous acid formation) on BAL fluid proteins have been detected in patients with ARDS at significantly elevated levels compared to ventilated and normal control groups, findings suggestive of a role for this oxidant in lung injury seen in these patients [84].

It is now clear that RNS are formed in a variety of inflammatory disease states where NO may be formed in excess. Upregulation of inducible NOS leads to increased formation of NO. Under such conditions, where there are high levels of both NO and O_2^-, $ONOO^-$ formation is favoured. This reaction is very fast and 'out competes' SOD enzymes, and occurs at a much faster rate than iron catalysed $\cdot OH$ formation. Promoting some to suggest that $ONOO^-$ is chiefly responsible for the oxidative damage seen in pathological conditions (reviewed in [2]). $ONOO^-$ is a powerful oxidant, but supportive evidence for its formation *in vivo* comes mainly from measurement of products formed due to its action as a nitrating species, in particular its ability to nitrate tyrosine residues [98]. The precise mechanism of the nitration reaction is unclear, but may involve an iron-dependent reaction in which nitronium ions are formed and react with tyrosine [98] or via the formation of a reactive intermediate with carbon dioxide [99, 100]. Macrophages [101], neutrophils [102], and cultured vascular endothelium [103], have all been implicated as sources of $ONOO^-$. In addition nitrotyrosine has been detected by immunohistochemistry in lung slices [104] and by high-pressure liquid chromatography (HPLC) in BAL fluid proteins from patients with ARDS [84].

The mechanisms of $ONOO^-$ mediated lung injury are varied, and may include its ability as an oxidant to cause lipid peroxidation [105], glutathione depletion [106] and other forms of $\cdot OH$-like damage. It can nitrate lung surfactant proteins (SP-A) leading to a decreased ability to aggregate lipids [107] and decreased mannose binding ability [108] resulting in impaired surfactant function. It may also impair sodium transport [109] and surfactant synthesis by alveolar type II cells [110]. All these adverse effects might be exacerbated by the use of inhaled NO therapy, which is sometimes used as a treatment for pulmonary hypertension [111]. Indeed, numerous studies in animals have demonstrated damage and dysfunction associated with inhaled NO treatment [111].

3.5. Antioxidants

The extracellular iron-binding and iron-oxidising anti-oxidant proteins transferrin and caeruloplasmin, are compromised in patients with ARDS [112, 113] and free redox active iron can be detected in the plasma of some patients [114]. Likewise in BAL fluid of patients with ARDS, abnormalities in transferrin and caeruloplasmin are present [115]. Recently, redox active iron has been demonstrated in normal BAL fluid, and elevated levels of transferrin iron saturation have been found in BAL fluid from patients with ARDS [23]. Deficiencies in these antioxidants may therefore contribute to increased oxidative damage and nitration, via iron catalysed mechanisms, in these patients. Interestingly, plasma levels of the intracellular iron-binding protein ferritin have been shown to be a predictive mortality factor in ARDS [116]. Reduced glutathione contains a thiol group, it reacts with oxidants such as H_2O_2, hypochlorous acid, and $ONOO^-$, and protects proteins from aldehydic modification [117], and is a cofactor for the antioxidant protein glutathione peroxidase. Extracellular levels of glutathione are low except in lung lining fluid, but in patients with ARDS this is not the case as most of the glutathione is oxidised [118], suggestive of increased oxidative stress in the lungs of these patients. In plasma, glutathione levels are very low, but there are other high molecular mass thiol containing proteins (mainly albumin) which perform similar antioxidant functions, levels of which are reduced in patients with ARDS [119]. Other plasma and lipid phase antioxidants such as ascorbic acid and vitamin E are similarly reduced in these patients [120, 121]. To compensate for this deficiency in antioxidant levels treatment regimes involving the use of exogenous antioxidants such as N-acetylcysteine have been employed with limited success [122].

3.6. Other Lung Diseases

ROS and RNS have been implicated in many other respiratory diseases including asthma and chronic obstructive pulmonary disease (COPD), in which iron [123], inflammatory cell activation [124] and ROS [124] production are implicated (for review see [125]). XOD formation may also contribute to oxidative stress in these patients [126]. The underlying mechanism of asthma is at present unclear, but ROS formed by inflammatory cells are implicated [127]. Further, lung cells recovered from asthmatics can generate increased amounts of ROS and have reduced antioxidant (SOD) activity [127], other antioxidants are also reduced in the plasma of these patients (glutathione peroxidase) [128]. Elevated levels of inducible NOS and NO [129] are also seen, raising the possibility of ONOO⁻ production in these patients. In addition, inhaled oxidant pollution gases are implicated in asthma (see previous sections), as are particulate air pollution products (PM10s). Recent findings show that these particles exhibit oxidant activity [130].

Patients with cystic fibrosis experience elevated oxidative stress due to chronic lung inflammation, and inadequate absorption of dietary antioxidants. Increased levels of markers of oxidative damage to lipids and DNA are found in such patients [131, 132], which in the case of lipids correlates with pulmonary dysfunction. Markers of RNS formation are elevated in the lungs of patients with idiopathic pulmonary fibrosis implicating such species in the disease process [133]. Paraquat poisoning causes damage to pulmonary tissue via the redox cycling activity of this herbicide which results in the formation ROS capable of damaging DNA [134].

4. ROS and RNS as Second Messengers

NO is a known second messenger, but recently other RNS/ROS have been attributed roles in intracellular signal transduction pathways. Many cellular processes including apoptosis [135], are thought to be regulated by subtoxic levels of ROS/RNS. Indeed the anti-apoptotic gene *bcl-2* has been shown to operate by lowering intracellular ROS production [136, 137]. The level of oxidative stress is critical in the signalling process, low concentrations of H_2O_2 will induce apoptosis, but higher concentrations lead to unwanted cell death via necrosis [138], similar findings are seen with other

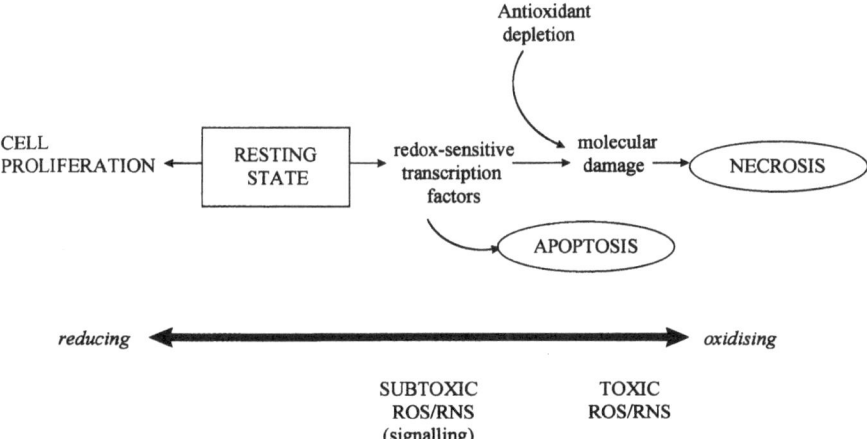

Figure 3. The role of ROS and RNS as second messengers in determining cellular fate are illustrated.

ROS and RNS (for reviews see 139). Transcription factors such as AP-1 [140], and NFκB [141, 142] are redox-sensitive and can be activated by ROS/RNS, apoptosis may ultimately be regulated by mechanisms such as these (see Fig. 3).

5. Concluding Remarks

The direct measurement of oxidants and the detection of specific markers of oxidative damage in both acute and chronic lung injury, are suggestive of the production of ROS and RNS in these disease states. However, in humans the role of these species as contributors or consequential agents to disease processes still remains to be elucidated. In animal models the evidence is more obvious as both oxidants and antioxidants have been shown to exhibit profound and opposing effects in the lung. Much recent interest has centred on the contribution of ROS and RNS, at sublethal levels, to lung function and heart disease. It is now apparent that at low levels, many reactive species can act as second messenger molecules and may be involved in many regulatory steps that determine cellular fate. Understanding these redox regulatory processes may lead to a better understanding of the role of ROS and RNS in lung injury and other disease processes.

6. References

1 Gutteridge JMC (1993) Free radicals in disease processes: a complication of cause and consequence. *Free Rad Res* 19: 141–158
2 Muijsers RBR, Folkerts G, Henricks PAJ, Sadeghi-Hashjin G, NijKamp FP (1997) ONOO⁻: a two-faced metabolite of nitric oxide. *Life Sci* 60: 1833–1845
3 Bannister WH, Bannister JV (1988) Isolation and characteristation of superoxide dismutase: a personal history and tribute to Joe McCord and Irwin Fridovich. *Free Rad Biol Med* 5: 371–376
4 Halliwell B, Gutteridge JMC (1990) Role of free radicals and catalytic metal ions in human disease: an overview. *Methods Enzymol* 186: 1–85
5 Beckman JS, Beckman TW, Chan J, Marshall PA, Freeman BA (1990) Apparent hydroxyl radical production by peroxynitrite: Implications for endothelial injury from and superoxide. *Proc Nat Acad Sci* 87. 1620–1624
6 Candeias LP, Patel KB, Stratford MR, Wardman P (1993) Free hydroxyl radicals are formed on reaction between the neutrophil-derived species superoxide anion and hypochlorous acid. *FEBS Letts* 33: 151–153
7 Pryor WA, Squadrito GL (1995) The chemistry of peroxynitrite: a product from the reaction of nitric oxide with superoxide. *Am J Physiol* 268: L699–L722
8 Candeias LP, Stratford MR, Wardman P (1994) Formation of hydroxyl radicals on reaction of hypochlorous acid with ferrocyanide, a model iron (II) complex. *Free Rad Res* 20: 241–249
9 Doelman CJ, Bast A (1990) Oxygen radicals in lung pathology. *Free Rad Bio Med* 9: 381–400
10 Hanley N, Kozumbo W, Costa D et al (1993) Induction of DNA single strand breaks in lung cells by ozone exposure *in vivo* and *in vitro*. *Am Rev Respir Dis* 147: A670
11 Cross CE, Motchnik PA, Bruener BA, Jones DA, Kaur H, Ames BN, Halliwell B (1992) Oxidative damage to plasma constituents by ozone. *FEBS Letts* 298: 269–272
12 Weiss SJ (1989) Tissue destruction by neutrophils. *N Engl J Med* 320: 365–376

13 Heinecke JW, Li W, Francis GA, Goldstein JA (1993) Tyrosyl radical generated by myeloperoxidase catalyzes the oxidative cross-linking of proteins. *J Clin Invest* 91: 2866–2872

14 van der Vliet A, Eiserich JP, Halliwell B, Cross CE (1997) Formation of reactive nitrogen species during peroxidase-catalysed oxidation of nitrite. A potential additional mechanism of nitric oxide-dependent toxicity. *J Biol Chem* 272: 7617–7625

15 Eiserich JP, Cross CE, Jones AD, Halliwell B, van der Vliet A (1996) Formation of nitrating and chlorinating species by reaction of nitrite with hypochlorous acid. A novel mechanism for nitric oxide-mediated modification. *J Biol Chem* 271: 19199–19208

16 Rawls H, Van Santen P (1997) Singlet oxygen: A possible source of the original hydroperoxides in fatty acids. *Ann NY Acad Sci* 171: 135–137

17 Cueto R, Squadrito GL, Bermudez E, Pryor WA (1992) Identification of heptanal and nonenal in bronchoalveolar lavage from rats exposed to low levels of ozone. *Biochem Biophys Res Comm* 188: 129–134

18 Radi R, Beckman JS, Bush KM, Freeman BA (1991) Peroxynitrite-induced membrane lipid peroxidation: The cytotoxic potential of superoxide and nitric oxide. *Arch Biochem Biophys* 288: 481–487

19 Panasenko OM, Evgina SA, Aidyraliev RK, Sergienko VI, Vladimrov YA (1994) Peroxidation of human blood lipoproteins induced by exogenous hypochlorite or hypochlorite generated in the system of myloperoxidase $^+H_2O_2^+$ Cl^-. *Free Rad Biol Med* 16: 143–148

20 Fukahori M, Ichimori K, Ishida H, Nakagawa H, Okino H (1994) Nitric oxide reversibly suppresses xanthine oxidase activity. *Free Rad Res* 21: 203–212

21 Brooks EC, Mahr NN, Radisavljevic Z, Jacobson ED, Terada LS (1997) Attenuates and xanthine oxidase exaggerates lung damage-induced gut injury. *Am J Physiol* 272: G845–G852

22 Strand V, Rak S, Svartengren M, Bylin G (1997) Nitrogen dioxide exposure enhances asthmatic reaction to inhaled allergen in subjects with asthma. *Am J Respir Crit Care Med* 155: 881–887

23 Beckman J, Tsai J-H (1994) Reactions and diffusion of nitric oxide and peroxynitrite. *The Biochemist* Oct/Nov 8–10

24 Blough N, Zafiriou O (1985) Reaction of superoxide with nitric oxide to form peroxynitrite in alkaline aqueous solutions. *Inorg Chem* 24: 3502–3504

25 Xia Y, Dawson VL, Dawson TM, Snyder SH, Zweier JL (1996) Nitric oxide synthase generates superoxide and nitric oxide in arginine-depleted cells leading to peroxynitrite-mediated cellular injury. *Proc Natl Acad Sci USA* 93: 6770–6774

26 Radi R, Beckman JS, Bush K, Freeman BA (1991) Peroxynitrite oxidation of sulfhydryls: The cytotoxic potential of superoxide and nitric oxide. *J Biol Chem* 266: 4244–4250

27 Gatti RM, Radi R, Augusto O (1994) Peroxynitrite-mediated oxidation of albumin to the protein-thiyl free radical. *FEBS Letts* 348: 287–290

28 Ischiropoulos H, Zhu L, Chen J, Tsai M, Martin JC, Smith CD, Beckman JS (1992) Peroxynitrite mediated tyrosine nitration catalysed by superoxide dismutase. *Arch Biochem Biophys* 298: 431–437

29 Rubbo AB, Barnes KM, Freeman BA, Radi R (1996) Peroxynitrite-dependent tryptophan nitration. *Chem Res Toxicol* 9: 390–396

30 Butler AR, Rhodes P (1997) Chemistry, analysis, and biological roles of S-nitrosothiols. *Anal Biochem* 249: 1–9

31 Singh RJ, Hogg N, Joseph J, Kalyanaraman B (1996) Mechanism of nitric oxide release from S-nitrosothiols. *J Biol Chem* 271: 18596–18603

32 Davidson CA, Kaminski PM, Wolin MS (1997) NO elicits prolonged relaxation of bovine pulmonary arteries via endogenous peroxynitrite generation. *Am J Physiol* 273: L437–L444

33 Guidot DM, Repine MJ, Hybertson BM, Repine JE (1995) Inhaled nitric oxide prevents neutrophil-mediated, oxygen radical-dependent leak in isolated rat lungs. *Am J Physiol* 269: L2–L5

34 Gutierrez HH, Nieves B, Chumley P, Rivera A, Freeman BA (1996) Nitric oxide regulation of superoxide-dependent lung injury: oxidant-protective actions of endogenously produced and exogenously administered nitric oxide. *Free Rad Biol Med* 21: 43–52

35 Nossuli TO, Reid H, Scalia R, Lefer AM (1997) Peroxynitrite reduces myocardial infarct size and preserves coronary endothelium after ischemia and reperfusion in cats. *Circulation* 96: 2317–2324

36 Bernard GR, Artigas A, Brigham KL, Carlet J, Falke K, Hudson L et al (1994) The American-European consensus on ARDS. *Am J Respir Crit Care Med* 149: 818–824

37 Pittet JF, Mackersie RC, Martin TR, Matthay MA (1997) Biological markers of acute lung injury: prognostic and pathogenic significance. *Am J Respir Crit Care Med* 155: 1187–1205

38 Gerschman R, Gilbert D, Nye S et al (1954) Oxygen poisioning and x-radiation: A mechanism in common. *Science* 199: 623–626

39 Jackson R (1990) Molecular, pharmacologic, and clinical aspects of oxygen induced lung injury. *Clin Chest Med* 1: 73–86

40 Cross CE, Van der Viliet A, O'Neill C, Eiserich J (1994) Reactive oxygen species and the lung. *Lancet* 344: 930–933

41 Deneke S, Fanburg B (1980) Normobaric oxygen toxicity of the lung. *N Engl J Med* 303: 76–86

42 Balaan M, Bowman L, Dedhia H, Miles P (1995) Hyperoxia-induced alterations of rat alveolar lavage composition and properties. *Exp Lung Res* 21: 141–156

43 Clerch L, Massaro D (1993) Tolerance of rats to hyperoxia: Lung antioxidant enzyme gene expression. *J Clin Invest* 91: 499–508

44 Frank L, Summerville J, Massaro D (1980) Protection from oxygen toxicity with endotoxin. Role of the endogenous antioxidant enzymes of the lung. *J Clin Invest* 65: 1104–1110

45 White C, Ghezzi P, Dinarello C, Caldwell S, McMurty I, Repine J (1987) Recombinant tumour necrosis factor/cachectin and interleukin 1 pretreatment decreases lung oxidised glutathione accumulation, lung injury and mortality in rats exposed to hyperoxia. *J Clin Invest* 79: 1868–1873

46 Erzurum S, Danel C, Gillssen A, Chu CS, Trapnell BC, Crystal RG (1993) *In vivo* antioxidant gene expression in human airway epithelium of normal individuals exposed to 100% oxygen. *J Appl Physiol* 75: 1256–1262

47 Fleming R, Whitman I, Gitlin J (1991) Induction of caeruloplasmin gene expression in rat lung during inflammation and hyperoxia. *Am J Physiol* 260: L68–L74

48 Town I, Phillips G, Murdoch E, Holgate S, Kelly F (1993) Temporal association between pulmonary inflammation and antioxidant induction following hyperoxic exposure of the preterm guinea-pig. *Free Rad Res Communs* 18: 211–223

49 Nozik-Grayck E, Piantadosi CA, van Adelsberg J, Alsper SL, Huang YC (1997) Protection of perfused lung from oxidant injury by inhibitors of anion exchange. *Am J Physiol* 273: L296–L304

50 McCord J (1985) Oxygen-derived free radicals in postischaemic tissue injury. *N Engl J Med* 312: 159–163

51 Ferrari R (1994) Oxygen free radicals at myocardial level: effects of ischaemia and reperfusion. In: Armstrong D (ed). Free radicals in diagnostic medicine. A systems approach to laboratory technology, clinical correlations, and antioxidant therapy. New York and London: Plenum Press, 99–122

52 Granger D, Hollwarth M, Parks D (1986) Ischaemia-reperfusion injury: Role of oxygen derived free radicals. *Physiol Scand Suppl* 548: 47–63

53 Ward A, McBurney A, Lunec J (1994) Evidence for the involvement of oxygen-derived free radicals in ischaemia-reperfusion injury. *Free Rad Res* 20: 21–28

54 Parks D, Granger N (1986) Xanthine oxidase: biochemistry, distribution and physiology. *Acta Physiol Scand* 54: 87–99

55 Wakabayashi Y, Fujita H, Morita I, Kawagushi H, Murota S (1995) Conversion of xanthine oxidase in bovine carotid artery endothelial cells induced by activated neutrophils: involvement of adhesion molecules. *Biochim Biophys Acta* 1265: 103–109

56 Xia Y, Zweier JL (1995) Substrate control of free radical generation from xanthine oxidase in the postischemic heart. *J Biol Chem* 270: 18797–18803

57 Quinlan GJ, Lamb NJ, Tilly R, Evans TW, Gutteridge JMC (1997) Plasma hypoxanthine levels in ARDS: implications for oxidative stress, morbidity and mortality. *Am J Respir Crit Care Med* 155: 479–484

58 Grum C, Ragsdale R, Ketani L, Simon R (1987) Plasma xanthine oxidase activity in patients with adult respiratory distress syndrome. *J Crit Care* 2: 22–26

59 Tate R, Vanbenthuysen K, Shasby D, McMurtry IF, Repine JE (1982) Oxygen radical mediated permeability oedema and vasoconstriction in isolated perfused rabbit lungs. *Am Rev Respir Dis* 126: 802–806

60 Johnson K, Fantone J, Kaplan J, Ward PA (1981) *In vivo* damage of rat lungs by oxygen metabolits. *J Clin Invest* 67: 983–993
61 Faggioni R, Gatti S, Demitri M, Delgado R, Echtenacher B, Gnocchi P et al (1994) Role of xanthine oxidase and reactive oxygen intermediates in LPS and TNF-induced pulmonary oedema. *J Lab Clin Med* 123: 394–399
62 Kurosaki M, Li Calzi M, Scanziani E, Garattini E, Terao M (1995) Tissue- and cell-specific expression of mouse xanthine oxidoreductase gene *in vivo*: Regulation by bacterial LPS. *Biochem J* 306: 225–234
63 Sarnesto A, Linder N, Raivio KO (1996) Organ distribution and molecular forms of human xanthine dehydrogenase/xanthine oxidase protein. *Lab Invest* 74: 48–56
64 Adachi T, Fukushima T, Usami Y, Hirano K (1993) Binding of human xanthine oxidase to sulphated glycosaminoglycans on the endothelial-cell surface. *Biochem J* 289: 523–527
65 Nielsen VG, Tan S, Weinbroum A, McCammon AT, Samuelson PN, Gelman S et al (1996) Lung injury after hepatoenteric Ischemia-reperfusion injury: role of xanthine oxidase. *Am J Respir Crit Care Med* 154: 1364–1369
66 Phan S, Gannon D, Varani J, Ryan U, Ward P (1989) Xanthine oxidase activity in rat pulmonary artery endothelial cells and its alteration by activated neutrophils. *Am J Pathol* 134: 1201–1211
67 Zweier J, Kuppusamy P, Thompson-Gorman S, Klunk D, Lutty G (1994) Measurement and characterisation of free radical generation in reoxygenated human endothelial cells. *Am J Physiol* 266: C700–C708
68 Ward P (1991) Mechanisms of endothelial cell injury. *J Lab Clin Med* 118: 421–426
69 Till G, Friedl H, Ward P (1991) Lung injury and complement activation: Role of neutrophils and xanthine oxidase. *Free Rad Biol Med* 10: 379–386
70 Moores H, Beehler C, Hanley M, Shanley PF, Stevens EE, Repine JE et al (1994) Xanthine oxidase promotes neutrophil sequestration but not injury in hyperoxic lungs. *J Appl Physiol* 76: 941–945
71 Shenkar R, Abraham E (1996) Plasma from hemorrhaged mice activates CREB and increases cytokine expression in lung mononuclear cells through a xanthine oxidase-dependent mechanism. *Am J Respir Cell Mol Biol* 14: 198–206
72 Shenkar R, Schwartz MD, Terada LS, Repine JE, McCord J, Abraham E (1996) Hemorrage activates NK-kappa B in murine lung mononuclear cells *in vivo*. *Am J Physiol* 270: L729–L735
73 Babior B (1984) The respiratory burst of phagocytes. *J Clin Invest* 73: 599–601
74 Thannickal VJ, Fanburg BL (1995) Activation of H_2O_2 – generating NADH oxidase in human lung fibroblasts by transforming growth factor *beta* 1. *J Biol Chem* 270: 30334–30338
75 Kelly F, Rickett G, Philips G (1992) Magnitude of hyperoxic stress and degree of lung maturity determine the nature of pulmonary antioxidant response in the guinea-pig. *Free Rad Res Communs* 17: 335–347
76 Wizemann T, Laskin D (1994) Enhanced phagocytosis, chemotaxis, and production of reactive oxygen intermediates by interstitial lung macrophages following acute endotoxemia. *Am J Respir Cell Mol Biol* 11: 358–365
77 Wang W, Suzuki Y, Tanigaki T, Rank D, Raffin T (1994) Effect of the NADPH oxidase inhibitor apocynin on septic lung injury in guinea-pigs. *Am J Respir Crit Care Med* 150: 1449–1452
78 Wyman M, Tscharner V, Deranleau D, Baggiolini M (1987) Chemiluminescence detection of hydrogen peroxide produced by human neutrophils during the respiratory burst. *Anal Biochem* 165: 371–378
79 Baldwin S, Simon R, Grum C, Ketai LH, Boxer LA, Devall LJ et al (1986) Oxidant activity in expired breath of patients with adult respiratory distress syndrome. Lancet 1: 11–14
80 Sznajder J, Fraiman A, Hall J, Sanders SW, Schmidt G, Crawford G et al (1989) Increased hydrogen peroxide in the expired breath of patients with acute hypoxemic respiratory failure. *Chest* 96: 602–612
81 Mathru M, Rooney M, Dries D, Hirsch LJ, Barnes L, Tobin MJ et al (1994) Urine hydrogen peroxide during adult respiratory distress syndrome in patients with and without sepsis. *Chest* 105: 232–236
82 Sibille Y, Reynolds H (1990) Macrophages and polymorphonuclear neutrophils in lung defence and injury. *Am Rev Respir Dis* 141: 471–501

83 Gutteridge JMC, Mumby S, Quinlan GJ, Chung KF, Evans TW (1996) Pro-oxidant iron is present in human pulmonary epithelial lining fluid: implications for oxidative stress in the lung. *Biochem Biophys Res Communs* 220: 1024–1027

84 Lamb NJ, Gutteridge JMC, Baker CS, Evans TW, Quinlan GJ (1999) Oxidative damage to proteins of bronchoalveolar lavage fluid protein in patients with ARDS. Evidence for neutrophil mediated hydroxylation, nitration and chlorination. *Crit Care Med* in press

85 Demling H, Lalonde C, Jin L, Ryan P, Fox R (1986) Endotoximia causes increased lung tissue lipid peroxidation in unanesthetized sheep. *J Appl Physiol* 60: 2094–2100

86 Ward PA, Till GO, Hatherill JR, Annesley TM, Kunkel R (1985) systemic complement activation, lung injury, and the products of lipid peroxidation. *J Clin Invest* 76: 517–527

87 Richard C, Lemonnier F, Thibault M, Couturier M, Auzepy P (1990) Vitamin E deficiency and lipperoxidation during adult respiratory syndrome. *Crit Care Med* 18: 4–9

88 Lefevre G, Brunet F, Bonneau C et al (1994) Human polymorphonuclear leukocyte metabolism and lipopreoxidation during adult respiratory distress syndrome treated by extracorporeal carbon dioxide removal. *Pathophysiology* 1: 13–19

89 Baouali AB, Aube H, Maupoil V, Blettery B, Rochette L (1994) Plasma lipid peroxidation in critically ill patients: importance of mechanical ventilation. *Free Rad Biol Med* 16: 223–227

90 Esterbauer H, Schauer R, Zollner H (1991) Chemistry and biochemistry of 4-hydroxynonenal, malonaldehyde and related aldehydes. *Free Rad Biol Med* 11: 81–128

91 Schaur RJ, Dussing G, Kink E, Schauenstein E, Posch W, Kukovetz E et al (1994) The lipid peroxidation product 4-hydroxy-2-nonenal is formed by – and is able to attract – rat neutrophils *in vivo*. *Free Rad Res* 20: 365–373

92 Quinlan GJ, Lamb NJ, Evans TW, Gutteridge JMC (1996) Plasma fatty acid changes and increased lipid peroxidation in patients with adult respiratory distress syndrome. *Crit Care Med* 24: 241–246

93 Olafsdottir K, Ryrfeldt A, Atzori L, Berggren M, Moldeus P (1991) Hydroperoxide-induced broncho- and vasoconstriction in the isolated rat lung. *Exp Lung Res* 17: 615–627

94 Pacifici E, Mcleod L, Peterson H, Sevanian A (1994) Linoleic acid hydroperoxide-induced peroxidation of endothelial cell phospholipids and cytotoxicity. *Free Rad Biol Med* 17: 285–295

95 Pacifici E, Mcleod L, Sevanian A (1994) Lipid hydroperoxide-induced peroxidation and turnover of endothelial phospholipids. *Free Rad Biol Med* 17: 297–309

96 Vissers CM, Thomas C (1997) Hypochlorous acid disrupts the adhesive properties of subendothelial matrix. *Free Rad Biol Med* 23: 401–411

97 Merritt A, Amirkanian J, Helbock H, Halliwell B, Cross C (1993) Reduction of the surface-tension-lowering ability of surfactant after exposure to hypochlorous acid. *Biochem J* 295: 19–22

98 Ischiropoulos H, Zhu L, Chen J, Tsai M, Martin JC, Smith CD et al (1992) Peroxynitrite mediated tyrosine nitration catalysed by superoxide dismutase. *Arch Biochem Biophys* 298: 431–437

99 Denicola A, Freeman BA, Trujillo M, Radi R (1996) Peroxynitirte reaction with carbon dioxide/bicarbonate: kinetics and influence on peroxynitrite-mediated oxidations. *Arch Biochem Biophys* 333: 49–58

100 Pryor WA, Lemercier JN, Zhang H, Uppu RM, Squadrito GL (1997) The catalytic role of carbon dioxide in the decomposition of peroxynitrite. *Free Rad Biol Med* 23: 331–338

101 Ischiropoulos H, Zhu L, Beckman J (1992) Peroxynitirte formation from activated rat alveolar macrophages. *Arch Biochem Biophys* 298: 446–451

102 Carreras M, Pargament G, Catz S, Poderoso J, Boveris A (1994) Kinetics of nitric oxide and hydrogen peroxide production and formation of peroxynitrite during the respiratory burst of human neutrophils. *FEBS Letts* 341: 65–68

103 Kooy N, Royall J (1994) Antagonist-Induced peroxynitrite production by endothelial cells. *Arch Biochem Biophys* 310: 353–359

104 Kooy N, Royall J, Ye Y, Kelly D, Beckman J (1995) Evidence for *in vivo* peroxynitrite production in human acute lung injury. *Am J Respir Crit Care Med* 151: 1250–1254

105 Radi R, Beckman J, Bush K, Freeman B (1991) Peroxynitrite-induced membrane lipid peroxidation: The cytotoxic potential of superoxide and nitric oxide. *Arch Biochem Biophys* 288: 481–487

106 Radi R, Beckman J, Bush K, Freeman B (1991) Peroxynitrite oxidation of sulfhydryls: The cytotoxic potential of superoxide and nitric oxide. *J Biol Chem* 266: 4244–4250
107 Haddad IY, Zhu S, Ischiropoulos H, Matalon S (1996) Nitration of surfactant protein A results in decreased ability to aggregate lipids. *Am J Physiol* 270: L281–L288
108 Zhu S, Haddad IY, Matalon S (1996) Nitration of surfactant protein A (SP-A) tyrosine residues results in decreased mannose binding ability. *Arch Biochem Biophys* 333: 282–290
109 Hu P, Ischiropoulos H, Beckman JS, Matalon S (1994) Peroxynitrite inhibition of oxygen consumption and sodium transport in alveolar type II cells. *Am J Physiol* 266: L628–L634
110 Haddad IY, Zhu S, Crow J, Barefield E, Gadilhe T, Matalon S (1996) Inhibition of alveolar type II cell ATP and surfactant synthesis by nitric oxide. *Am J Physiol* 270: L898–L906
111 Matalon S, DeMarco V, Haddad IY, Myles C, Skimming JW, Schurch S et al (1996) Inhaled nitric oxide injures the pulmonary surfactant systems of lambs *in vivo*. *Am J Physiol* 270: L273–L280
112 Kresek-Staples J, Kew R, Webster R (1992) Caeruloplasmin and transferrin levels are altered in serum and bronchoalveolar lavage fluid of patients with adult respiratory distress syndrome. *Am Rev Respir Dis* 145: 1009–1015
113 Gutteridge JMC, Quinlan GJ, Mumby S, Heath A, Evans TW (1994) Primary plasma antioxidants in adult respiratory distress syndrome patients: Changes in iron-oxidising, iron-binding, and free radical-scavenging proteins. *J Lab Clin Med* 124: 263–273
114 Gutteridge JMC, Quinlan GJ, Evans TW (1994) Transient iron-overload with bleomycin-detectable iron in the plasma of patients with adult respiratory distress syndrome. *Thorax* 49: 707–710
115 Lykens M, Davis B, Pacht E (1992) Antioxidant activity of bronchoalveolar lavage fluid in the adult respiratory distress syndrome. *Am J Physiol* 262: L169–L175
116 Conelly KG, Moss M, Parsons PE, Moore EE, Moore FA, Giclas PC et al (1997) Serum ferritin as a predictor of the acute respiratory distress syndrome. *Am J Respir Crit Care Med* 155: 21–25
117 O'Neill C, Halliwell B, van der Vliet A, Davis PA, Packer L, Tritschler H et al (1994) Aldehyde-induced protein modifications in human plasma: Protection by glutathione and dihydrolipoic acid. *J Lab Clin Med* 124: 359–370
118 Bunnell E, Pacht ER (1993) Oxidised glutathione is increased in the alveolar fluid of patients with the adult respiratory distress syndrome. *Am Rev Respir Dis* 148: 1174–1178
119 Quinlan GJ, Evans TW, Gutteridge JMC (1994) Oxidative damage to plasma proteins in adult respiratory distress syndrome. *Free Rad Res* 20: 289–298
120 Cross C, Forte T, Stocker R, Louie S, Yamamoto Y, Ames BN et al (1990) Oxidative stress and abnormal cholesterol metabolism in patients with adult respiratory distress syndrome. *J Lab Clin Med* 115: 396–404
121 Leff J, Parson P, Day C, Taniguchi N, Jochum M, Fritz H et al (1993) Serum antioxidants as predictors of adult respiratory distress syndrome in patients with sepsis. *Lancet* 341: 777–780
122 Bernard GR, Wheeler AP, Arons MM, Moris PE, Paz HL, Russell JA et al (1997) A trial of antioxidants N-acetylcysteine and procysteine in ARDS. The antioxidant in ARDS study group. *Chest* 112: 164–172
123 Dekhuijzen PN, Aben KK, Dekker I, Aarts LP, Wielders PL, van Herwaarden CL et al (1996) Increased exhalation of hydrogen peroxide in patients with stable and unstable chronic obstructive pulmonary disease. *Am J Respir Crit Care Med* 154: 813–816
124 Calhoun WJ, Bush RK (1990) Enhanced reactive oxygen species metabolism of airspace cells and airway inflammation follow antigen challenge in human astham. *J Allergy Clin Immunol* 86: 306–313
125 Repine JE, Bast A, Lankhorst I (1997) Oxidative stress in chronic obstructive pulmonary disease. Oxidative Stress Study Group. *Am J Respir Crit Care Med* 156: 341–357
126 Pinamonti S, Muzzoli M, Chicca MC, Papi A, Ravenna F, Fabbri LM et al (1996) Xanthine oxidase activity in bronchoalveolar lavage fludi from patients with chronic obstructive pulmonary disease. *Free Radic Biol Med* 21: 147–155
127 Smith LJ, Shamsuddin M, Sporn PH, Denenberg M, Anderson J (1997) Reduced super-oxide dismutase in lung cells of patients with astham. *Free Radic Biol Med* 22: 1301–1307

128 Kadrabova J, Mad'aric A, Kovacikova Z, Podivinsky F, Ginter E, Gazdik F (1996) Selenium status is decreased in patients with intrinsic asthma. *Biol Trace Elem Res* 52: 241–248

129 Hamid Q, Springall DR, Riveros-Moreno V, Chanez P, Howarth P, Redington A et al (1993) Induction of nitric oxide synthase in asthma. *Lancet* 342: 8886–8887

130 Li XY, Gilmour PS, Donaldson K, MacNee W (1996) Free radical activity and proinflammatory effects of particulate air pollution (PM10) *in vivo* and *in vitro*. *Thorax* 51: 1216–1222

131 Brown RK, Wyatt H, Price JF, Kelly FJ (1996) Pulmonary dysfunction in cystic fibrosis is associated with oxidative stress. *Eur Respir J* 9: 334–339

132 Brown RK, McBurney A, Lunec J, Kelly FJ (1995) Oxidative damage to DNA in patients with cystic fibrosis. *Free Radic Biol Med* 18: 801–806

133 Saleh D, Barnes PJ, Giaid A (1997) Increased production of the potent oxidant peroxynitrite in the lungs of patients with idiopathic pulmonary fibrosis. *Am J Respir Crit Care Med* 155: 1763–1769

134 Ali S, Jain SK, Abdulla M, Athar M (1996) Paraquat induced DNA damage by reactive oxygen species. *Biochem Mol Biol Int* 39: 63–67

135 Sarafian TA, Bredesen DE (1994) Is apoptosis mediated by reactive oxygen species? *Free Radic Res* 21: 1–8

136 Kane DJ, Sarafian TA, Anton R, Hahn H, Gralla EB, Valentine JS et al (1993) Bcl-2 inhibition of neural death: decreased generation of reactive oxygen species. *Science* 262: 1274–1277

137 Hockenbery DM, Oltvai ZN, Yin XM, Milliman CL, Corsmeyer SJ (1993) Bcl-2 functions in an antioxidant pathway to prevent apoptosis. *Cell* 75: 241–251

138 Lennon SV, Martin SJ, Cotter TG (1991) Dose-dependent induction of apoptosis in human tumour cell lines by widely diverging stimuli. *Cell Prolif* 24: 203–214

139 Sen CK, Packer L (1996) Antioxidant and redox regulation of gene transcription. *FASEB J* 10: 709–720

140 Abate C, Patel L, Rauscher FJ, Curran T (1990) Redox regulation of fos and jun DNA-binding activity *in vitro*. *Science* 249: 1157–1161

141 Staal FJ, Roederer M, Herzenberg LA, Herzenberg LA (1990) Intracellular thiols regulate activation of nuclear factor kappa B and transcription of human immunodeficiency virus. *Proc Natl Acad Sci* 87: 9943–9947

142 Schreck R, Rieber P, Baeuerle PA (1991) Reactive oxygen intermediates as apparently widely used messengers in the activation of the NF-κ B transcription factor and HIV-1. *EMBO J* 10: 2247–2258

Role of Endogenous Nitric Oxide in the Lung

Nitric Oxide in Pulmonary Processes:
Role in Physiology and Pathophysiology of Lung Disease
ed. by M. G. Belvisi and J. A. Mitchell
© 2000 Birkhäuser Verlag Basel/Switzerland

CHAPTER 3
Non-Adrenergic Non-Cholinergic Neurotransmission in the Airways: Role of Nitric Oxide

Maria G. Belvisi[1] and Alan Gibson[2]

[1] *Pharmacology Department, Rhône-Poulenc Rorer Research and Development, Rainham Road South, Dagenham, Essex RM10 7XS, UK*
[2] *Pharmacology Group, Biomedical Sciences Division, King's College London, Manresa Road, Chelsea, London SW3 6LX, UK*

1   Introduction
2   Inhibitory (Relaxant) Mechanisms
2.1   Amphibians and Reptiles
2.2   Birds
2.3   Mammals
2.3.1 Guinea-pig
2.3.2 Rabbit
2.3.3 Dog
2.3.4 Cat
2.3.5 Sheep
2.3.6 Pig
2.3.7 Cow
2.3.8 Horse
2.4   Non-human Primates
2.5   Human
3   Non-Adrenergic, Non-Cholinergic (NANC) Mechanisms
3.1   Involvement of VIP in NANC Relaxant Responses in the Airways
3.2   Involvement of NO in NANC Relaxant Responses in the Airways
3.2.1 Guinea-pig
3.2.2 Cat
3.2.3 Pig
3.2.4 Rabbit
3.2.5 Horse
3.2.6 Ferret
3.2.7 Human
4   Distribution of NANC Responses in the Human Respiratory Tract
5   Nature of the Neurotransmitter
6   Functional Significance of the NANC Response
7   NANC Inhibitory Pathways in Disease
8   Conclusions
9   References

1. Introduction

Autonomic nerves regulate several aspects of airway function [1]. However, for the purposes of this chapter, we will focus on the role of nitric oxide (NO)-containing nerves in the control of airway smooth muscle function. Neural control of airway smooth muscle is very complex since in addition to cholinergic and adrenergic innervation there is a non-adrenergic non-cholinergic (NANC) innervation. The existence of a NANC nervous system in the gastrointestinal tract, which controls gut motility, sphincters and secretions had previously been established in vertebrates from fish to humans [2]. The airways develop embryologically from the foregut and so the existence of NANC nerves in the respiratory tract was not an unexpected finding.

On the whole most experiments in the literature describing patterns of innervation in the airways have centred on developing *in vitro* systems of measuring smooth muscle relaxation. In this manner the effects of electrical field stimulation (EFS), which stimulates all nerves in a preparation, on isometric tension development by the trachealis or bronchial smooth muscle have been determined in the presence or absence of various drugs. From these experiments it was elucidated that the smooth muscle of mammalian airways receives a dual contractile and relaxant innervation [3, 4] (see Fig. 1). In general neural relaxation of airway smooth muscle is achieved via activation of adrenergic and NANC neural pathways [5]. However, the sympathetic innervation to airway smooth muscle is species-dependent and may be sparse or even absent [6]. Moreover, in humans, sympathetic nerves innervate bronchial blood vessels, submucosal glands and parasympathetic ganglia and there are few, if any, nerve fibres supplying the airways smooth muscle [7]. Therefore, at least in human airways the major neural bronchodilator pathway is the NANC system (see Fig. 1). This chapter will discuss the evidence that NO is the NANC neurotransmitter involved in neurally mediated relaxation of airways smooth muscle. Since in inflammatory airway diseases such as asthma, changes in bronchial smooth muscle tone can occur very rapidly, it has been suggested that this could be due to a defect in the autonomic control of the airways smooth muscle [8]. This could manifest itself as an increase in the constrictor and a decrease in the dilator control of the airways. Therefore, if the NANC dilator innervation is dysfunctional in inflammatory conditions, its absence may lead to exaggerated bronchoconstriction [4].

Studies in animals have provided valuable information on the neural control of the respiratory tract and many of these studies have taken place on dogs, cats and rodents with few studies performed on human airways until the last few years. These experiments have highlighted an obvious variability in the innervation of the lung among species of animals, and any extrapolation between species in terms of either their physiological responses or the anatomical distribution of the nerves should be viewed with caution. In this chapter we illustrate the intra-species and regional differences in the relaxant innervation and the possible physiological and morphological changes that may be seen in the relaxant innervation to the respiratory tract under pathophysiological conditions.

2. Inhibitory (Relaxant) Mechanisms

2.1. Amphibians and Reptiles

The first studies investigating the inhibitory bronchodilator neural system in the lung were carried out in amphibians and reptiles [9, 10]. The lungs of the lizard and the toad have been studied using pharmacological and histochemical techniques. These studies provided evidence which suggested the existence of an inhibitory system with pre-ganglionic fibres present in the vagus and ganglion cells within the lung. In contrast to other species, it seems that the predominant inhibitory pathways in the lizard were the adrenergic fibres since noradrenaline evoked bronchodilation and adrenergic blocking agents significantly reduced, but did not abolish, nerve mediated relaxation [10]. This residual response was later confirmed to be non-adrenergic since it was not blocked in tissues pre-treated with 6-hydroxydopamine [11–13]. In addition, morphological studies in amphibians demonstrated the existence of large opaque vesicles (80–200 nm in diameter) within autonomic nerve terminals in the respiratory tract suggestive of the NANC inhibitory system [11].

2.2. Birds

The majority of studies on the neural innervation in birds have been carried out on the domestic chicken. Physiological studies have been carried out on the major bronchus of the chicken in vitro. EFS of this preparation in vitro elicited a primary response that was relaxant. However, although adrenergic agonists, either administered to the animal [14] or added to airway smooth muscle in vitro, evoked relaxations, ultrastructural studies have failed to demonstrate axon profiles characteristic of adrenergic nerves [15]. Furthermore, the relaxant response obtained in response to EFS was not blocked by propranolol [16]. Interestingly, the chicken bronchus only produced a contraction (atropine-sensitive) when the muscle was relaxed prior to the EFS stimulus [16]. Therefore, from these studies it was suggested that the major bronchus of the chicken is controlled by NANC inhibitory fibres that are dominant over the cholinergic constrictor response, a situation that is the reverse of that found in most species including human [17].

Following the above mentioned studies on amphibians, reptiles and birds the presence of the NANC inhibitory system was also detected in mammalian airways where it was first demonstrated in the guinea-pig [18–22].

2.3. Mammals

2.3.1. Guinea-pig: This species has been used extensively in pharmacological studies involving the mechanisms contributing to neural relaxation of the airways. Most studies suggest that parasympathetic, adrenergic and NANC nerves innervate guinea-pig airway smooth muscle with the cholinergic system being dominant. The adrenergic inhibitory nerves have been demonstrated physiologically to be more frequent in the proximal portions of the trachea [19]. This has been confirmed by morphological studies which have demonstrated the proximal localisation of the adrenergic nerves and also showed a complete lack of adrenergic fibres in the distal airways [22]. It was presumed that this lack of adrenergic dilator fibres in the distal airways would be compensated for by an increased NANC innervation to the lower airways but functional data did not support this hypothesis. However, in contrast to the findings of Coburn and Tomita [19] other studies have shown that the relative contribution of the two inhibitory neural inputs to the total relaxation response appeared to be similar in all regions of the guinea-pig trachea [23]. Furthermore, this study also demonstrated that both adrenergic and NANC inhibitory responses were frequency-dependent and that adrenergic nerves were activated at lower frequencies than NANC nerves.

The first evidence to suggest the existence of NANC inhibitory nerves in guinea-pig airways came from studies of EFS stimulated tracheal smooth muscle [19–21, 24]. Coburn and Tomita [19] demonstrated a biphasic response to EFS that consisted of an initial contraction followed by a relaxation. The contractile response was prevented by atropine whereas the relaxation response was not affected by muscarinic receptor antagonists and only partially inhibited by β-adrenoceptor blockade or by reserpine pretreatment establishing the existence of a NANC response in this species. The existence of NANC inhibitory nerves in guinea-pig trachea was also described in studies were luminal pressure changes were measured in a tracheal tube preparation after transmural stimulation. Neurally evoked contractile responses were inhibited by atropine and inhibitory responses were reduced, but not abolished by propranolol, guanethidine (adrenergic neurone blocker) or by pretreatment of the animals with 6-hydroxydopamine (which depletes catecholamines). These relaxations were blocked by tetrodotoxin indicating that these NANC responses were neural in origin [20, 21].

Other investigators studied the inhibitory innervation of an *in situ* cervical tracheal tube preparation in which vagal and sympathetic nerves could be selectively stimulated. In addition, the preparation allowed for stimulation of the cervical tracheal directly via transmural electrodes. These studies suggested that adrenergic relaxations (elicited via sympathetic nerve stimulation) accounted for 60–80% and NANC relaxations (elicited by vagal nerve stimulation) accounted for the residual (20–40%) of the relaxation response elicited via transmural stimulation [25]. This data also confirmed an earlier study which suggested that the NANC inhibitory system in the guinea-pig trachea receives pre-ganglionic innervation from the vagus nerve [26]. In contrast, other investigators found that the NANC nerves are the major inhibitory neural input to airway smooth muscle and that these responses were more evident at higher frequencies of stimulation [27]. Importantly, the NANC relaxant response has also been demonstrated *in vivo* in this species [28].

The precise anatomical pathways of the NANC innervation have not been determined and there may be species differences. However, most information has been gathered from studies undertaken in guinea-pig airways. The guinea-pig trachea receives NANC relaxant innervation from at least two extrinsic sources [29]. These two vagal pathways that serve the rostral portion of the guinea-pig trachea include a hexamethonium-sensitive relaxant innervation with pre-ganglionic fibres carried by the recurrent laryngeal nerves and capsaicin-sensitive vagal pathways carried by the superior laryngeal nerves. These pathways traverse through ganglia associated with the oesophagus [29]. Autonomic neurons often contain multiple transmitter substances. This co-transmission probably is a mechanism via which nerves can achieve precise control over a target organ. This has given rise to the common assumption that the NANC transmitter substance is colocalised with acetylcholine (ACh) (and possibly vasoactive intestinal peptide (VIP)) in post-ganglionic parasympathetic neurons. However, Canning and Undem [29] have suggested that the cholinergic contractile response and the NANC relaxation response of guinea-pig trachea are differentially sensitive to oesophageal removal. Therefore, it is now in doubt as to whether the NANC transmitter and ACh are in fact co-localised.

2.3.2. Rabbit: NANC relaxant responses, evoked by EFS, can also be demonstrated in rabbit tracheal smooth muscle but not in bronchial smooth muscle or lung parenchymal strips [30, 31]. In the same studies, rat tracheal smooth muscle did not exhibit NANC inhibitory responses to EFS.

2.3.3. Dog: Most studies in the dog have been carried out in isolated tracheal or bronchial strips *in vitro* in the presence and absence of adrenergic receptor antagonists. On the whole these studies suggest that the principle inhibitory innervation in dog airways is adrenergic and that the NANC nerves are either absent or have no significant functional role in regulating airway tone in this species [32–34].

2.3.4. Cat: Neural relaxation responses have been demonstrated in isolated segments of cat trachea and bronchi pre-contracted with 5-hydroxytryptamine (5-HT) [35]. These experiments suggested that both adrenergic and NANC nerves contributed to the relaxant response evoked by EFS. Moreover, experiments performed in the cat were among the first to demonstrate that the NANC inhibitory system could be demonstrated *in vivo* [36, 37] by stimulation of efferent vagal nerves. This response can be inhibited by the ganglion blocker hexamethonium, indicating that nerves containing the NANC transmitter have a pre-ganglionic parasympathetic origin [36]. Inhalation of capsaicin or mechanical stimulation of the larynx induces a similar bronchodilator response in cats after pre-treatment with atropine and propranolol indicating that reflex activation of these pathways is possible [38, 39].

2.3.5. Sheep: The autonomic innervation of sheep airway smooth muscle has also been studied by examining responses to EFS in isolated segments of the airway *in vitro* in the presence of adrenoceptor blockade. These studies suggested that sheep airways are innervated by both sympathetic and NANC inhibitory nerves with the adrenergic nerve population being more pronounced in the trachea compared to the bronchi [40].

2.3.6. Pig: Initially, experimental evidence pointed to the absence of NANC nerves in porcine airways. In these experiments the ganglion stimulant dimethylphenylpiperazinium bromide (DMPP), evoked frequency-related relaxations in the pig trachea *in vivo* that were completely blocked by propranolol. In addition, supramaximal bilateral vagal nerve stimulation failed to elicit airway smooth muscle relaxation following administration of propranolol [41]. Therefore, these authors concluded that NANC inhibitory nerves are not present in porcine airways. However, more recently, NANC relaxation responses have been demonstrated after EFS in porcine tracheal smooth muscle [42].

2.3.7. Cow: In the bovine trachea where there is little resting tone it is difficult to demonstrate a neural inhibitory response in an already relaxed preparation. Therefore, experiments in which investigators have examined a NANC inhibitory response *in vitro* have usually used preparations which have high tone. In these experiments Cameron et al. [43] demonstrated the existence of NANC inhibitory nerves in isolated bovine trachea.

2.3.8. Horse: In equine tracheal smooth muscle which has been pre-treated with indomethacin, atropine, phentolamine, EFS evoked a frequency-dependent relaxation response [44]. Following the addition of propranolol to the tissue baths, EFS still caused a frequency-dependent relaxation but the magnitude of the relaxation was less at each frequency in the trachea. These observations suggest the presence of both sympathetic and NANC inhibitory innervation in trachea of horses with an equal importance of each inhibitory system at this level. This response was mainly limited to the trachea and central bronchi with no detectable nerve supply to the peri-

pheral bronchi [45]. Interestingly, this response is absent in the third generation airways of horses with recurrent obstructive disease (heaves) [44].

2.4. Non-human Primates

The baboon [46] and rhesus monkey [47] also have a NANC inhibitory
system as the major inhibitory pathway in the relaxation of airway smooth
muscle. In this way primates are very similar to humans with cholinergic
excitatory constrictor nerves and NANC inhibitory nerves with no evidence
for the existence of adrenergic nerves functioning in the control of airway
smooth muscle tone. Therefore, because the pattern of innervation in non-
human primates seems to be identical to that in humans they may be the
species of preference for studying any abnormalities. Previously, most
investigators have studied neural control in the guinea-pig which in addition to the NANC system also has an adrenergic system [48, 49] or the dog
which lacks NANC innervation to the airway smooth muscle [33, 50].

2.5. Human

The existence of a NANC system was first reported by Richardson and
Béland [17]. These workers demonstrated that EFS of isolated tracheal or
bronchial strips evoked a biphasic response which consisted of a cholinergic contractile response and a relaxant response, in the presence of atropine, that was unaffected by propranolol and partially blocked by tetrodotoxin (TTX) (Fig. 1). These findings were later confirmed by other workers
[27, 31, 51, 52]. Moreover, these responses can be elicited in both large and
small airways, in humans down to an internal diameter of 0.5 mm [53, 54].
Furthermore, these NANC relaxant responses have also been described *in
vivo* in humans by reflex stimulation of the larynx [55–57]. These studies
involve stimulation of the laryngeal afferent pathways with capsaicin or
mechanical irritation. Capsaicin inhalation induces a transient bronchoconstrictor response in normal subjects [58] but following cholinergic inhibition with ipratropium bromide and β-adrenoceptor blockade with propranolol, capsaicin causes a bronchodilator response in the presence of
increased bronchomotor tone induced by leukotriene D_4 (LTD$_4$) [56]. This
bronchodilator response is transient (< 2 min) and does not totally reverse
the bronchoconstrictor effect of LTD$_4$. This is in contrast to studies in cats
[36, 59], where the bronchodilator effect lasted for several minutes which
may suggest the involvement of different transmitter substances mediating
the NANC response in the two species. This bronchodilator response
appeared to be neural in origin as capsaicin-induced bronchodilator responses were blocked by local anaesthesia of the airway mucosa [56]. In
similar experiments Ichinose et al. [57] demonstrated a bronchodilator re-

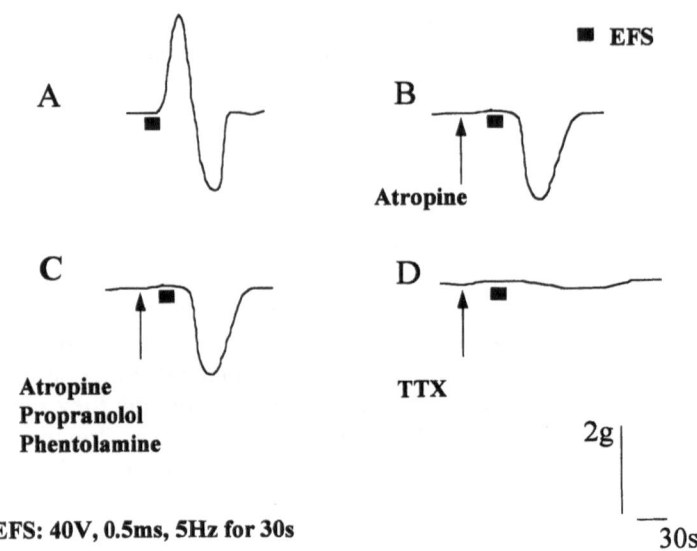

EFS: 40V, 0.5ms, 5Hz for 30s

Figure 1. Schematic diagram describing the response of human airway tracheal smooth muscle to electrical field stimulation (EFS: 40 V, 0.5 ms, 5 Hz for 30 s). *In vitro* organ bath systems allow the measurement of airway smooth muscle tone on EFS which stimulates all the nerves in the preparation. In these experiments the tissue can be electrically stimulated and changes in isometric tension evaluated. From these experiments it has been elucidated that human smooth muscle receives a dual contractile and relaxant innervation (A). The contractile response is cholinergic in nature as it is blocked by the muscarinic receptor antagonist atropine (B). The relaxant response is non-adrenergic non-cholinergic in nature as it is not blocked by α and β-adrenoceptor antagonists (C). However, the response is neural in nature as it is blocked by tetrodotoxin (D).

sponse to capsaicin inhalation in normal subjects after muscarinic and β-adrenoceptor blockade in airways constricted with prostaglandin F2α. Again, this NANC dilator response appeared to be transient and as described for cat airways *in vivo* the response was blocked by hexamethonium. Interestingly, localisation studies using fluorescence histochemical techniques have failed to reveal the presence of adrenergic nerves in tracheal or bronchial smooth muscle. Therefore, it seems that the NANC system provides the primary inhibitory control over human airways that, like baboon and monkey airways, seem to lack functional adrenergic innervation.

However, contradictory results have been obtained by Hutás et al. [60] who demonstrated that β-adrenoceptor blockade, in the absence of atropine, partially or completely blocked the neural relaxant response. These findings lead to the suggestion that the relaxant response before atropine was mainly due to the activation of adrenergic nerves and that NANC relaxation responses are only evident after muscarinic receptor blockade.

3. NANC Mechanisms

As described above, the first conclusive evidence that pointed to the existence of a NANC relaxant response in airway smooth muscle came with the development of potent adrenoceptor antagonists. Neural relaxation responses evoked by EFS in guinea-pig trachea were not altered in the presence of the muscarinic antagonist atropine and were only partially inhibited by propranolol [19]. This response had stimulus characteristics similar to NANC inhibitory nerves described in other tissues such as the gut. Subsequently, NANC bronchodilator responses have been demonstrated in airways smooth muscle *in vitro* by EFS in human, guinea-pig, cat, ferret, sheep, horse, mouse, cow, and pig [61]. NANC relaxations can also be demonstrated *in situ* [25] or *in vivo* by electrical stimulation of the cervical vagus nerve [36, 37] and by reflex stimulation of the larynx [55–57]. The relaxant response is abolished by TTX and therefore is assumed to be neural in origin. In several species, both adrenergic and NANC pathways coexist, but in human airways, the NANC response is the only neural bronchodilator mechanism [47]. In contrast, the dog [32–34] and rat [30] airways appear to lack a functional NANC relaxant response. However, the neural relaxant response is not always consistent throughout the airways in either the density of innervation or receptor population [31]. In human airways the NANC relaxant response is greatly reduced in the peripheral compared to central airways [4, 54].

Although identification of the mediators of this NANC response has been the subject of much research, the identity of the putative neurotransmitter or neurotransmitters has remained obscure until recently. Several candidates have been proposed to be mediators involved in the NANC response. γ-amino-n-butyric acid (GABA), opiates and the prostaglandins were thought to be unlikely candidates for the role of NANC transmitter. GABA failed to mimic the effects of nerve stimulation, and naloxone (opioid receptor antagonist) and indomethacin (an inhibitor of prostaglandin production) failed to reduce or abolish the inhibitory response in bovine trachea [43]. More promising candidates have included adenosine-5'-triphosphate (ATP), and, more recently, VIP and NO. The reason these specific mediators were investigated to assess their involvement in the NANC relaxant response in the airways was because they have also been implicated in NANC neural relaxation responses of the gastrointestinal and genitourinary tract [62].

3.1. Involvement of VIP in NANC Relaxant Responses in the Airways

VIP is a 28 amino acid peptide, with a wide distribution in the peripheral nervous system, which was among the first peptides to be detected in the respiratory tract [63]. VIP-immunoreactive nerve fibres innervating airway smooth muscle have been demonstrated in many species including humans

[5, 64–72]. Furthermore, VIP is a potent relaxant of airways smooth muscle *in vitro*, an effect which is not altered by propranolol or indomethacin [52, 73–76]. Several lines of evidence have implicated VIP as a neurotransmitter of NANC bronchodilator nerves in the airways but this seems to be species dependent [3, 4]. However, the role of endogenously released VIP is uncertain, since there are no potent and selective antagonists available. Two VIP antagonists have been described, [AC-Tyr[1], D-Phe[2]]-GRF (1-29)-NH$_2$ was found to be a VIP antagonist in rat pancreatic membranes [77], and [4-Cl-D-Phe[6], Leu[17]]-VIP a VIP antagonist both of guinea-pig pancreatic amylase secretion, and in colonic epithelial tumour cells [78]. In contrast, these antagonists had no effect on NANC relaxation responses to EFS in guinea-pig trachea *in vitro* and surprisingly they were also without effect on relaxation responses to VIP [78].

In the absence of a suitable antagonist for VIP, experiments have been performed to try to elucidate its role in neurotransmission using antibodies against VIP, desensitisation of VIP receptors and non-specific peptidases such as α-chymotrypsin which are known to degrade VIP. On the basis of experiments of this type VIP has been suggested as a candidate for the role of the neurotransmitter involved in NANC bronchodilator responses in the airways of several species. In fact, *in vitro* experiments have demonstrated that VIP is responsible for approximately 50% of the NANC relaxant response elicited by EFS in guinea-pig tracheal preparations *in vitro* [79, 80]. However, even after desensitisation or pretreatment of tissues with VIP antibody a major component of the NANC response was still evident suggesting that VIP may be involved in this response but not ruling out the possibility of the involvement of other transmitter substances.

The evidence that has been presented in favour of VIP being involved in NANC neurotransmission is less convincing in all other species studied. VIP is a potent relaxant of cat isolated tracheal and bronchial smooth muscle [81] and causes bronchodilation in the cat *in vivo* [82]. Moreover, studies have demonstrated that VIP desensitisation [74] and incubation with VIP anti-serum [81] reduced the NANC relaxant response in feline airways. These results would seem to indicate that VIP is at least partly responsible for the NANC relaxant response in cat airways. However, in contrast, there is evidence arguing against a role for VIP as the NANC transmitter in cat airways. Firstly, although α-chymotrypsin abolished responses to exogenous VIP in cat trachea [82] there was no effect on the NANC relaxant response [83]. Secondly, both VIP desensitisation and VIP antserum did not affect NANC dilator responses in cat airways [84].

Interestingly, recent evidence suggests that in cat trachea, EFS in the presence of atropine and guanethidine, elicited a monophasic NANC relaxation. By contrast NANC relaxation elicited in the peripheral airway was biphasic, which comprised of an initial fast component followed by a second slower component [85]. This secondary component of the NANC response in the peripheral airways was greatly attenuated by α-chymotrypsin. Hence, these results suggest that at least two neurotransmitters, VIP and another transmitter (NO, see below), are involved in NANC neurotransmission and that the contribution of these two transmitter substances to the NANC response differs in the central and peripheral airway of the cat [85].

VIP also has a relaxant effect on human airway smooth muscle *in vitro* [52, 73, 76, 86] and it has been suggested that VIP may be the neurotransmitter responsible for NANC relaxant responses. However, phosphoramidon, an inhibitor of neutral endopeptidase, significantly potentiated relaxations to low concentrations of VIP with no effect on NANC responses [73]. In addition, relaxations evoked by VIP were abolished by α-chymotrypsin but NANC responses were unaffected in human tracheal and bronchial smooth muscle [53, 73, 76, 87]. These data support the view that VIP does not mediate any component of the NANC relaxant response in human airways. This is somewhat surprising as it has been demonstrated that there are large numbers of VIP-immunoreactive nerves in human airway smooth muscle [68]. However, the role of VIP in neurally evoked relaxation will remain elusive until definitive studies evaluating the effect of selective VIP receptor antagonists on NANC relaxations are performed.

3.2. Involvement of NO in NANC Relaxant Responses in the Airways

NO formed from L-arginine by NO synthase (NOS) is released from a wide variety of cells [88]. Several isoforms of NOS have now been isolated, purified, cloned and expressed [89]. The isoform present in endothelial cells is a 135 kDa protein located in the membrane fraction [90] whereas neuronal or brain NOS is a 155 kDa protein located in the soluble fraction [91–93]. Bacterial lipopolysaccharide (LPS) or cytokines induce macrophages, vascular smooth muscle cells, endothelial cells, neutrophils, pulmonary epithelial cells [94, 95] and other cell types to express a different isoform of NOS (inducible (i) NOS) [88, 89]. Endogenously produced NO may play an integral role in many physiological and pathophysiological events in the lung. It seems to be involved in the neural NANC bronchodilator system in human airways, in vasodilator mechanisms, in the regulation of airway and pulmonary blood flow, and is known to be produced as a consequence of the inflammatory process [96]. All isoforms of NOS are inhibited by guanidino nitrogen-substituted L-arginine analogues such as N^G monomethyl-L-arginine (L-NMMA) and N^G nitro-L-arginine (L-NA). These compounds have been used as tools to demonstrate the role of NO in numerous physiological and pathophysiological events.

NOS inhibitors have been shown to inhibit the NANC neural relaxation response evoked by EFS in guinea-pig trachea *in vitro* by approximately 50% [80, 97] suggesting a role for NO in neurotransmission. Similar results have been observed in human, cat, pig and horse airways (4) although, in contrast to guinea-pig airways, the inhibition evoked by NOS inhibitors was almost complete. Experimental evidence suggests that certain substances (hydroquinone, superoxide anions) reduce relaxations to exogenous NO but not to NANC nerve stimulation. Therefore, it is still in doubt as to whether it is NO itself that is released as the NANC transmitter or NO attached to a carrier molecule (e.g. released as a nitrosothiol; see below).

3.2.1. Guinea-pig: The peptidase-resistant component of the NANC relaxation response to EFS, evoked in pre-contracted tissue, is attenuated in a concentration-dependent manner by L-NA or N-nitro-L-arginine methylester (L-NAME) [76, 80, 97]. The inhibition observed was approximately 89% but this was of relaxations elicited by low stimulation frequencies (4 Hz) [97]. However, in some reports, L-NAME completely abolished NANC relaxation responses at lower frequencies of stimulation (1 Hz) [80]. In addition, L-NAME was more potent than L-NMMA in reducing NANC relaxations. The reason for this potency difference is not clear but it may be that L-NMMA is less effective as it can also act as a substrate for NOS [98] or that it is due to an effect other than inhibition of the enzyme. In fact, L-NMMA, but not L-NAME, has recently been shown to inhibit the endothelial cell L-arginine transporter [99] and so may inhibit its own transport into the cell. The effect of these NOS inhibitors is stereoselective since D-NA and D-NMMA are without effect [80, 97]. The inhibitory effects of L-NA and L-NMMA are partially reversed by L-arginine but not D-arginine [76, 80, 97]. There are several reasons why reversal by L-arginine is only partial. L-NAME and L-arginine may have different abilities to access intact cells. These enantiomer-specific effects are similar to those which have been observed in other tissues that exhibit NANC relaxant responses such as the anococcygeus muscle [100, 101]. NOS inhibitors do not affect responses to sodium nitroprusside or isoprenaline, more evidence suggesting that a component of the NANC relaxation response in guinea-pig trachea is mediated by NO or an NO-related compound.

Interestingly, there is some evidence in other organs e.g. gastrointestinal tract, that VIP stimulates the release of NO from gastric muscle cells, so that NO acts as an indirect transmitter of relaxation [102]. However, in the airways, L-NA or L-NAME have no effect on relaxation responses to VIP [76, 80, 97]. Therefore, it is unlikely that NO is released as a secondary event by the release of VIP from airway nerves.

More evidence implicating NO in the neural control of airway tone comes from immunohistochemical studies describing the presence of the enzyme NOS in nerve fibres that project to the airways. In the guinea-pig, the origin of NOS containing nerves has been demonstrated, by NOS-immunoreactivity and NADPH diaphorase staining, to be extrinsic ganglia (jugular, nodose, stellate ganglia) with no positive staining in the intrinsic parasympathetic ganglia [103].

The release of the NANC transmitter in guinea-pig trachea is Ca^{2+}-dependent since relaxant responses to NANC stimulation are reduced or abolished at low frequencies of stimulation by ω-conotoxin which inhibits Ca^{2+} influx through neuronal N-type channels [80, 104]. With respect to the classical neurotransmitters, this could suggest that exocytotic release of transmitter is taking place. However, this may not be the case for NO as constitutive NOS contained in neurons is a Ca^{2+}-dependent enzyme and therefore the Ca^{2+} entry may be purely to activate the enzyme within the nerve terminals.

3.2.2. Cat: In the cat trachea, the NOS inhibitor L-NAME completely inhibited NANC responses as measured as changes in isometric force of contraction, evoked by EFS in tissues precontracted with 5-HT [84]. A tenfold greater concentration of L-arginine, the substrate for NOS, reversed this inhibitory response. These results suggest that the NANC response evoked by EFS in cat trachea is mediated primarily by NO.

In contrast, other workers have demonstrated that NOS inhibitors failed to effect NANC relaxation responses evoked by EFS of cat intrapulmonary bronchi pre-contracted with 5-HT at concentrations which abolished ACh-induced vascular relaxation in cat femoral artery and thoracic aorta [105]. In addition, NOS inhibitors had no effect on NANC relaxant responses evoked by vagal stimulation in mechanically ventilated cats in which airways tone had been elevated by 5-HT (105). These results, in contrast to Fisher et al. [84] do not appear to support a role for NO as a mediator of the NANC relaxant response in cat airways.

More recently data has been presented which suggests that at least two neurotransmitters are involved in NANC neurotransmission [106]. These workers have demonstrated that EFS applied to the tracheal smooth muscle during contraction induced by 5-HT in the presence of atropine and guanethidine elicited a monophasic NANC relaxation. By contrast, NANC relaxation elicited in peripheral airway was biphasic, comprising an initial fast component which was blocked by L-NAME followed by a second slow component which was not affected by L-NAME [85]. These results indicate that at least two neurotransmitters, possibly NO or NO-containing compounds and VIP, are involved in NANC neurotransmission and the distribution of the two components differs in the central and peripheral airways.

3.2.3. Pig: In pig tracheal smooth muscle, which has been pre-contracted with carbachol and where isometric force of contraction is monitored, EFS evokes a frequency-dependent relaxation response which is NANC in origin [42]. This NANC response is completely inhibited by NOS inhibitors and reversed by L-arginine in a stereospecific manner [107]. In addition, in the presence of an NOS inhibitor VIP, the nicotinic cholinoceptor agonist DMPP and isoprenaline relaxed carbachol-induced tone in pig trachea implying that none of the aforementioned agents relax tracheal smooth muscle via a mechanism involving NO. These results seem to indicate that NO may be a transmitter involved in NANC neurotransmission in pig trachea. In fact, nerves immunoreactive for constitutive NOS have been localised in the bronchial wall of the pig adjacent to blood vessels, submucosa and smooth muscle [3].

3.2.4. Rabbit: NANC relaxant responses, evoked by EFS, can also be demonstrated in rabbit smooth muscle but not in bronchial smooth muscle or in lung parenchymal strips [31, 108].

3.4.5. Horse: In equine tracheal smooth muscle which has been pre-treated with indomethacin, atropine, phentolamine and propranolol, EFS evoked a frequency-dependent NANC relaxation response *in vitro* [44]. This NANC relaxant innervation is mainly limited to the trachea and main bronchi. Interestingly, this response is absent in the third generation airways of horses with recurrent obstructive disease (heaves). Recently, it has been demonstrated that the NANC relaxation response is completely abolished by inhibitors of NOS suggesting that the NANC response is mediated by NO [45].

3.2.6. Ferret: NOS and VIP have been localised in a subpopulation of neurons within the plexus of the ferret trachea. The nerve cell bodies were located in specific ganglia and in the nerve fibres associated with tracheal smooth muscle and blood vessel walls [109]. However, there is no functional evidence, as yet, for a NANC relaxant response.

3.2.7. Human: There is a prominent NANC response in human airways *in vitro* which is blocked in a concentration-dependent manner by the NOS inhibitor L-NAME [73, 87]. This would seem to indicate that NO is the only demonstrable mediator involved in the NANC response in human tracheal smooth muscle. In these experiments, L-NAME had no significant effect on relaxation response curves to sodium nitroprusside (SNP) in human tracheal and bronchial smooth muscle demonstrating that L-NAME inhibits NOS and does not act via blockade of NO-dependent responses or by inhibition of any responses that are guanosine monophosphate (cGMP)-dependent [73, 76]. L-NAME was also without effect on relaxation responses to VIP and isoprenaline [76] which is in agreement with the data described for guinea-pig airways. D-NAME was ineffective at producing inhibition of the NANC response and the inhibitory effect of L-NAME was partially reversed by L-arginine but not D-arginine [73, 87]. These effects which are enantiomer specific, are similar to those described in guinea-pig trachea [80, 97].

NANC relaxant responses may also be evoked by EFS in human peripheral bronchioles (0.5 to 2 mm inner diameter) and central airways (5 to

12 mm inner diameter) [53, 54]. Ellis and Undem [53] have suggested that the NANC innervation is quantitatively similar between central and peripheral airways. However, these authors did not compare NANC responses evoked by EFS in trachea and main bronchi. Other investigators have suggested that the NANC response diminishes as the size of the airway decreases [52]. NOS inhibitors seem to inhibit NANC relaxant responses to EFS in human bronchial smooth muscle *in vitro* [53, 76] and 3-morpholinosydnonimine (SIN-1), an NO donor, relaxes both central and peripheral airways [53] suggesting that NANC responses may be mediated by NO. Ellis and Undem [53] have demonstrated that there was almost complete inhibition by L-NA of the TTX-sensitive portion of the NANC relaxant response in human peripheral and central airways pre-contracted with histamine (3 µM). This study is in agreement with studies on NANC responses of human tracheal smooth muscle [73]. In contrast, Bai and Bramley [76] found that L-NAME only inhibited approximately 50% of the neurally-mediated airways smooth muscle relaxation in human bronchi [76]. This study seems to suggest that a large TTX-sensitive residual relaxation persists after NOS inhibition in human bronchi. However, in this later study, the tissues were pre-contracted with methacholine before NANC responses were elicited and therefore atropine was not added to the bathing medium during the course of the experiment. The omission of atropine from the experiment could lead to a certain amount of functional antagonism being produced which may have reduced the magnitude of the inhibitory effect. Alternatively, in these experiments, ACh release from cholinergic nerve terminals could be acting at muscarinic cholinoceptors to release other neurotransmitters/mediators which may also have the ability to relax human airways smooth muscle. Finally, differences between studies may just simply reflect differences in tissue viability, the age group studied, the medical history of the patient or the time from organ removal to the start of the experiment.

NO activates soluble guanylyl cyclase after binding to its haem moiety to initiate a three dimensional change in the shape of the enzyme which increases activity and consequently the production of cGMP. The rise in cGMP can initiate a whole series of events including relaxation of smooth muscle [110], but the mechanism by which this happens is unknown. However, it appears that neurally mediated NANC relaxations in human trachea are associated with a concomitant selective elevation of cGMP, but not cyclic adenosine monophosphate (cAMP) levels, which is inhibited by L-NAME [111]. This confirms the hypothesis that the L-arginine-NO-cGMP pathway, and not VIP, is responsible for mediating the NANC relaxant response in this tissue.

It is not certain from where the NO is formed or the location of the NOS enzyme. However, the NO released on EFS does not appear to be localised in the epithelium as its removal has no effect on the NANC response evoked by EFS at least in guinea-pig airways [112, 113]. Recently, in human trachea obtained at autopsy, neuronal NOS-immunoreactivity has been described in nerve fibres present in airway smooth muscle, around submucosal glands and blood vessels [114] and in some cases NOS is co-localised with VIP. In addition, the density of neuronal NOS-immunoreactivity is reduced from proximal to distal airways and these data correlate with the functional data demonstrating a reduced NANC relaxation response in peripheral compared to central airways [54]. Therefore, in view of the extensive array of studies describing the localisation of neuronal NOS in neurons within the airways of several species [109, 103, 114, 115], and its correlation with functional data, it is more likely that NO is released from nerves to evoke an NANC relaxant response rather than another neurotransmitter substance inducing the release of NO from another cell type e.g. endothelial, epithelial or airway smooth muscle cells.

4. Distribution of NANC Responses in the Human Respiratory Tract

In human airways *in vitro* NANC responses evoked by EFS were progressively reduced from main airways (trachea/main bronchi) through peripheral airways (3–10 mm) to distal airways (< 3 mm) [54]. This functional decrease was associated with a decrease in the NOS-immunoreactive nerve density suggesting that the NANC neural relaxations are reduced going down the tracheobronchial tree apparently due to a decrease in the density of the 'nitrergic' innervation [54]. In contrast, Ellis and Undem [53] found no significant difference between NANC relaxations in human central (5–12 mm internal diameter) compared to peripheral (0.5–2 mm internal diameter) airways. However, responses in the smaller airways were not compared with those in the larger airways (trachea) where the differences may have been more profound.

The reduction in NANC responses down the human tracheobronchial tree observed by Ward et al. [54] in human airways are also consistent with a number of studies in other species. In feline airways both *in vivo* [36] and *in vitro* [75], the NANC response is reduced in distal bronchi. Similar results were found for the NO-mediated NANC response in equine airways [44, 116]. In guinea-pig airways NANC relaxant responses were obtained in trachea but not bronchial smooth muscle [117]. Undem et al. [118], however, showed that when the non-cholinergic contractions were inhibited by capsaicin desensitisation and the tone raised with histamine, NANC relaxations could be elicited by EFS in the mainstem bronchi. This data is supported by anatomical studies demonstrating the existence of NOS positive nerves in the peripheral bronchi of the guinea-pig [114]. However, the NANC relaxant response to EFS in the guinea-pig trachea is still more prominent in the cervical compared to the thoracic trachea [119]. Reduced NANC responses have also been demonstrated in rabbit, monkey [31] and bovine [120] distal bronchi.

Therefore, results obtained in several different mammalian species all seem to support the theory that NANC nerves exhibit their primary influence on airways located in the conducting airways rather than the gas exchange regions of the lung. However, the functional significance of this pattern of innervation is unclear.

5. Nature of the Neurotransmitter

As described in the previous section, there is now substantial evidence that the L-arginine/NO system generates the neurotransmitter responsible for NANC relaxations in smooth muscle of the respiratory, gastrointestinal, and urogenital tracts [121, 122]. However, while this so-called 'nitrergic' neurotransmission process has provided a long-awaited explanation for the atropine-resistant parasympathetic relaxations first described some 100 years ago by Langley and Anderson [123], it has also challenged several of the existing dogma relating to neurotransmission; thus, the neurotransmitter is not stored, but is synthesised and released on demand, and release appears to occur by simple diffusion rather than by vesicular stimulus/secretion coupling. In addition, during the early investigations into nitrergic neurotransmission it became clear that a number of NO-scavengers (superoxide anions, hydroquinone, and carboxy-PTIO) could profoundly inhibit relaxations to exogenous NO, but had little or no effect on responses to nitrergic nerve stimulation [124–129]; these discrepancies were at variance with the criterion of mimicry usually expected between the putative transmitter (NO) and the nerve-mediated response, and questioned the whole concept of nitrergic neurotransmission. Consequently, there has been a substantial effort to resolve this issue, and a number of possible explanations have been considered [130].

One possibility was that the NO radical generated by NOS would interact with a protective, carrier molecule prior to release into the junctional gap; this NO-adduct would be stable and resistant to attack by NO-scavengers. Nitrosothiols have been considered as the most likely transmitter candidates, and several physiologically relevant nitrosothiols (S-nitroso-glutathione; S-nitroso-cysteine; S-nitroso-coenzyme A) were found to relax nitrergically innervated tissues [125, 131–133], including airways smooth muscle [129, 134, 135]. However, while nitrosothiols do mimic the ability of nitrergic stimulation to relax these tissues, this is perhaps not unexpected since they are all NO-donors. There is as yet no direct, convincing evidence that a nitrosothiol is the substance actually released from the nerves. Indeed, it has been shown that the chemical reaction of NO with cysteine occurs only slowly at neutral pH [128], and none of the nitrosothiols studied to data show true parallelism with the nitrergic transmitter [128, 131, 133]. It has been suggested that the nature of the chemical entity released from the nitrergic nerves may vary among tissues, and even within the same tissue under different experimental conditions [121].

A second potential explanation has been provided by Wood and Garth-waite [136]. Mathematical analysis of the diffusion characteristics of NO (rapid and relatively unhindered by membrane barriers) indicated that in-activation of the radical would have very little effect on its biological actions, at least over short distances (up to 200 μm). Thus, NO-scavengers would have a much greater effect on the actions of exogenous NO than on NO released from endogenous sources, adjacent to the target tissue. It is likely that this property of NO, again unique to the nitrergic neurotransmission process, does indeed provide an explanation for the lack of effect of NO-scavengers in certain circumstances. However, these calculations were based on the assumption that the half-life of NO lies in the range 0.5–5 sec; it has been argued that the NO-scavenger carboxy-PTIO would reduce the half-life of NO to around 70 μsec and that this would be sufficient to limit its actions [137]. Thus, the validity of this explanation may depend on the reaction kinetics between NO and the NO-scavenger.

Recent experimental findings have indicated a third possible explanation for the lack of mimicry. It has been proposed that the neurotransmitter released from the nitrergic nerves is indeed free radical NO, but that the reactive radical is protected from scavenger attack by 'guardian' molecules within the tissue, which do not interact with the NO itself, but with poten-tial scavengers [138–141]. Such 'guardian' molecules might include superoxide dismutase (SOD; protects NO from superoxide anions), α-toco-pherol (protects NO from carboxy-PTIO), reduced glutathione (protects NO from hydroquinone) and ascorbate (protects NO from superoxide anions, hydroquinone and carboxy-PTIO) [141]. Indeed, it has been demonstrated that in tissues in which SOD function has been depressed using the copper chelating agent diethyldithiocarbamate, nitrergic relaxa-tions do become sensitive to inhibition by superoxide anion generating agents such as pyrogallol and duroquinone [139, 140]. α-Tocopherol, re-duced glutathione, and ascorbate can protect exogenous NO [141], but it has yet to be demonstrated that depletion of these antioxidant systems leads to increased vulnerability of the nitrergic transmitter to attack. Neverthe-less, it does seem that the redox environment of the tissue acts to shield neurotransmitter NO from interaction with scavenger molecules; exogen-ous NO, on the other hand, would be vulnerable to attack before reaching the protection of the tissue. Again, this is an important new aspect of nitrergic neurotransmission. Not only would the antioxidant 'guardian' molecules allow neuronallygenerated NO to traverse the junctional gap and reach its target guanylyl cyclase in the smooth muscle cytosol, but they would also prevent the formation of potentially toxic metabolites. For instance, NO can react rapidly with superoxide anions to form the highly toxic peroxynitrite [142–145]; such a reaction would be prevented by suf-ficient tissue levels of SOD and ascorbate. A corollary of this would be that reduced tissue antioxidant status could have serious pathophysiological consequences. Thus, the balance of evidence now suggests that free radical

NO does act as the principal neurotransmitter released from nitrergic nerves. However, its contribution may depend on the tissue under investigation and on the experimental conditions used [121]. Recent work with cat trachea [129] has shown that the NO-scavenger carboxy-PTIO only partially suppressed the NOS-generated component of the relaxation to field stimulation, suggesting that both free radical NO, and other NO-containing substances, contribute to NANC relaxation in this tissue.

In conclusion, investigations into the nature of the neurotransmitter actually released from the nitrergic nerves has identified several unique aspects of this novel neurotransmission process which must be taken into account when interpreting experimental results: it is possible that the nature of the transmitter may vary among tissues, depending on available carriers; the biophysical characteristics of NO, certainly in terms of its diffusion, may give rise to misleading results; and, the antioxidant status of the tissue might have important consequences for the efficacy and safety of NO when it functions as a neurotransmitter.

6. Functional Significance of the NANC Response

The exact role of the NANC relaxant response in health and disease has not yet been defined, however, there are several theories which have been put forward to explain the purpose of this phenomenon. Firstly, and probably the most obvious explanation is that the NANC inhibitory system may play an important physiological role in the regulation of bronchomotor tone [4]. Alternatively Coburn and Tomita [19] hypothesised that may be important in the control of the cough reflex. Finally, a more heretical explanation that has been put forward is that the NANC relaxant response is an innocuous response remaining from a primitive inhibitory system that has been conserved through the evolutionary process [146].

7. NANC Inhibitory Pathways in Disease

The NANC bronchodilator nerves are the only neural relaxant pathway in human airways therefore it is important to determine whether there is any defect in the ability of these nerves to function in diseased airways. In fact, it has been suggested that a defective function of the NANC nerves may contribute to bronchoconstriction and bronchial hyperresponsiveness in asthma [147]. On the basis of experiments performed in animals it seemed as though this hypothesis could be true. Inasmuch as NANC nerve stimulation potently inhibited antigen-induced bronchoconstriction and the increase in arterial plasma histamine in cats [148] suggesting that the transmitter substances responsible for the NANC dilator response prevent the release of mediators such as histamine from activated sensitised mast cells

[149]. Furthermore, the same workers also demonstrated that the broncho-dilator action of VIP and the neural relaxation response were reduced after allergen exposure and that the protease inhibitor, leupeptin, abolished the allergen induced NANC dysfunction in sensitised cats [150]. These results would seem to indicate that NANC relaxation is less effective in sensitised animals due to the degradation of the putative NANC neurotransmitter, such as VIP, by proteases released during the allergic response. VIP and related peptides are degraded by mast cell proteases such as tryptase and chymase [151]. This possible increase in mast cell proteases found in al-lergic conditions may contribute to bronchial hyperresponsiveness and to the decreased VIP-immunoreactivity seen in nerves in asthmatic airways [152], as mast cells are often found in close association with nerves [153]. However, these observations may be more relevant in structures (e.g. human pulmonary vessels rather than airways) and species (guinea-pig and cat airways) that receive a NANC innervation which is mediated by a neuropeptide which is susceptible to peptidases such as VIP. More recent-ly it has also been demonstrated that airway allergic inflammation also affects NANC relaxant responses mediated by NO in tissues from antigen exposed guinea-pigs [154]. This defect in the NANC relaxant response did not appear to be due to a decrease in the number of NOS-containing nerves but rather the scavenging of neural NO during the diffusion process from nerve endings to the effective sites of airway smooth muscle (see Fig. 2).

However, in human airways *in vitro* NANC responses do not appear to be impaired in airways of patients with chronic airflow limitation [155]. Moreover, airways from mild asthmatic patients have been found to have a normal NANC response [156]. In addition, airways from patients who died during severe asthma attacks showed similar NANC inhibitory responses to control airways from non-asthmatic subjects [157]. In agreement with the *in vitro* data other investigators demonstrated that the degree of bronchodilator response observed in mild asthmatic patients was of similar duration and magnitude as that seen in normal subjects, suggesting that the NANC bronchodilator system was functioning in mild asthmatic sub-jects [55, 147].

A reduction in VIP-immunoreactivity has recently been reported in the airways of asthmatic patients with severe disease [152]. This loss of VIP may be due to the presence of human tryptase secreted from airway mast cells. However, more recently, preliminary data has emerged suggesting no difference in VIP-immunoreactivity in nerves from biopsy samples from normals and mild asthmatics [158]. If VIP was the neurotransmitter of NANC nerves in human airways this data may suggest that there could be a decrease in the NANC dilator response in asthma according to the sever-ity of the disease. However, as yet, there is no conclusive data implicating a role for VIP in NANC neurotransmission, at least in the nerves innervat-ing the airway smooth muscle, in human airways.

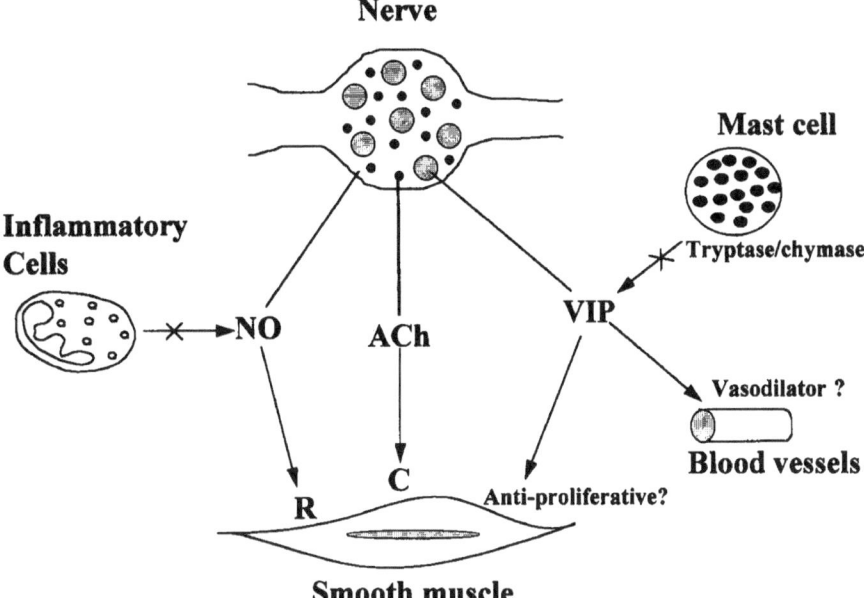

Figure 2. Schematic diagram describing the release of multiple transmitter substances (acetyl-choline, [ACh], vasoactive intestinal peptide [VIP], nitric oxide [NO]) from airway nerves. VIP and NO may be stored together or in different nerves and released on nerve stimulation to evoke relaxation (R) and act as a functional 'brake' for cholinergic nerve-induced bronchoconstriction by counteracting the constrictor (C) action of ACh on airway smooth muscle. There is no neural control of airway tone (at least in human airway) exerted due to the release of VIP. This may be because, in human airways, VIP may be broken down by mast cell tryptase and chymase or it may be that VIP-containing nerves are more important for controlling the proliferative actions of airway smooth muscle. Alternatively, it could be that VIP has a role as a neural vasodilator. In human airways, where nitrergic neurotransmission is dominant, mediators such as superoxide anions from activated inflammatory cells may rapidly degrade NO leading to unopposed cholinergic bronchoconstriction.

In contrast to asthmatic airways, NANC responses were significantly reduced in tissues from patients with cystic fibrosis compared to NANC responses in normal donor tissue [159]. It is possible that 'nitrergic' neurotransmission is impaired in inflammatory diseases of the airways, as production of superoxide anions by inflammatory cells, such as neutrophils and eosinophils, would lead to a rapid degradation of neurally released NO. This abnormality in the airway NANC innervation of cystic patients may lead to exaggerated bronchoconstrictor responses. Since the 'nitrergic' innervation appears to be dysfunctional in some inflammatory diseases it was tempting to suggest that NO functions as an endogenous braking mechanism in the airways and that its absence may therefore lead to exaggerated bronchoconstriction. We investigated the effect of NOS inhibition (i.e. effectively removing NANC relaxation responses) on cholinergic constrictor responses evoked by EFS in human donor tissue from trachea to peripheral airways. L-NAME produced a concentration-dependent enhancement of cholinergic neural constrictor responses to EFS with no effect on cumulative concentration-response curves to ACh in guinea-pig and human airways [160–162]. In human airways, L-NAME evoked maximal enhancement of cholinergic contractile responses in main airways and this became smaller in segmental and subsegmental airways suggesting that the NO-mediated NANC response was less prominent in lower airways [163] and recently we have demonstrated this to be the case [54]. The mechanism of this modulation was determined by studying the effects of endogenously released NO on ACh release evoked by EFS from strips of human tracheal smooth muscle that had been denuded of epithelium. Overflow of ^{3}H, evoked by EFS, in tissues previously loaded with [^{3}H]-choline, which seems to be a good marker for measurement of neuronally-evoked ACh release, is not affected by NOS inhibitors [163]. Therefore, it seems that endogenous NO does not modulate cholinergic contractile responses by pre-junctional inhibition of ACh release from the nerve terminal. In conclusion, it would appear that NO is probably modulating cholinergic neurotransmission post-junctionally by functional antagonism of ACh at the level of the airway smooth muscle which could, in theory, oppose cholinergic bronchoconstriction (see Fig. 2).

8. Conclusions

In this chapter we have illustrated the species differences in the neural control of the relaxation of airway smooth muscle. This serves to remind us of the problems which might be encountered when studying neural relaxation responses in animal airways and extrapolating the findings to the human condition.

In terms of the criteria for defining whether a substance is a neurotransmitter it seems that NO differs radically from the classical neurotransmitters such as ACh and noradrenaline. However, the criteria that are satisfied by NO for neurotransmitter status in the airways are as follows. The enzyme that is involved in the synthesis of NO from L-arginine has now been localised in neurons in the airways. Secondly, exogenously administered NO itself or alternatively nitrodilators have been shown to relax airway smooth muscle and therefore NO is able to mimic the effects of NANC nerve stimulation. Furthermore, inhibition of NO formation with an NOS inhibitor results in the attenuation of the nerve evoked relaxation of airway smooth muscle. However, this is where the similarity to classical neurotransmitter substances seems to end. The most difficult concept to reconcile, in terms of the classical ideas of neurotransmission is the absence of a conventional stimulus-secretion coupling mechanism as the release of NO does not appear to involve vesicular, quantal release of neurotransmitter.

However, although this substance seems an unlikely candidate, in that it is a gas which is not stored in synaptic vesicles or released by exocytosis, and which does not act at typical cell membrane associated receptors, NO may prove to have a more widespread and fundamental role than most classical neurotransmitters. The discovery of NO as a transmitter substance revolutionises the classical pharmacological basis for neurotransmission and may lead to the identification of other equally unlikely candidates.

In conclusion, the NANC bronchodilator mechanism has been identified as the predominant system in the neural control of human airway smooth muscle relaxation. However, the precise physiological or pathophysiological role of this system remains to be defined. The identification of a disruption in this pathway in tissue from patients with airway inflammation is interesting but the mechanism behind this dysfunction and the consequences of this are unknown and warrants further study.

9. References

1 Barnes PJ (1992) Modulation of neurotransmission in airways. *Physiological Reviews* 72: 699–729
2 Burnstock G (1972) Purinergic nerves. *Pharmacol Rev* 24: 247–324
3 Belvisi MG, Bai TR (1994) Inhibitory non-adrenergic non-cholinergic innervation of airways smooth muscle: Role of nitric oxide. In: Raeburn D, Giemybycz MA (eds) Airways Smooth Muscle: Structure, Innervation and Neurotransmission. Basel: Birkhäuser Verlag, 157–187
4 Belvisi MG, Ward JK, Mitchell JA, Barnes PJ (1995) Nitric oxide as neurotransmitter in human airways. *Archives Internationales de Pharmacodynamie et Thérapie* 329: 97–110
5 Ellis JL, Undem BJ (1994) Pharmacology of non-adrenergic, non-cholinergic nerves in airway smooth muscle. *Pulmonary Pharmacology* 7: 205–223
6 Mann SP (1971) The innervation of mammalian bronchial smooth muscle, the localisation of catecholamines and cholinesterases. *Histochem J* 3: 319–331
7 Richardson J, Béland J (1976) Non-adrenergic inhibitory nervous system in human airways. *J Appl Physiol* 41: 764–771
8 Barnes PJ (1986) Neural control in health and disease. *Am Rev Respir Dis* 134: 1289–1314
9 Burnstock G, Wood MJ (1967) Innervation of the lungs of the sleepy lizard (*Trachysaurus regosus*). II. Physiology and pharmacology. *Comp Biochem Physiol* 22: 815–831
10 Wood MJ, Burnstock G (1967) Innervation of the lungs of the toad (*Bufo marinus*). I. Physiology and Pharmacology. *Comp Biochem Physiol* 22: 755–766
11 Robinson PM, Mclean JR, Burnstock G (1971) Ultrastructural identification of non-adrenergic inhibitory nerve fibres. *J Pharmacol Exp Ther* 179: 149–160
12 Berger PJ (1973) Autonomic innervation of the visceral and vascular smooth muscle of the lizard lung. *Comp Gen Pharmacol* 4: 1–10
13 Burnstock G (1975) Comparative studies of purinergic nerves. *J Exp Zool* 194: 103–134
14 Fedde MR, Burger RE, Kitchell R (1961) The influence of the vagus nerve on respiration. *Poult Sci* 40: 1401–1407
15 Cook RD, King AS (1969) Observations on the ultrastructure of the smooth muscle and its innervation in the avian lung. *J Anat* 105: 202–208
16 Richardson JB (1979) Nerve supply to the lungs. *Am Rev Respir Dis* 119: 785–802
17 Richardson JB, Béland J (1976) Nonadrenergic inhibitory nervous system in human airways. *J Appl Physiol* 41: 764–771
18 Bando TX, Shindo N, Shimo Y (1973) Non-adrenergic inhibitory nerves in tracheal smooth muscle in guinea-pig. *Proc J Physiol Soc Jpn* 35: 508–509
19 Coburn RF, Tomita T (1973) Evidence for nonadrenergic inhibitory nerves in the guinea-pig trachealis muscle. *Am J Physiol* 224: 1072–1080

20 Coleman RA (1973) Evidence for a non-adrenergic inhibitory nervous pathway in guinea-pig trachea. *Br J Pharmacol* 48: 360–361

21 Coleman RA, Levy GP (1974) A non-adrenergic inhibitory nervous pathway in guinea-pig trachea. *Br J Pharmacol* 52: 167–174

22 O'Donnell SR, Saar N (1973) Histochemical localisation of adrenergic nerves in the guinea-pig trachea. *Br J Pharmacol* 47: 707–710

23 Kalenburg S, Satchell DG (1979) The inhibitory innervation of the guinea-pig trachea: a study of its adrenergic and non-adrenergic components. *Clin Exp Pharmacol Physiol* 6: 53–64

24 Richardson JB, Bouchard T (1975) Demonstration of a non-adrenergic inhibitory nervous system in the trachea of the guinea-pig. *J Allergy Clin Immunol* 56: 473–480

25 Yip P, Palambini B, Coburn RF (1981) Inhibitory innervation of the guinea-pig trachealis muscle. *J Appl Physiol* 50: 373–382

26 Hammarström M, Sjöstrand NO (1979) Pathways for excitatory and inhibitory innervation to the guinea-pig tracheal smooth muscle. *Experimentia* 35: 64–65

27 Taylor JF, Paré PD, Schellenburg RR (1984) Cholinergic and non-adrenergic mechanisms in human and guinea-pig airways. *J Appl Physiol* 56: 958–965

28 Chesrown SE, Venugoplan CS, Gold WM, Drazen JM (1980) *In vivo* demonstration of non-adrenergic inhibitory innervation of the guinea-pig trachea. *J Clin Invest* 65: 314–320

29 Canning BJ, Undem BJ (1993) Relaxant innervation of the guinea-pig trachealis: demonstration of capsaicin-sensitive and insensitive vagal pathways. *J Physiol* 460: 719–739

30 Satchell D (1982) Non-adrenergic non-cholinergic nerves in mammalian airways: their function and the role of purines. *Comp Biochem Physiol* 72: 189–196

31 Doidge JM, Satchell DG (1982) Adrenergic and nonadrenergic inhibitory nerves in mammalian airways. *J Autonomic Nervous System* 5: 83–99

32 Suzuki H, Morita K, Kuriyama H (1976) Innervation and properties of the smooth muscle of the dog trachea. *Jpn J Physiol* 26: 303–320

33 Russell J (1980) Noradrenergic inhibitory innervation of canine airways. *J Appl Physiol* 48: 16–22

34 Kannan MS, Daniel EE (1980) Structural and functional study of control of canine tracheal smooth muscle. *Am J Physiol* 238: C27–C33

35 Altiere RJ, Szarek JL, Diamond L (1984) Neural control of relaxation in cat airways smooth muscle. *J Appl Physiol* 57: 1536–1544

36 Diamond L, O'Donnell M (1980) A non-adrenergic vagal inhibitory pathway to feline airway. *Science* 208: 185–188

37 Irvin CG, Boileau R, Tremblay J, Martin RR, Macklem PT (1980) Bronchodilatation: Noncholinergic, nonadrenergic mediation demonstrated *in vivo* in the cat. *Science* 207: 791–792

38 Szarek JL, Gillespie MN, Altiere RJ, Diamond L (1986) Reflex activation of the non-adrenergic non-cholinergic inhibitory system in feline airway. *Am Rev Respir Dis* 133: 159–162

39 Inoue H, Ichinose M, Miura M, Katsumata U, Takishima T (1989) Sensory receptors and reflex pathways of non-adrenergic inhibitory nervous system in feline airway. *Am Rev Respir Dis* 139: 1175–1178

40 Sheller JR, Brigham KL (1982) Bronchomotor responses of isolated sheep airways to electrical field stimulation. *J Appl Physiol* 53: 1088–1093

41 Leff AR, Munoz NM, Tallet J, David AC, Cavigelli MA, Garrity ER (1985) Autonomic response characteristics of porcine airway smooth muscle *in vivo*. *J Appl Physiol* 58: 1176–1188

42 Kannan MS, Johnson DE (1992) Functional innervation of pig tracheal smooth muscle: neural and non-neural mechanisms of relaxation. *J Pharmacol Exp Ther* 260: 1180–1184

43 Cameron AR, Johnston CF, Kirkpatrick CT, Kirkpatrick MCA (1983) The quest for the inhibitory neurotransmitter in bovine tracheal smooth muscle. *Q J Exp Physiol* 68: 413–426

44 Broadstone RV, Leblanc PH, Derksen FJ, Robinson NE (1991) *In vitro* responses of airway smooth muscle from horses with recurrent airway obstruction. *Pulm Pharmacol* 4: 191–202

45 Yu M, Wang Z, Robinson NE, Leblanc PH (1994) Inhibitory nerve distribution and mediation of NANC relaxation by nitric oxide in horse airways. *J Appl Physiol* 76: 339–344

46 Middendorf WF, Russell JA (1980) Innervation of airway smooth muscle in the baboon: evidence for a nonadrenergic inhibitory system. *J Appl Physiol Respir Environ Exercise Physiol* 48: 947–956

47 Richardson JB (1981) Nonadrenergic inhibitory innervation of the lung. *Lung* 159: 315–322

48 Rikimaru A, Sudoh M (1971) Innervation of the smooth muscle of the guinea-pig trachea. *Jpn J Smooth Muscle Res* 7: 35–44

49 Foster RW, O'Donnell SR (1975) Evidence that adrenergic nerves are responsible for the active uptake of norepinephrine in the guinea-pig isolated trachea. *Br J Pharmacol* 53: 109–112

50 Ind PW (1994) Role of the sympathetic nervous system and endogenous catecholamines in the regulation of airways smooth muscle tone. In: Raeburn D, Giembycz MA (eds) Airway Smooth Muscle: Structure, Innervation and Neurotransmission. Basel: Birkhäuser Verlag, 29–41

51 Davis C, Kannan MS, Jones TR, Daniel EE (1982) Control of human enzyme smooth muscle: *in vitro* studies. *J Appl Physiol* 53: 1080–1087

52 Palmer JBD, Cuss FMC, Barnes PJ (1986) VIP and PHM and their role in non-adrenergic inhibitory responses in isolated human airways. *J Appl Physiol* 61: 1322–1328

53 Ellis JL, Undem BJ (1992) Inhibition by L-N^G-nitro-L-arginine of nonadrenergic noncholinergic relaxations of human isolated central and peripheral airways. *Am Rev Respir Dis* 146: 1543–1547

54 Ward JK, Barnes PJ, Springall DR, Abelli L, Tadjkarimi S, Yacoub MH et al (1995) Distribution of human i-NANC bronchodilator and nitric oxide-immunoreactive nerves. *Am J Respir Cell Mol Biol* 13: 175–184

55 Michoud M-C, Amyot R, Jeanneret-Grosjean A, Couture J (1988) Reflex decrease of histamine-induced bronchoconstriction after laryngeal stimulation in humans. *Am Rev Respir Dis* 136: 616–622

56 Lammers J-W, Minette M, McCusker M, Chung KF, Barnes PJ (1988) Nonadrenergic bronchodilator mechanisms in normal human subjects *in vivo*. *J Appl Physiol* 64: 1817–1822

57 Ichinose M, Inoue H, Miura M, Takishima T (1988) Nonadrenergic bronchodilation in normal subjects. *Am Rev Respir Dis* 138: 31–34

58 Fuller RW, Dixon CMS, Barnes PJ (1985) The bronchoconstrictor response to inhaled capsaicin in humans. *J Appl Physiol* 85: 1080–1085

59 Irvin CG, Martin RR, Macklem PT (1982) Nonpurinergic nature and efficacy of nonadrenergic bronchodilation. *J Appl Physiol* 52: 562–569

60 Hutás I, Hadházy P, Debreczeni L, Vizi ES (1981) Relaxation of human isolated bronchial smooth muscle. *Lung* 159: 153–161

61 Barnes PJ, Baraniuk JN, Belvisi MG (1991) Neuropeptides in the respiratory tract. *Am Rev Respir Dis* 144: 1187–1198

62 Burnstock G, Campbell G, Satchell DG, Smythe A (1970) Evidence that adenosine triphosphate or a related nucleotide is the transmitter substance released by non-adrenergic inhibitory nerves in the gut. *Br J Pharmacol* 40: 668–675

63 Sundler F, Ekblad E, Grunditz T, Håkanson R, Uddman R (1988) Vasoactive intestinal peptide in the peripheral nervous system. *Ann New York Acad Sci* 527: 143–167

64 Uddman R, Alumets J, Densert O, Håkånson R, Sundler F (1978) Occurrence and distribution of VIP nerves in the nasal mucosa and tracheobronchial wall. Acta Otolaryngol 86: 443–448

65 Dey RD, Shannon WA, Said SI (1981) Localisation of VIP-immunoreactive nerves in airways and pulmonary vessels of dogs, cats and human subjects. Cell Tissue Res 220: 231–238

66 Ghatei MA, Sheppard MN, O'Shaughnessy DJ, Adrian TE, McGregor GP, Polak JM et al (1982) Regulatory peptides in the mammalian respiratory tract. *Endocrinology* 111: 1248–1254

67 Lundberg JM, Fahrenkrug J, Hökfelt T (1984) Co-existence of peptide histidine isoleucine (PHI) and VIP in nerves regulating blood flow and bronchial smooth muscle tone in various mammals including man. *Peptides* 5: 593–598

68 Laitinen A, Partanen M, Hervonen A, Pelto-Huikko M, Laitinen LA (1985) VIP-like immunoreactive nerves in human respiratory tract. *Histochemistry* 82: 313–319

69 Uddman R, Sundler F (1987) Neuropeptides in the airways: a review. *Am Rev Respir Dis* 136: S3–8

70 Dey RD, Hoffpauir J, Said SI (1988) Co-localisation of vasoactive intestinal peptide- and substance P-containing nerves in cat bronchi. *Neuroscience* 24: 275–281

71 Dey RD, Altemus JB, Michalkiewicz M (1991) Distribution of vasoactive intestinal peptide- and substance P-containing nerves originating from neurons of airway ganglia in cat bronchi. *J Comp Neurol* 304: 330–340

72 Bowden JJ, Gibbins IL (1992) Vasoactive intestinal peptide and neuropeptide Y co-exist in non-noradrenergic sympathetic neurons to guinea-pig trachea. *J Autonomic Nervous System* 38: 1–20

73 Belvisi MG, Stretton CD, Miura M, Verleden GM, Tadjkarimi S, Yacoub MH et al (1992) Inhibitory NANC nerves in human tracheal smooth muscle: a quest for the neurotransmitter. *J Appl Physiol* 73: 2505–2510

74 Ito Y, Takeda K (1982) Non-adrenergic inhibitory nerves and putative neurotransmitters in the smooth muscle of cat trachea. *J Physiol* 330: 497–511

75 Altiere RJ, Diamond L (1984) Comparison of vasoactive intestinal peptide and iso-proterenol relaxant effects in isolated cat airways. *J Appl Physiol* 56: 986–992

76 Bai TR, Bramley AM (1993) Effect of an inhibitor of nitric oxide synthase on neural relaxation of human bronchi. *Am J Physiol: Lung Cell Mol Physiol* 8: L425–L430

77 Waelbroeck M, Robberecht P, Coy DH, Camus J-C, De Neef P, Christophe J (1985) Interaction of growth hormone-releasing factor (GRF) and 14 GRF analogues with vasoactive intestinal peptide (VIP) receptors of rat pancreas. Discovery of [AC-Tyr^1, D-Phe^2]-GRF(1-29)-NH$_2$ as a VIP antagonist. *Endocrinol* 116: 2643–2649

78 Pandol SJ, Dharmsathaphorn K, Schoeffield MS, Vale W, Rivier J (1986) Vasoactive intestinal peptide receptor antagonist [4-Cl-D-Phe^6, Leu^{17}]-VIP. *Am J Physiol* 250: G553–G557

79 Ellis JL, Farmer SG (1989) The effects of vasoactive intestinal (VIP) antagonists, and VIP and peptide histidine isoleucine antisera on non-adrenergic, non-cholinergic relaxations of tracheal smooth muscle. *Br J Pharmacol* 96: 513–520

80 Li CG, Rand MJ (1991) Evidence that part of the NANC relaxant response of guinea-pig trachea to electrical field stimulation is mediated by nitric oxide. *Br J Pharmacol* 102: 91–94

81 Hakoda H, Xie ZQ, Aizawa H, Inoue H, Hirata M, Ito Y (1991) Effects of immunisation against VIP on neurotransmission in cat trachea. *Am J Physiol* 261: L341–L348

82 Altiere RJ, Diamond L (1984) Relaxation of cat tracheobronchial and pulmonary arterial smooth muscle by vasoactive intestinal peptide: lack of influence of peptidase inhibitors. *Br J Pharmacol* 82: 321–328

83 Altiere RJ, Diamond L (1985) Effect of α-chymotrypsin on the non-adrenergic non-cholinergic inhibitory system in cat airways. *Eur J Pharmacol* 114: 75–78

84 Fisher JT, Anderson JW, Waldron MA (1993) Nonadrenergic noncholinergic neurotransmitter of feline trachealis: VIP or nitric oxide. *J Appl Physiol* 74: 31–39

85 Takahashi N, Tanaka H, Abdullah N, Jing L, Inoue R, Ito Y (1995) Regional difference in the distribution of L-NAME-sensitive and -insensitive NANC relaxations in cat airway. *J Physiol* 488: 709–720

86 Raffestin B, Cerrina J, Boullet C, Labat C, Benveniste J, Brink C (1985) Response and sensitivity of isolated human pulmonary muscle preparations to pharmacological agents. *J Pharmacol Exp Ther* 233: 186–194

87 Belvisi MG, Stretton CD, Yacoub MH, Barnes PJ (1992) Nitric oxide is the endogenous neurotransmitter of bronchodilator nerves in humans. *Eur J Pharmacol* 210: 221–222

88 Nathan CF (1992) Nitric oxide as a secretory product of mammalian cells. *FASEB J* 6: 3051–3064

89 Forstermann U, Schmidt HHHW, Pollock JS, Sheng H, Mitchell JA, Warner TD et al (1991) Isoforms of nitric oxide synthase: Characterisation and purification from different cell types. *Biochem Pharmacol* 42: 1849–1857

90 Pollock JS, Forstermann U, Mitchell JA, Warner TD, Schmidt HH, Nakane M et al (1991) Purification and characterisation of particulate endothelium-derived relaxant factor synthase from cultured and native bovine aortic endothelial cells. *Proc Natl Acad Sci (USA)* 88: 10480–10484

91 Bredt DS, Snyder SH (1990) Isolation of nitric oxide synthetase, a calmodulin-requiring enzyme. *Proc Natl Acad Sci (USA)* 87: 682–685

92 Schmidt HHHW, Pollock JS, Nakane M, Gorsky LD, Forstermann U, Murad F (1991) Purification of a soluble isoform of guanylyl cyclase-activating-factor synthase. *Proc Natl Acad Sci* 88: 365–369

93 Mitchell JA, Sheng H, Forstermann U, Murad F (1991) Characterisation of NO synthase in non-adrenergic non-cholinergic nerve containing anoccocygeus. *Br J Pharmacol* 104: 289–291

94 Hamid Q, Springall DR, Riveros-Moreno V, Chanez P, Howarth P, Redington A et al (1993) Induction of nitric oxide synthase in asthma. *Lancet* 342: 1510–1513

95 Robbins RA, Barnes PJ, Springall DR, Warren JB, Kwon OJ, Buttery LD et al (1994) Expression of inducible nitric oxide synthase in human bronchial epithelial cells. *Biochem Biophys Res Commun* 203: 209–218

96 Barnes PJ, Belvisi MG (1993) Nitric oxide and lung disease. *Thorax* 48: 1034–1043

97 Tucker JF, Brave SR, Charalambous L, Hobbs A, Gibson AJ (1990) L-N^G-nitro arginine inhibits nonadrenergic, noncholinergic relaxations of guinea-pig tracheal smooth muscle. *Br J Pharmacol* 100: 663–664

98 Hecker M, Mitchell JA, Harris HJ, Katsura M, Thiemermann C, Vane JR (1990) Endothelial cells metabolize N^G-monomethyl-L-arginine to L-citrulline and subsequently to L-arginine. *Biochem Biophys Res Commun* 167: 1037–1043

99 Bogle RG, Moncada S, Pearson JD, Mann GE (1993) Identification of inhibitors of nitric oxide synthase that do not interact with the endothelial cell L-arginine transporter. *Br J Pharmacol* 105: 768–770

100 Li CG, Rand MJ (1989) Evidence for a role of nitric oxide in the NANC-mediated relaxations in rat anococcygeus muscle. *Clin Exp Physiol Pharmacol* 16: 933–938

101 Li CG, Rand MJ (1990) Nitric oxide and vasoactive intestinal polypeptide mediate non-adrenergic, non-cholinergic inhibitory transmission to smooth muscle of the rat gastric fundus. *Eur J Pharmacol* 191: 303–309

102 Grider JJ, Murthy KS, Jin JG, Makhlouf GM (1992) Stimulation of nitric oxide from muscle cells by VIP: Pre-junctional enhancement of VIP release. *Am J Physiol* 262: G774–G778

103 Fischer A, Mundel P, Mayer B, Preissler U, Philippin B, Kummer W (1993) Nitric oxide synthase in guinea-pig lower airway innervation. *Neurosci Letts* 149: 157–160

104 De Luca A, Li CG, Rand J, Reid JJ, Thaina P, Wong-Dusting HK (1990) Effects of ω-conotoxin GVIA on autonomic neuroeffector transmission in various tissues. *Br J Pharmacol* 101: 437–447

105 Diamond L, Lantta J, Thompson D, Altiere RJ (1992) Nitric oxide synthase inhibitors fail to affect cat airway nonadrenergic noncholinergic inhibitory (NANCI) responses. *Am Rev Resp Dis* 145: A382

106 Jing L, Inoue R, Tashiro K, Takahashi S, Ito Y (1995) Role of nitric oxide in inhibitory and modulation of excitatory neuroeffector transmission in cat airway. *J Physiol* 481: 225–237

107 Kannan MS, Johnson DE (1992) Nitric oxide mediated the neural non-adrenergic, non-cholinergic relaxation of pig tracheal smooth muscle. *Am J Physiol* 262: L511–L514

108 Fame TM, Loader JE, Graves J, Colasurdo GN, Larsen GL (1993) Decrease in the airways' non-adrenergic, non-cholinergic inhibitory system in allergen sensitised rabbit. *Am Rev Respir Dis* 147: A285

109 Dey RD, Mayer B, Said SI (1993) Colocalisation of vasoactive intestinal peptide and nitric oxide synthase in neurons of the ferret trachea. *Neurosci* 54: 839–843

110 Rapoport RM, Murad F (1983) Agonist induced endothelium-dependent relaxation in rat thoracic aorta may be mediated through cGMP. *Circ Res* 52: 352–357

111 Ward JK, Barnes PJ, Tadjkarimi S, Yacoub MH, Belvisi MG (1995) Neural relaxation in human tracheal smooth muscle (HTSM) is mediated by an increase in cGMP: further evidence for the role of nitric oxide. *J Physiol* 483: 525–536

112 Watson NJ, Maclagan J, Barnes PJ (1993) Vagal control of guinea-pig tracheal smooth muscle: lack of involvement of VIP or nitric oxide. *J Appl Physiol* 74: 1964–1971

113 Rhoden KJ, Barnes PJ (1989) Epithelial modulation of NANC and VIP-induced responses: role of neutral endopeptidase. *Eur J Pharmacol* 171: 247–250

114 Fischer A, Hoffman B (1996) Nitric oxide synthase in neurons and nerve fibres of lower airways and vagal sensory ganglia of man. *Am J Respir Crit Care Med* 154: 209–216

115 Hassall CJS, Saffrey MJ, Burnstock G (1993) NADPH-diaphorase activity by guinea-pig paratracheal neurons. *Neuro Report* 4: 49–52
116 Yu M, Robinson NE, Wang Z (1993) Regional distribution of nitroxidergic and adrenergic nerves in equine airway smooth muscle. *Am Rev Respir Dis* 147: A286
117 Grundstrom N, Andersson RGG, Wikberg JES (1981) Pharmacological characterisation of the autonomic innervation of guinea-pig tracheobronchial smooth muscle. *Acta Pharmacol Scand* 49: 150–157
118 Undem BJ, Myers AC, Barthlow H et al (1990) Vagal innervation of the guinea-pig bronchus. *J Appl Physiol* 69: 1336–1346
119 Ellis JL, Undem BJ (1990) Non-adrenergic, non-cholinergic contractions in the electrically field stimulated guinea-pig trachea. *Br J Pharmacol* 101: 875–880
120 Palmer JBD, Sampson AP, Barnes PJ (1985) Cholinergic and non-adrenergic inhibitory responses in bovine airways: distribution and functional association. *Am Rev Respir Dis* A283
121 Rand MJ, Li CG (1995) Nitric oxide as a neurotransmitter in peripheral nerves: Nature of transmitter and mechanism of transmission. *Annu Rev Physiol* 57: 659–682
122 Rand MJ, Li CG (1995) Nitric oxide in the autonomic and enteric nervous systems. In: Vincent SR (ed) Nitric oxide in the nervous system. London: Academic Press 229–279
123 Langley JN, Anderson HK (1895) The innervation of the pelvic and adjoining viscera. *J Physiol* 19: 71–139
124 Gillespie JS, Sheng H (1990) The effects of pyrogalol and hydroquinone on the response to NANC nerve stimulation in the rat anococcygeus and the bovine retractor penis. *Br J Pharmacol* 99: 194–196
125 Hobbs AJ, Tucker JF, Gibson A (1991) Differentiation by hydroquinone of relaxations induced by exogenous and endogenous nitrates in non-vascular smooth muscle: Role of superoxide anions. *Br J Pharmacol* 104: 645–650
126 Barbier AJM, Lefebvre RA (1992) Effect of LY83583 on relaxation induced by non-adrenergic, non-cholinergic nerve stimulation and exogenous nitric oxide in the rat gastric fundus. *Eur J Pharmacol* 219: 331–334
127 Knudsen MA, Svane D, Tottrup A (1992) Action profiles of nitric oxide, S-nitroso-L-cysteine, SNP, and NANC responses in oppossum lower esophageal sphincter. *Amer J Physiol* 262: G840–846
128 Liu X, Gillespie JS, Martin W (1994) Non-adrenergic, non-cholinergic relaxation of the bovine retractor penis muscle: Role of S-nitrosothiols. *Br J Pharmacol* 111: 1287–1295
129 Tanaka H, Jing L, Takahashi S, Ito Y (1996) The possible role of nitric oxide in relaxations and excitatory neuroeffector transmission in the cat airway. *J Physiol* 493: 785–791
130 Gibson A, Brave SR, McFadzean I, Tucker JF, Wayman C (1995) The nitrergic transmitter of the anococcygeus – NO or not? *Arch Int Pharmacodyn Ther* 329: 39–51
131 Gibson A, Babbedge R, Brave SR, Hart SL, Hobbs AJ, Tucker JF et al (1992) An investigation of some S-nitrosothiols, and of hydroxy-arginine, on the mouse anococcygeus. *Br J Pharmacol* 107: 715–721
132 Barbier AJM, Lefebvre RA (1994) Influence of S-nitrosothiols and nitrate tolerance in the rat gastric fundus. *Br J Pharmacol* 111: 1280–1286
133 Rand MJ, Li CG (1993) Differential effects of hydroxocobalamin on relaxations induced by nitrosothiols in rat aorta and anococcygeus muscle. *Eur J Pharmacol* 241: 249–254
134 Jansen A, Drazen J, Osborne JA, Brown R, Loscalzo JP, Stamler JS (1992) The relaxant properties in guinea-pig airways of S-nitrosothiols. *J Pharmacol Exp Ther* 261: 154–160
135 Mathews WR, Kerr SW (1993) Biological activity of S-nitrosothiols – The role of nitric oxide. *J Pharmacol Exp Ther* 267: 1529–1537
136 Wood J, Garthwaite J (1994) Models of the diffusional spread of nitric oxide: implications for neural nitric oxide signalling and its pharmacological properties. *Neuropharmacology* 33: 1235–1244
137 Rand MJ, Li CG (1995) Discrimination by the NO-trapping agent, carboxy-PTIO, between NO and the nitrergic transmitter but not between NO and EDRF. *Br J Pharmacol* 116: 1906–1910
138 Brave SR, Gibson A, Tucker JF (1993) The inhibitory effects of hydroquinone on nitric oxide-induced relaxation of the mouse anococcygeus are prevented by native thiols. *Br J Pharmacol* 109: 10P

139 Martin W, McAllister KHM, Paisley K (1994) NANC neurotransmission in the bovine retractor penis muscle is blocked by superoxide anion following inhibition of superoxide dismutase with diethyldithiocarbamate. *Neuropharmacology* 33: 1293–1301

140 Lilley E, Gibson A (1995) Inhibition of relaxations to nitrergic stimulation of the mouse anococcygeus by duroquinone. *Br J Pharmacol* 116: 3231–3236

141 Lilley E, Gibson A (1996) Antioxidant protection of NO-induced relaxations of the mouse anococcygeus against inhibition by superoxide anions, hydroquinone and carboxy-PTIO. *Br J Pharmacol* 119: 432–438

142 Radi R, Beckman JS, Bush KM, Freemans BA (1991) Peroxynitrite oxidation of sulfhydryls. *J Biol Chem* 266: 4244–4250

143 van der Vliet A, Smith D, O'Neil CA, Kaur H, Darley-Usmar V, Cross CE et al (1994) Interactions of peroxynitrite with human plasma and its constituents: oxidative damage and antioxidant depletion. *Biochem J* 303: 295–301

144 Villa LM, Salas E, Darley-Usmar V, Radomski MW, Moncada S (1994) Peroxynitrite induces both vasodilatation and impaired vascular relaxation in the isolated perfused rat heart. *Proc Natl Acad Sci USA* 91: 12383–123887

145 Bolanos JP, Heales SJR, Land JM, Clark JB (1995) Effect of peroxynitrite on the mitochondrial respiratory chain: differential susceptibility of neurons and astrocytes in primary culture. *J Neurochem* 64: 1965–1972

146 Diamond L, Altiere RJ (1989) Airway nonadrenergic noncholinergic inhibitory nervous system. In: Kaliner M, Barnes PJ (eds) Lung Biology in Health and Disease. The Airways: neural control in health and disease. Marcel Dekker: New York, 343–394

147 Lammers J-WJ, Barnes PJ, Chung KF (1992) Nonadrenergic, non-cholinergic airway inhibitory nerves. *Eur Respir J* 5: 239–246

148 Miura M, Inoue H, Ichinose M, Kimura K, Katsumata U, Takishima T (1990) Effect of nonadrenergic, noncholinergic inhibitory nerve stimulation on the allergic reaction in cat airways. *Am Rev Respir Dis* 141: 29–32

149 Undem BJ, Dick EC, Buckner CK (1983) Inhibition by vasoactive intestinal peptide of antigen-induced histamine release from guinea-pig minced lung. *Eur J Pharmacol* 88: 247–250

150 Miura M, Kimura K, Takahashi T, Inoue H, Takishima T (1990) Possible mechanisms of the antigen-induced dysfunction of nonadrenergic, noncholinergic inhibitory nervous system. *Am Rev Respir Dis* 141: A387

151 Tam EK, Caughey GH (1990) Degradation of airway neuropeptides by human lung typtase. *Am J Respir Cell Mol Biol* 3: 27–32

152 Ollerenshaw Jarvis D, Woolcock A, Sullivan C, Scheibner T (1989) Absence of immunoreactive vasoactive intestinal polypeptide in tissue from the lungs of patients with asthma. *N Engl J Med* 320: 1244–1248

153 Kakuta Y, Stead RH, Perdue MH, Marshall JS, Bienenstock J (1989) Micro-anatomical relationship of mast cells and nerves in rat lung and trachea. *Am Rev Respir Dis* 139: A118

154 Miura M, Yamauchi H, Ichinose M, Ohuchi Y, Kageyama N, Tomaki M et al (1997) Impairment of neural nitric oxide-mediated relaxation after antigen exposure in guinea-pig airways. *Am J Respir Crit Care Med* 156: 217–222

155 Taylor SM, Paré P, Armour CL, Hogg JC, Schellenburg RR (1985) Airway reactivity in chronic obstructive pulmonary disease. Failure of *in vivo* methacholine responsiveness to correlate with cholinergic, adrenergic, or non-adrenergic responses *in vitro*. *Am Rev Respir Dis* 132: 30–35

156 Belvisi MG, Ward JK, Tadjkarimi S, Yacoub MH, Barnes PJ (1993) Inhibitory NANC nerves in human airways: differences in disease and after extrinsic denervation. *Am Rev Respir Dis* 147: A286

157 Bai TR (1990) Abnormalities in airway smooth muscle in fatal asthma. *Am Rev Respir Dis* 141: 552–557

158 Howarth P, Springall DR, Redington AE, Djukanovic R, Holgate ST, Polak JM (1995) Neuropeptide-containing nerves in endobronchial biopsies from asthmatic and non-asthmatic subjects. *Am J Respir Cell Mol Biol* 13: 288–296

159 Belvisi MG, Ward JK, Springall DR, Tadjkarimi S, Yacoub MH, Polak JM et al (1994) Nitrergic innervation in the airways of patients with cystic fibrosis. *Am J Respir Med* and *Crit Care Med* 149: A675

160 Belvisi MG, Miura M, Stretton CD, Barnes PJ (1993) Endogenous vasoactive intestinal peptide and nitric oxide modulate cholinergic neurotransmission in guinea-pig trachea. *Eur J Pharmacol* 231: 97–102

161 Brave SR, Hobbs AJ, Gibson A, Tucker JF (1991) The influence of L-N^G-nitro-arginine on field stimulation-induced contractions and acetylcholine release in guinea-pig isolated smooth muscle. *Biochem Biophys Res Commun* 179: 1017–1022

162 Belvisi MG, Stretton CD, Barnes PJ (1991) Nitric oxide as an endogenous modulator of cholinergic neurotransmission in guinea-pig airways. *Eur J Pharmacol* 198: 219–221

163 Ward JK, Belvisi MG, Fox AJ, Miura M, Tadjkarimi S, Yacoub MH et al (1993) Modulation of cholinergic bronchoconstrictor responses by endogenous nitric oxide and vasoactive intestinal peptide in human airways *in vitro. J Clin Invest* 92: 736–742

Nitric Oxide in Pulmonary Processes:
Role in Physiology and Pathophysiology of Lung Disease
ed. by M. G. Belvisi and J. A. Mitchell
© 2000 Birkhäuser Verlag Basel/Switzerland

CHAPTER 4
Localisation of Nitric Oxide Synthases in the Lung

Axel Fischer

*Institute for Anatomy and Cell Biology, Justus-Liebig-University, Aulweg 123,
D-35385 Giessen, Germany*

1   Introduction
2   Methods to Localise Nitric Oxide Synthases (NOS)
2.1 NADPH-Diaphorase-Histochemistry
2.2 Immunohistochemistry
2.3 *In-Situ*-Hybridisation
3   Localisation of NOS Isoforms
3.1 Neuronal NOS
3.2 Inducible NOS
3.3 Endothelial NOS
4   Localisation of NOS in Lung Disease
4.1 Inflammation
4.2 Pulmonary Hypertension
4.3 Tumors
5   Acknowledgements
6   References

1. Introduction

Nitric oxide synthases (NOSs) had been localised in neuronal and non-neuronal tissues for many years before they had been identified. This paradox was possible, because the histochemical technique of NADPH-diaphorase staining had been used to label subpopulations of neurons without knowing what their function was. About 25 years after the first description of the NADPH-diaphorase histochemistry, it became clear that the neurons labeled with this histochemical technique were identical to the neurons immunoreactive for neuronal NOS. Also the other isoforms that were cloned and sequenced from endothelial cells and macrophages display NADPH-diaphorase activity. Since the domain that generates nitric oxide (NO) from L-arginine is different from the domain of the enzyme that is responsible for the NADPH-diaphorase activity, which has also been found in other enzymes, it has been concluded that the NADPH-diaphorase shows a more widespread distribution than the NOS isoforms. However, each of the three isoforms of NOS has subsequently been found in several cells types other than the tissues from which they had originally been cloned. Thus, in some cell types in the respiratory tract the presence of all isoforms has been reported. Similarly, the initial discrimination between constitutive and inducible isoforms is less distinct than originally thought, since a constitutive expression of inducible NOS and an induction of the constitutive isoforms has been demonstrated. This differential expression of the NOS isoforms is even more complex under pathophysiological conditions such as airway inflammation in bronchial asthma or chronic infections in cystic fibrosis. Modern morphological techniques have contributed to our current view on the localisation of NOS isoforms and its functional implications, particularly through the description of the subcellular localisation. Indirect evidence for the effects of NO in the lung comes from localisation studies of the target molecule of NO, soluble guanylyl cyclase, which generates cyclic guanosine monophosphate (cGMP) as an intracellular messenger molecule.

In the present chapter, these morphological techniques will be introduced briefly and the results obtained for each of the isoforms will be discussed in detail. Finally, morphological alterations with regard to the distribution of the NOS isoforms in inflamed lungs and their pathophysiological implications will be reviewed.

2. Methods to Localise NOS

2.1. NADPH-Diaphorase Histochemistry

The NADPH-diaphorase histochemical reaction is based on the property of the flavoprotein to catalyze the electron transfer to unspecific acceptors such as tetrazolium dyes, resulting in a dark blue formazan deposition. By a peculiar phenomenon, in paraformaldehyde-fixed tissues the NADPH-diaphorase activity of other enzymes is lost, whereas the activity of the NADPH-diaphorase domain of the NOS is unaffected [1]. Although described already earlier [2], the occurrence of subpopulations of NADPH-diaphorase stained neurons was first reported by Thomas and Pearse [3]. Since then, an indirect and a direct NADPH-diaphorase technique has been described. Due to the unspecific labelling observed with the indirect method [4, 5], only the direct method as described by Hope and Vincent [6] should be used. Despite some reports on differences between the location of neuronal NOS and NADPH-diaphorase in the cat spinal cord [7], it is still generally accepted that neuronal NOS and NADPH-diaphorase are identical [8–11].

The NADPH-diaphorase technique can also be used for electronmicroscopy, although the use of the modified tetrazolium salt 2-(2′-benzothiazolyl)-5-styryl-3-(4′-phtalhydrazidyl) tetrazolium chloride (BSPT) as an electron acceptor has been recommended [12].

2.2. Immunohistochemistry

The success of immunohistochemical techniques depends on the primary antisera. For the generation of antisera, the availability and choice of the antigens used for immunisation is most critical. The first antisera to NOS isoforms were raised against purified proteins extracted from tissues. Since polyclonal antisera contain a mixture of antibodies directed against several epitopes of the purified protein [13], the immunohistochemical labeling results often are better than with monoclonal antibodies. However, due to the 50–60% structural homology between the NOS isoforms, cross-reactivity has to be determined by Western Blot analysis, though it cannot be fully excluded. In practice, most of the immunohistochemical studies in the respiratory tract were performed using polyclonal antisera against purified proteins [14–17]. After the three isoforms of NOS had been cloned and sequenced, antibodies to synthetic peptides from the deduced amino acid sequences were raised. These antisera offer the theoretical advantage of a higher specificity, although the peptides do not necessarily form epitopes that resemble the natural proteins. Several of these antisera have successfully been used for immunohistochemistry [14, 18].

Only few studies on the ultrastructural localisation of NOS isoforms in the lung have been published. In principle, anti-NOS antisera could be used for pre- and for postembedding immunohistochemistry. The studies published so far for the lung have used preembedding techniques [19–21].

2.3. In situ *Hybridisation*

Once the isoforms of NOS had been cloned, cDNAs were available to identify the NOS mRNA expressing cells. In these first studies, *in situ* hybridisation was used to correlate mRNA and protein expression in neuronal [22] and non-neuronal tissues [23]. These studies have confirmed a high degree of co-expression of NOS mRNAs and proteins, although *in situ* hybridisation occasionally appears to be difficult, because for the NOS proteins only a low level of synthesis is required. In another approach, *in situ* hybridisation has been employed using probes directed against a common sequence of the three NOS isoforms in order to reveal the presence of all isoforms [24].

Finally, *in situ* hybridisation is very useful tool to assess changes in the expression of NOS in pathophysiological conditions. The induction of increased expression of NOS mRNA has been shown in the nervous system in response to axotomy or inflammation [25, 26].

3. Localisation of NOS Isoforms

3.1. *Neuronal NOS*

Neuronal NOS has been localised to the airway innervation of humans [17, 18, 27, 33], as well as of other species such as rat [17], mouse [28] guinea-pig [16, 29], ferret [30, 31], frog [32] and pig [18]. Substantial species dif-

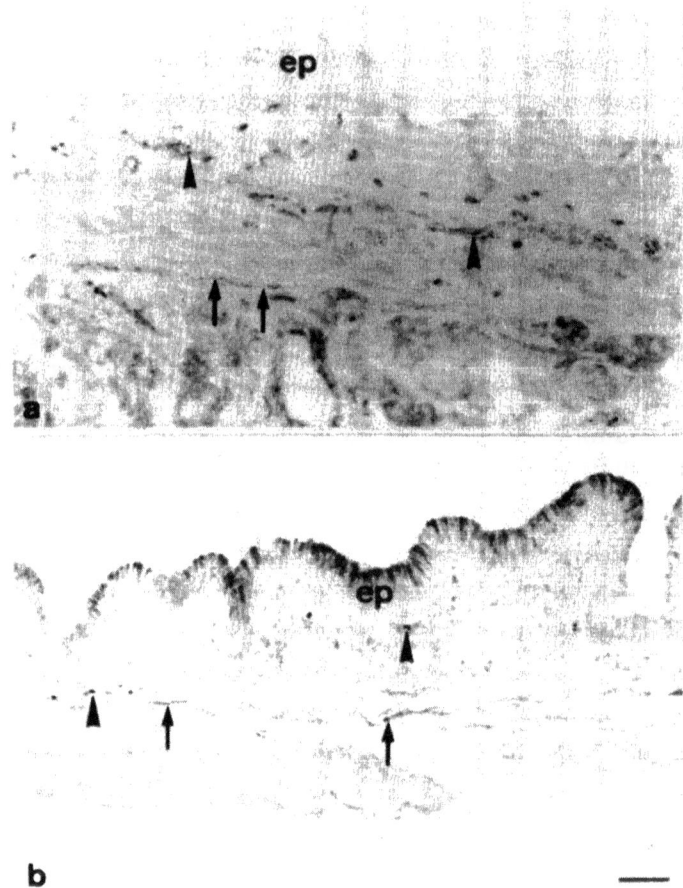

Figure 1. NADPH-diaphorase staining of normal and inflamed human bronchi. (a) In a bronchus from a healthy lung donor, NADPH-diaphorase staining is seen in nerve fibers (arrows) and in endothelial cells (arrowheads). The respiratory epithelium (ep) is devoid of labeling. (b) In the chronically inflamed bronchus of a patient suffering from cystic fibrosis, in addition to nerve fibers (arrows and endothelial cells (arrowheads), staining is also seen in the respiratory epithelium (ep). Scale bar represents 50 μm.

ferences became apparent with regard to the extent of the innervation and the origin of nerve fibers. In human airways, nerve fibers containing neuronal NOS were shown both by immunohistochemistry and NADPH-diaphorase histochemistry (Fig. 1) [17, 27, 33]. These nerve fibers are present in the airway smooth muscle, where NO has been shown to be the major mediator for the neural smooth muscle relaxation [34, 35]. The density of these nerve fibers decreases from trachea to small bronchi [27], which is associated with a reduced neural bronchodilation [33, 36] mediated by the inhibitory non-adrenergic, non-cholinergic (iNANC) system [for review 37].

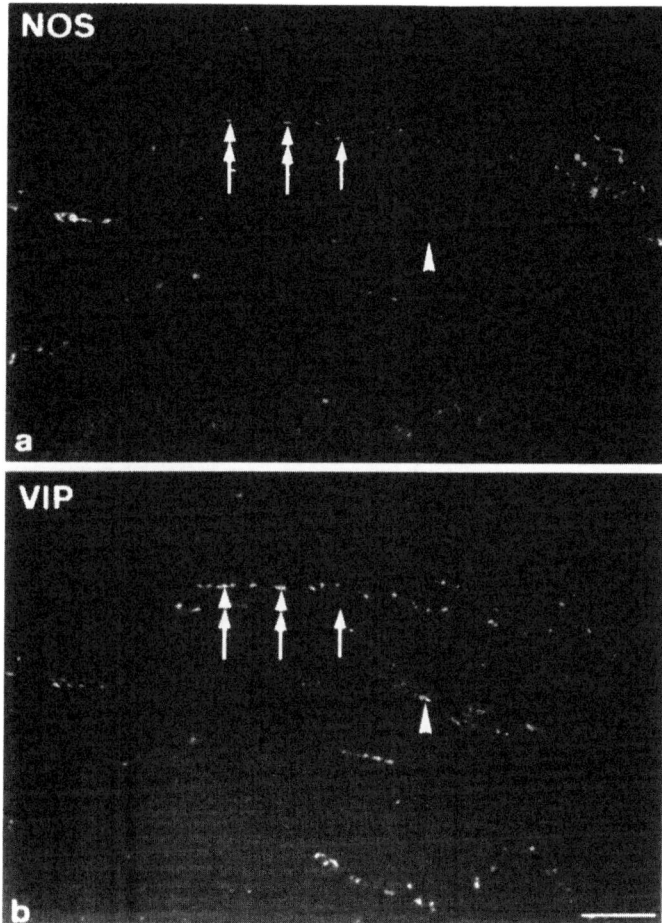

Figure 2. Localisation of (a) neuronal nitric oxide synthase (NOS)-immunoreactivity in nerve fibers in the airway smooth muscle in a human bronchus and correlation with (b) vasoactive intestinal peptide (VIP). Using a confocal laser scanning microscope, in these thin optical sections NOS appears to be frequently colocalised with VIP (double arrows), but NOS can also be seen without VIP (arrow) and VIP without NOS (arrowhead). Scale bar represents 20 μm.

Co-localisation with vasoactive intestinal peptide (VIP) is frequently observed (Fig. 2; 38]. In human airways, NOS-containing nerve fibers are present around submucosal glands [27], although their functional role for the regulation of glandular secretion is not clear yet. In the guinea-pig, this type of nerve fibre has not been found, however a substantial number of nerve fibers immunoreactive for NOS were found in the lamina propria (Fig. 4) and occasionally also in the respiratory epithelium [16]. In the lamina propria, NO was shown to have potent effects on blood vessels, in the regulation of plasma extravasation [39].

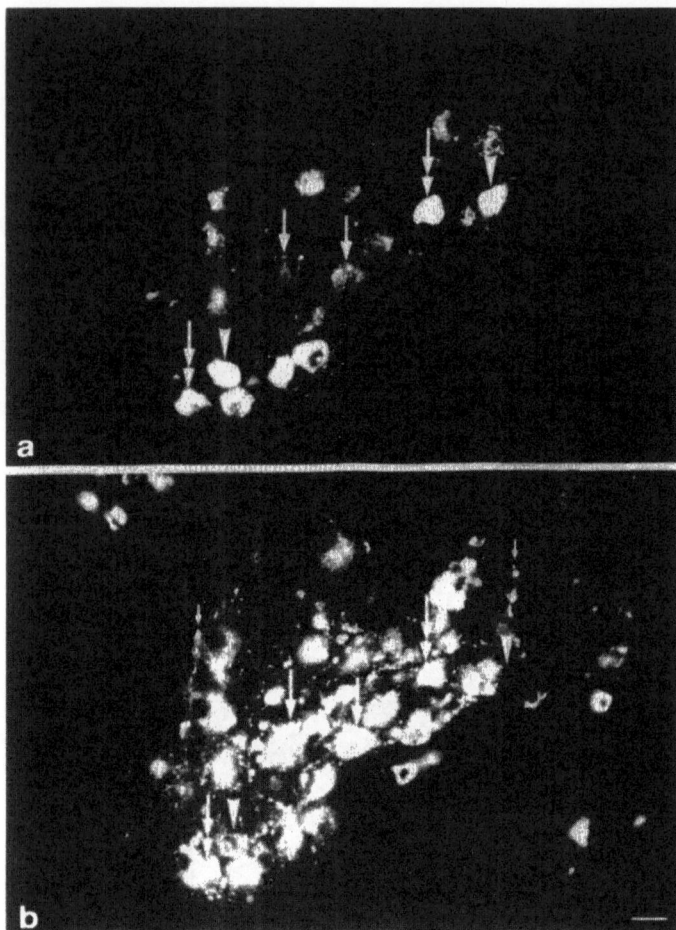

Figure 3. Most of the cell bodies of the (a) neuronal nitric oxide synthase (NOS)-immuno-
reactive nerve fibres of human airways are localised in the local parasympathetic ganglia.
Many of the cells are also immunoreactive for (b) vasoactive intestinal peptide (VIP; double
arrowheads). Some of the cells display either NOS (arrowhead)- or VIP (arrow)-immunoreac-
tivity. Note the VIP-immunoreactive nerve fibers (small arrows) innervating the cell bodies.
Scale bar represents 20 μm.

The cell bodies of these neurons innervating the airways of humans [18,
27], ferrets [30, 31] and piglets [18] has been localised predominantly to
the local parasympathetic ganglia (Fig 4). Contradictory results have been
reported for guinea-pig airways. Shimosegawa et al. [29] have reported
some NADPH-diaphorase stained neurons innervating the airways, whereas
in studies of our laboratory [16, 40, 41], NOS immunoreactivity was only
seen in neurons related to the pulmonary artery and vein, while the airway
intrinsic ganglia were devoid of NOS staining. In this species, a projection
of the relaxant innervation from the adjacent oesophagus was demonstrat-

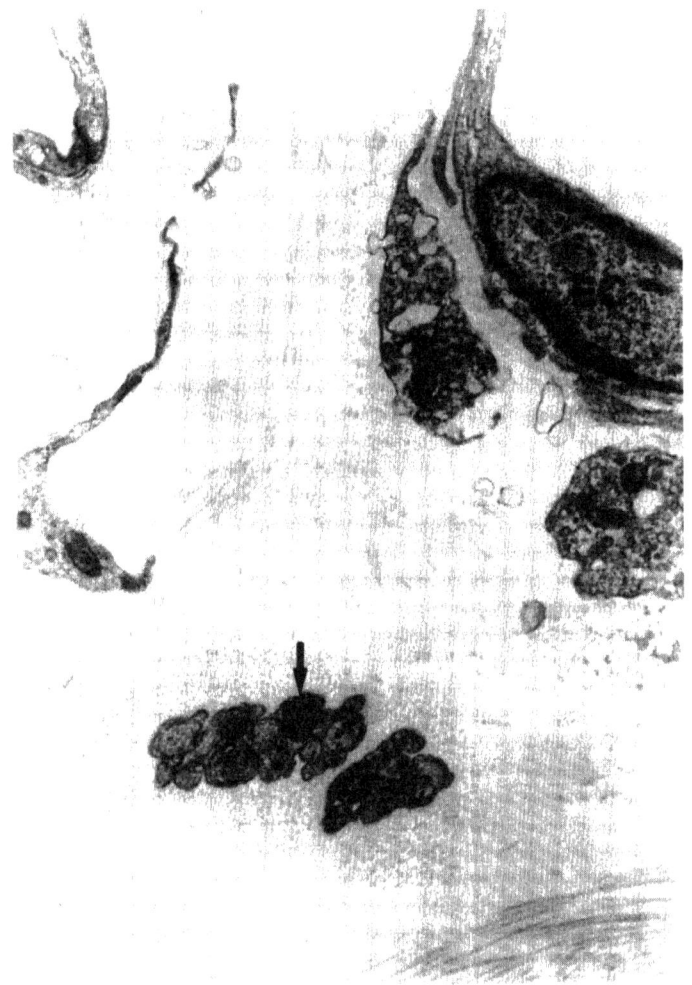

Figure 4. Electron microscopic micrograph of a guinea-pig bronchus. A nerve fiber bundle in the lamina propria innervates a mucosal blood vessel, endothelial cell (EC). The nerve fiber contains several axons, only one axon is immunoreactive for neuronal nitric oxide synthase (arrow). Magnification × 14500.

ed [42, 43]. Additional sources [44] of NOS immunoreactive nerve fibers were shown in vagal sensory and sympathetic ganglia [45, 46]. NOS immunoreactive neurons have been demonstrated in vagal sensory ganglia in humans [27, 47, 48] and in rats [49], although in these species a projection to the airways has not been demonstrated. NO in sensory neurons could act as a neuromediator both at the peripheral and at the central ending [50].

A substantial NOS immunoreactive innervation has also been reported for the trunks of the guinea-pig pulmonary artery and vein [51] as well as for the pulmonary vessels with smaller diameters [52].

The subcellular localisation of the neuronal isoform of NOS in the airway innervation has not been clarified so far. In the central nervous system, early reports have identified the NOS activity in the cytosolic fraction after preparative centrifugation [for review see 53]. However, in the N-terminus of neuronal NOS, a PDZ-domain has been identified, which is responsible for a membrane attachment of neuronal NOS by interaction with the post synaptic density proteins (PSD) 95 and 93 [54]. Ultrastructural studies to localise NOS using colloidal gold markers on postembedding or ultra thin cryostat sections have been reported for the gastrointestinal tract [55], but not for the lung.

The presence of neuronal NOS has also been shown for non-neuronal tissues. In the respiratory epithelium of guinea-pig and rat, a constitutive NADPH-diaphorase staining and immunoreactivity for neuronal NOS has been shown [16, 17, 39]. Neuronal NOS was also demonstrated as a constitutive isoform in normal endothelial cells [56], and in pulmonary arteries and veins of rats at all ages over 50% of endothelial cells displayed a cytoplasmatic immunoreactivity [57].

3.2. Inducible NOS

The inducible isoform of NOS has been identified as a separate, calcium-independent isoform, which could only be detected after endotoxin treatment (Fig. 5) [58]. Although a constitutive NOS-/NADPH-diaphorase activity in macrophages has been reported, cloning and sequencing from macrophages [59–61] has revealed that the inducible NOS isoform is expressed de novo at the transcriptional level. Soon it became clear that this isoform is not only localised to macrophages, but it can be induced in many cells [for review see 62]. In the respiratory tract, expression of the inducible isoform has been reported for alveolar type II epithelial cells [63], lung fibroblasts [64], airway and vascular smooth muscle cells [65–67], airway respiratory epithelial cells [68–71], endothelial cells [72] and neutrophils [73]. The stimuli that cause transcriptional activation in these cells vary widely and include endogenous mediators (such as chemokines and cytokines) as well as exogenous factors such as bacterial toxins, virus infection, allergens, environmental pollutants (ozone, oxidative stress, silica), hypoxia, tumors etc. [74–76]. Even in diseases that are not related to the lung, e.g. intestinal reperfusion, inducible NOS has been shown to be upregulated [77]. The expression of inducible NOS in these cells in the lung can be prevented by glucocorticoids [78].

Under normal conditions, however, most investigators could not find an expression of the inducible isoform [79]. In respiratory epithelial cells of human lung, a 'constitutive' expression of the inducible isoform has been observed at the level of mRNA [80] and protein [17].

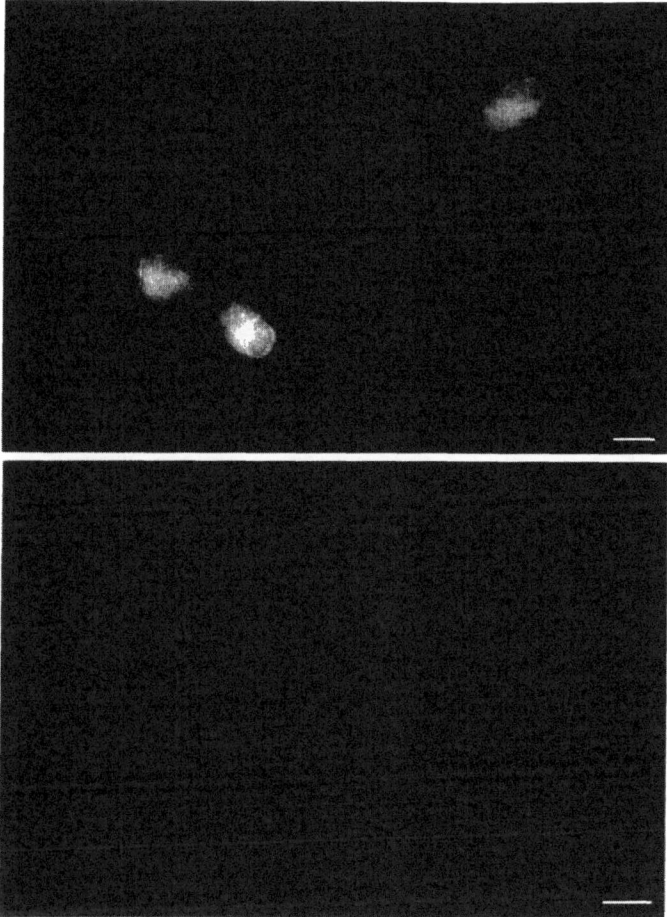

Figure 5. Alveolar macrophages from the guinea-pig express inducible nitiric oxide synthase after stimulation with lipopolysaccharide and interferon (upper panel). Unstimulated macrophages (lower panel) display no immunoreactivity. Scale bar represents 10 μm in the upper panel and 20 μm in the lower panel.

Biochemical studies have suggested a cytoplasmic localisation of inducible NOS [for review see 53]. Morphological observations on the ultrastructural location of the enzyme have not been reported to date.

3.3. Endothelial NOS

Soon after the identification of NO as a messenger molecule generated by endothelial cells [81, 82], a calcium- and L-arginine-dependent enzyme [83] has been proposed and more than 95% of its activity has been localised

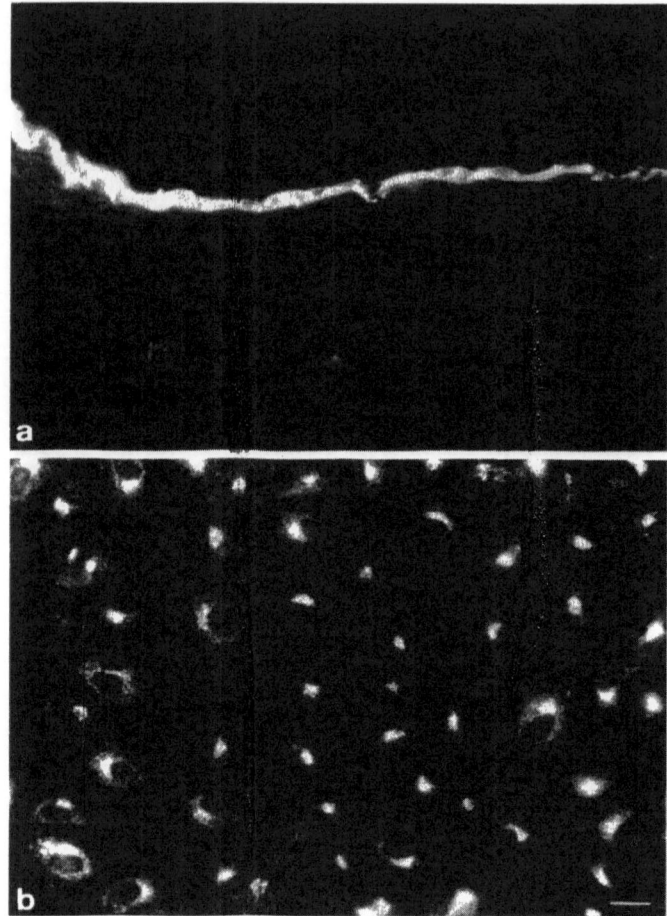

Figure 6. Immunohistochemical localisation of endothelial nitric oxide synthase in the guinea-pig pulmonary artery (a) and in cultured endothelial cells from porcine pulmonary artery (b). (a) Most of the endothelial cells display immunoreactivity for the endothelial isoform. (b) The cytoplasmatic, granular staining indicates that the endothelial isoform is located to the membrane of the Golgi apparatus. Scale bar represents 20 μm.

to the particulate fraction of the endothelial cells [84]. Indeed, when the enzyme had been cloned and sequenced [85–87], and specific antisera for the endothelial isoform of NOS had become available, abundant endothelial NOS immunoreactivity was demonstrated in endothelial cells of pulmonary vessels [Fig. 6]. In endothelial cells of submucosal blood vessels in the gastrointestinal tract, endothelial NOS has been localised to the Golgi apparatus and cytoplasmatic vesicles by immunohistochemistry at the electron microscopic level [88]. As demonstrated for endothelial cells from rat and bovine pulmonary artery, endothelial NOS is targeted to endothelial caveolae by palmitoylation [89].

Quantitative developmental studies of mRNA and protein expression as well as immunohistochemical examination have shown that the endothelial isoform increases during fetal development and reach a maximum at the time of birth followed by a postnatal decrease [90–93]. These changes have been largely attributed to the enzyme localised in endothelial cells and functionally been related to the changes in the pulmonary vascular resistance occurring at the transition from fetal to neonatal life.

In addition to the endothelial localisation, this isoform is constitutively expressed in respiratory epithelial cells [94]. Ultrastructural studies have revealed that endothelial NOS is localised at the basal membrane of ciliary microtubules [95], where it is thought to contribute to the regulation of ciliary beat frequence [96]. Thus, all three isoforms are localised to the respiratory epithelium [97] where they are cooperatively involved in the regulation of airway smooth muscle tone [98–101]. In other cells of the lung, for example in alveolar macrophages, the occurrence of the endothelial isoform has not been reported to date.

4. Localisation of NOS in Lung Disease

4.1. Inflammation

In lung diseases that are associated with acute or chronic inflammation, such as asthma [for review 102], bronchiectasis or cystic fibrosis, increased levels of NO were measured in the exhaled air [103, 104]. These increases have been attributed to an induction of the inducible isoform in the respiratory epithelium [105]. Characterisation of the enzyme activities, however, has shown that the increased activity is calcium-dependent [106], indicating that endothelial, neuronal or a recently reported calcium-dependent inducible isoform [107] could be involved. This is in line with earlier findings of an induction of a calcium-dependent NOS in the lung in response to Propionibacterium acnes and endotoxin treatment [108]. On the other hand, concomitant with the transcriptional induction of the calcium-independent isoform in endotoxin treated animals, there was a decrease in the mRNA levels of neuronal and endothelial NOS in the lung [109]. For airway nerves, plasticity of neuronal NOS expression [110] during development as well as plasticity of neuropeptide expression during allergic airway inflammation [111] has been described. However, the changes in NOS innervation, that have been observed in other models of peripheral inflammation [112, 113], axotomy [114] or after capsaicin treatment [115] have not been reported for the lung.

4.2. Pulmonary Hypertension

The potent vasorelaxant properties of NO have led to speculations that NOS deficiency may be involved in the pathophysiology of pulmonary hypertension. Indeed, in patients suffering from severe pulmonary hypertension with the typical signs of pathological alterations (thickening of the wall, plexiform lesions), there is an inverse correlation between the immunohistochemical expression of endothelial NOS in the endothelial cell layer and both the severity of the histological alterations and the total pulmonary resistance [116]. These findings indicate that the pulmonary vasoconstriction and the thickening of the arterial vessel wall could be caused by a reduced expression of endothelial NOS. In contast, in experimental models of pulmonary hypertension, when pulmonary vasoconstriction is induced by chronic hypoxia, an increased expression of NOS was observed by immunohistochemistry [67]. Interestingly, this increase is due to an induction of NOS in the endothelium and in the smooth muscle cells of the pulmonary resistance vessels and of the airways, which do not express NOS under normal conditions [66]. From this immunohistochemical absence of NOS in the small pulmonary arteries, NO appears to be relatively unimportant for the maintenance of the physiologically low pulmonary blood pressure. On the other hand, studies of exercise-induced pulmonary vasoconstriction in the presence of β-blockers have shown that endogenous NO actively dilates pulmonary vessels at rest [117]. From the studies that have been reported so far, the question whether reduced NOS expression contributes to the development of pulmonary hypertension or whether pulmonary hypertension leads to induction of NOS, cannot be answered at present.

4.3. Tumors

NO has cytotoxic effects and inhibitory effects on cell growth and proliferation. Both effects occur only at higher concentrations of NO. Thus, in the development of cancer or metastasis, impairment of NOS could be involved. Tumors themselves have been shown to produce NO [118] and mainly the neuronal and endothelial isoforms were found to be expressed in tumor cells by immunohistochemistry. In vitro, NO produced by tumor cells has been shown to inhibit cell growth. In vivo, however, a stimulation of tumor growth and metastasis was observed [119]. This is in contrast to the observation that tumor cells expressing NOS are less capable of forming metastases [120, 121]. Highly metastatic cells do not express NOS, but when they are transfected with the inducible isoform of NOS, the metastases were abrogated [122]. Taken together, the expression of NOS and the role of NOS in tumors and in lung metastases is still very controversial and the question whether NO is beneficial or harmful for tumor growth and production of metastasis cannot be answered at present.

5. Acknowledgements

Figure 2, Figure 4 and Figure 6b were kindly provided Mr. P. König, Prof. W. Kummer, and Dr. B. Höhler, Giessen, Germany.
Support from the DFG and the EU (BIOMED II) is gratefully acknowledged.

6. References

1 Matsumoto T, Kinoshita M, Toda N (1993) Mechanism of endothelium-dependent responses to vasoactive agents in isolated porcine coronary arteries. *J Cardiovasc Pharmacol* 21: 228–234
2 Cascarano J, Zweifach BW (1959) Factors influencing the histochemical demonstration of coenzyme-dependent dehydrogenase and diaphorase. *J Biophys Biochem Cytol* 5: 309–325
3 Thomas E, Pears AGE (1961) The fine localization of dehydrogenases in the nervous system. *Histochemie* 2: 266–282
4 Leeflang-de Pijper AM, Hülsmann WC (1974) Pitfalls in histochemical localization studies of NADPH generating enzymes or enzyme systems in the rat small intestine. *Histochemistry* 39: 143–153
5 Brüning G (1995) NADPH diaphorase is not inhibited by ethylendiaminetetraacetic acid and is not specific for nitric oxide synthase in the choroid plexus of rat and mouse. *Neurosci Lett* 185: 16–19
6 Hope BT, Vincent SR (1989) Histochemical characterization of neuronal NADPH-diaphorase. *J Histochem Cytochem* 37: 653–661
7 Vizzard MA, Erdman SL, Roppolo JR, Förstermann U, de Groat WC (1994) Differential localization of neuronal nitric oxide synthase immunoreactivity and NADPH-diaphorase activity in the cat spinal cord. *Cell Tissue Res* 278: 299–309
8 Bredt DS, Hwang PM, Glatt CE, Lowenstein C, Reed RR, Snyder SH (1991) Cloned and expressed nitric oxide synthase structurally resembles cytochrome P-450 reductase. *Nature* 351: 714–718
9 Dawson TD, Bredt DS, Fotuhi M, Hwang P, Snyder SH (1991) Nitric oxide synthase and neuronal NADPH diaphorase are identical in brain and peripheral tissues. *Proc Natl Acad Sci USA* 88: 7797–7801
10 Hope BT, Michael GJ, Knigge KM, Vincent SR (1991) Neuronal NADPH diaphorase is a nitric oxide synthase. *Proc Natl Acad Sci USA* 88: 2811–2814
11 Young HM, Furness JB, Shuttleworth CWR, Bredt DS, Snyder SH (1992) Co-localization of nitric oxide synthase immunoreactivity and NADPH-diaphorase staining in neurons of the guinea-pig intestine. *Histochemistry* 92: 375–378
12 Calka J, Wolf G, Schmidt W (1996) Induction of cytosolic NADPH-diaphorase/nitric oxide synthase in reactive microglia/macrophages after quinolinic acid lesions in the rat striatum: an electron and light microscopical study. *Histochem Cell Biol* 105: 81–89
13 Bredt DS, Snyder SH (1990) Isolation of nitric oxide synthase, a calmodulin-requiring enzyme. *Proc Natl Acad Sci USA* 87: 682–685
14 Schmidt HHHW, Gagne GD, Nakane M, Pollock JS, Miller MF, Murad F (1992) Mapping of neural nitric oxide synthase in the rat suggests frequent co-localization with NADPH-diaphorase but not with soluble guanylyl cyclase, and novel paraneuronal functions for nitrergic signal transduction. *J Histochem Cytochem* 40: 1439–1456
15 Springall DR, Riveros-Moreno V, Buttery L, Suburo A, Bishop AE, Merrett M et al (1992) Immunological detection of nitric oxide synthase(s) in human tissues using heterologous antibodies suggesting different isoforms. *Histochemistry* 98: 259–266
16 Fischer A, Mundel P, Mayer B, Preissler U, Phillippin B, Kummer W (1993) Nitric oxide synthase in guinea-pig lower airway innervation. *Neurosci Lett* 149: 157–160
17 Kobzik L, Bredt DS, Lowenstein CJ, Drazen J, Gaston B, Sugarbaker D et al (1993) Nitric oxide synthase in human and rat lung: immunocytochemical and histochemical localization. *Am J Respir Cell Mol Biol* 9: 371–377
18 Diaz de Rada O, Villaro AC, Montuenga LM, Martinez A, Springall DR, Polak JM (1993) Nitric oxide synthase-immunoreactive neurons in the human and porcine respiratory tract. *Neurosci Lett* 162: 121–124

19 Kummer W, Hauser-Kronberger C, Muss WH (1994) Preembedding immunocytochem-
    istry in transmission electron microscopy. In: Gu J, Hacker GW (eds) Modern analytical
    methods in analytical morphology. New York, London: Plenum Press; 187–201
20 Loesch A, Belai A, Burnstock G (1994) An ultrastructural study of NADPH-diaphorase
    and nitric oxide synthase in the perivascular nerves and vascular endothelium of the rat
    basilar artery. *J Neurocytol* 23: 49–59
21 Sosunov AA, Hassall CJS, Loesch A, Turmaine M, Burnstock G (1995) Ultrastructural
    investigation of nitric oxide synthase immunoreactive nerves associated with coronary
    blood vessels of rat and guinea-pig. *Cell Tissue Res* 280: 575–582
22 Bredt DS, Glatt CE, Hwang PM, Fotuhi M, Dawson TM, Snyder SH (1991) Nitric oxide
    synthase protein and mRNA are discretely localized in neuronal populations of the mam-
    malian CNS together with NADPH-diaphorase. *Neuron* 7: 615–624
23 Mundel P, Bachmann S, Baser M, Fischer A, Kummer W, Mayer B et al (1992) Expression
    of nitric oxide synthase in kidney macula densa cells. *Kidney Int* 42: 1017–1019
24 Torihashi S, Horowitz B, Pollock JS, Ward SM, Xue C, Kobayashi S et al (1996) Expres-
    sion of nitric oxide synthase in mucosal cells of the canine colon. *Histochem Cell Biol* 105:
    33–41
25 Verge VMK, Xu Z, Xu XJ, Wiesenfeld-Hallin Z (1992) Marked increase in nitric oxides
    synthase mRNA in rat dorsal root ganglia after peripheral axotomy: *in situ* hybridization
    and functional studies. *Proc Natl Acad Sci USA* 89: 11617–11621
26 Klimaschewski L, Obermüller N, Majewski M, Bachmann S, Heym C (1996) Increased
    expression of nitric oxide synthase in subpopulation of rat sympathetic neurons after
    axotomy – correlation with vasoactive intestinal peptide. *Cell Tissue Res* 285: 419–425
27 Fischer A, Hoffmann B (1996) Nitric oxide synthase in neurons and fibers of lower
    airways and in vagal sensory ganglia of man. *Am J Respir Crit Care Med* 154: 209–216
28 Grozdanovic Z, Baumgarten HG, Brüning G (1992) Histochemistry of NADPH-diaphor-
    ase, a marker for neuronal nitric oxide synthase, in the peripheral autonomic nervous
    system of the mouse. *Neuroscience* 48: 225–235
29 Shimosegawa T, Toyota T (1994) NADPH-diaphorase as a marker for nitric oxide synthase
    in neurons of the guinea-pig respiratory tract. *Am J Respir Crit Care Med* 150: 1402–1410
30 Dey RD, Mayer B, Said SI (1993) Colocalization of vasoactive intestinal peptide and nitric
    oxide synthase in neurons of the ferret trachea. *Neuroscience* 54: 839–843
31 Dey RD, Altemus JB, Rood A, Mayer B, Said SI, Coburn RF (1996) Neurochemical
    characterization of intrinsic neurons in ferret tracheal plexus. *Am J Respir Cell Mol Biol*
    14: 207–216
32 Bodegas ME, Villaro AC, Montuenga LM, Moncada S, Riveros-Moreno V, Sesma P (1995)
    Neuronal nitric oxide synthase immunoreactivity in the respiratory tract of the frog, Rana
    temporaria. *Histochem J* 27: 812–818
33 Ward JK, Barnes PJ, Springall DR, Abelli L, Tadjkarimi S, Yacoub MH et al (1995)
    Distribution of human i-NANC bronchodilator nitric oxide-immunoreactive nerves. *Am J
    Respir Cell Mol Biol* 13: 175–184
34 Li CG, Rand MJ (1991) Evidence that part of the NANC relaxant response of guinea-pig
    trachea to electrical field stimulation is mediated by nitric oxide. *Br J Pharmacol* 102:
    91–94
35 Belvisi MG, Stretton CD, Yacoub MH, Barnes PJ (1992) Nitric oxide is the endogenous neu-
    rotransmitter of bronchodilator nerves in human airways. *Eur J Pharmacol* 210: 221–222
36 Ellis JL, Undem BJ (1992) Inhibition by L-N^G-nitro-L-arginine of nonadrenergic-non-
    cholinergic-mediated relaxations of human isolated central and peripheral airways. *Am
    Rev Respir Dis* 146: 1543–1547
37 Stretton D (1991) Non-adrenergic non-cholinergic neural control of the airways. *Clin Exp
    Pharmacol Physiol* 18: 675–684
38 Kummer W, Fischer A, Mundel P, Mayer B, Hoba B, Philippin B et al (1992) Nitric oxide
    synthase in VIP-containing vasodilator nerve fibres in the guinea-pig. *NeuroReport*
    3: 653–655
39 Erjefält JS, Erjefält I, Sundler F, Persson CG (1994) Mucosal nitric oxide may tonically
    suppress plasma exudation. *Am J Respir Crit Care Med* 150: 227–232
40 Fischer A, Canning BJ, Kummer W (1996) Correlation of vasoactive intestinal peptide and
    nitric oxide synthase with choline acetyltransferase in the airway innvervation. *Ann N Y
    Acad Sci* 805: 717–722

41 Canning BJ, Fischer A (1997) Localization of cholinergic nerves in lower airways of guinea-pigs using antisera to choline acetyltransferase. *Am J Physiol* 272: L731–L738

42 Canning BJ, Undem BJ (1993) Relaxant innervation of the guinea-pig trachealis: demonstration of capsaicin-sensitive and -insensitive vagal pathways. *J Physiol* 460: 719–739

43 Canning BJ, Undem BJ (1993) Evidence that distinct neural pathways mediate parasympathetic contractions and relaxations of guinea-pig trachealis. *J Physiol* 471: 25–40

44 Kummer W, Fischer A, Kurkowski R, Heym C (1992) The sensory and sympathetic innervation of guinea-pig lung and trachea as studied by retrograde neuronal tracing and double-labelling immunohistochemistry. *Neuroscience* 49: 715–737

45 Olry R, Mayer B, Kummer W (1994) Nitric oxide synthase in the pre- and postganglionic axis of the sympathetic nervous system in the guinea-pig. In: Moncada S, Feelisch M, Busse R, Higgs EA (eds) Biology of Nitric Oxide. Part 2. London, Chapel Hill: Portland Press; 330–334

46 Fischer A, Mayer B, Kummer W (1996) Nitric oxide synthase in vagal sensory and sympathetic neurons innervating the guinea-pig trachea. *J Auton Nerv Syst* 56: 157–160

47 Kummer W, Fischer A, Mayer B (1992) Substance P and nitric oxide: Participation in airway innvervation. *Regul Peptides* S1: S92

48 Kummer W, Fischer A, Lang RE, Koesling D, Mayer B, Olry R (1994) Nitric oxide and guanylyl cyclases: correlation with neuropeptides. In: Baraniuk JN, Barnes PJ, Kaliner M, Kunkel GH (eds) Neuropeptides in respiratory medicine. New York: Marcel Dekker; 641–652

49 Aimi Y, Fujimura M, Vincent SR, Kimura H (1991) Localization of NADPH-diaphorase-containing neurons in sensory ganglia of the rat. *J Comp Neurol* 306: 382–392

50 Ruggiero DA, Mtui EP, Otake K, Anwar M (1996) Central and primary visceral afferents to nucleus tractus solitarii may generate nitric oxide synthase as a membrane-permeant neuronal messenger. *J Comp Neurol* 364: 51–67

51 Klimaschewski L, Kummer W, Mayer B, Couraud JY, Preissler U, Philippin B et al (1992) Nitric oxide synthase in cardiac nerve fibres and neurons of rat and guinea-pig heart. *Circ Res* 71: 1533–1537

52 Haberberger R, Schemann M, Sann H, Kummer W (1997) Innervation pattern of guinea-pig pulmonary vasculature depends on the vascular diameter. *J Appl Physiol* 82: 426–434

53 Förstermann U, Schmidt HHHW, pollock JS, Sheng H, Mitchell JA, Warner TD et al (1991) Isoforms of nitric oxide synthase: characterization and purification from different cell types. *Biochem Pharmacol* 42: 1849–1857

54 Brenman JE, Chao DS, Gee SH, McGee AW, Craven SE, Santillano DR et al (1996) Interaction of nitric oxide synthase with the postsynaptic density protein PSD-95 and alpha1-syntrophin mediated by PDZ domains. *Cell* 84: 757–767

55 Berezin I, Snyder SH, Bredt DS, Daniel EE (1994) Ultrastructural localization of nitric oxide synthase in canine small intestine. *Am J Physiol* 266: C981–989

56 Loesch A, Burnstock G (1995) Electron immunocytochemical localization of endothelial and neuronal isoforms of nitric oxide synthase in rat cerebral basilary artery. *Acta Neurobiol Exp* 55 (Suppl): 45

57 Loesch A, Burnstock G (1996) Ultrastructural localization of nitric oxide synthase and endothelin in rat pulmonary artery and vein during postnatal development and ageing. *Cell Tissue Res* 283: 355–365

58 Knowles RG, Merrett M, Salter M, Moncada S (1990) Differential induction of brain, lung and liver nitric oxide synthase by endotoxin in rat. *Biochem J* 270: 833–836

59 Lowenstein CJ, Glatt CS, Bredt DS, Snyder SH (1992) Cloned and expressed macrophage nitric oxide synthase contrasts with the brain enzyme. *Proc Natl Acad Sci USA* 89: 6711–6715

60 Lyons CR, Orloff GJ, Cunningham JM (1992) Molecular cloning and functional expression of an inducible nitirc oxide synthase from a murine macrophage cell line. *J Biol Chem* 267: 6370–6374

61 Xie Q, Cho H, Calaycay J, Mumford R, Swiderek T, Lee A, Ding T, Trosco T, Nathan C (1992) Cloning and characterization of inducible nitric oxide synthase from mouse macrophages. *Science* 256: 225–228

62 Nathan C (1992) Nitric oxide as a secretary product of mammalian cells. *FASEB J* 6: 3051–3064

63 Warner RL, Paine R 3rd, Christensen PJ, Marletta MA, Richards MK, Wilcosen SE et al (1995) Lung sources and cytokine requirements for *in vivo* expression of inducible nitric oxide synthase. *Am J Respir Cell Mol Biol* 12: 649–661

64 Jorens PG, Van Overveld FJ, Vermeire PA, Bult H, Herman AG (1992) Synergism between interleukin-1 beta and interferon-gamma, an inducer of nitric oxide synthase, in rat lung fibroblasts. *Eur J Pharmacol* 224: 7–12

65 Thomae KR, Geller DA, Billiar TR, Davies P, Pitt BR, Simmons RL et al (1993) Antisense oligodeoxynucleotide to inducible nitric oxide synthase inhibits nitric oxide synthesis in rat pulmonary artery smooth muscle cells in culture. *Surgery* 114: 272–277

66 Xue C, Rengasamy A, Le-Cras TD, Koberna PA, Dailey GC, Johns RA (1994) Distribution of NOS in normoxic vs. hypoxic rat lung: upregulation of NOS by chronic hypoxia. *Am J Physiol* 267: L667–L678

67 Griffith MJ, Liu S, Curzen NP, Messent M, Evans TW (1995) *In vivo* treatment with endotoxin induces nitric oxide synthase in rat main pulmonary artery. *Am J Physiol* 268: L509–518

68 Adcock IM, Brown CR, Kwon O, Barnes PJ (1994) Oxidative stress induces NF kappa B DNA binding and inducible NOS mRNA in human epithelial cells. *Biochem Biophys Res Commun* 199: 1518–1524

69 Hoffmann G, Grote J, Friedrich F, Mutz N, Schobersberger W (1995) The pulmonary epithelial cell line L2 as new model for an inducible nitric oxide synthase expressing distal airway epithelial cell. *Biochem Biophys Res Comm* 217: 575–583

70 Robbins RA, Barnes PJ, Springall DR, Warren JB, Kwon OJ, Buttery LD et al (1994) Expression of inducible nitric oxide synthase in human lung epithelial cells. *Biochem Biophys Res Commun* 203: 209–218

71 Robbins RA, Springall DR, Warren JB, Kwon OJ, Buttery LD, Wilson AJ et al (1994) Inducible nitric oxide synthase is increased in murine lung epithelial cells by cytokine stimulation. *Biochem Biophys Res Commun* 198: 835–843

72 Sato K, Miyakawa K, Takeya M, Hattori R, Yui Y, Sunamoto M et al (1995) Immunohistochemical expression of inducible nitric oxide synthase (iNOS) in reversible endotoxic shock studied by a novel monoclonal antibody against rat iNOS. *J Leuk Biol* 57: 36–44

73 Blackford JA Jr, Antonini JM, Castranova V, Dey RD (1994) Intracheal instillation of silica up-refulates inducible nitric oxide synthase gene expression and increases nitric oxide production in alveolar macrophages and neutrophils. *Am J Respir Cell Mol Biol* 11: 426–431

74 Goldman D, Cho Y, Zhao M, Casadevall A, Lee SC (1996) Expression of inducible nitric oxide synthase in rat pulmonary cryptococcus neoformans granulomas. *Am J Pathol* 148: 1275–1282

75 Yan ZQ, Hansson GK, Skoogh BE, Lotvall JP (1995) Induction of nitric oxide synthase in a model of alelrgic occupational asthma. *Allergy* 50: 760–764

76 Yeadon M, Price R (1995) Induction of calcium-independent nitric oxide synthase by allergen challenge in sensitized rat lung *in vivo. Br J Pharmacol* 116: 2545–2546

77 Turnage RH, Kadesky KM, Bartula L, Myers SI (1995) Intestinal reperfusion opregulates inducible nitric oxide synthase activity within the lung. *Surgery* 118: 288–293

78 Haddad EB, Liu SF, Salmon M, Robichaud A, Barnes PJ, Chung KF (1995) Expression of inducible nitric oxide synthase mRNA in Brown Norway rats exposed to ozone: effect of dexamethasone. *Eur J Pharmacol* 293: 287–290

79 Buttery LD, Evans TJ, Springall DR, Carpenter A, Cohen J, Polak JM (1994) Immunochemical localization of inducible nitric oxide synthase in endotoxin-treated rats. *Lab Invest* 71: 755–764

80 Guo FH, De Raeve HR, Rice TW, Stuehr DJ, Thunnissen FB, Erzurum SC (1995) Continuous nitric oxide synthesis by inducible nitric oxide synthase in normal human airway epithelium *in vivo. Proc Natl Acad Sci USA* 92: 7809–7813

81 Palmer RMJ, Ferridge AG, Moncada S (1987) Nitric oxide release accounts for the biological activity of endothelium-derived relaxing factor. *Nature* 327: 524

82 Moncada S, Radomski MW, Palmer RMJ (1988) Endothelium derived relaxing factor. Identification as nitric oxide and role in the control of vascular tone and platelet function. *Biochem Pharmacol* 37: 2495–2501

83 Palmer RMJ, Ashton DS, Moncada S (1988) Vascular endothelial cells synthesize nitric oxide from L-arginine. *Nature* 333: 664–666

84 Förstermann U, Pollock JS, Schmidt HHHW, Heller M, Murad F (1991) Calmodulin-dependent endothelium-derived relaxing factor/nitric oxide synthase activity is present in the particulate and cytosolic fractions of bovine aortic endothelial cells. *Proc Natl Acad Sci USA* 88: 1778–1792

85 Janssens SP, Schimouchi A, Quertermous T, Bloch DB, Bloch KD (1992) Cloning and expression of a cDNA encoding human endothelium-derived relaxing factor/nitric oxide synthase. *J Biol Chem* 267: 14519–14522

86 Nishida K, Harrison D, Navas J, Fisher A, Dockery S, Uematsu M et al (1992) Molecular cloning and characterization of the constitutive bovine aortic endothelial cell nitric oxide synthase. *J Clin Invest* 90: 2092–2096

87 Lamas S, Marsden PA, Li GK, Tempst P, Michel T (1992) Endothelial nitric oxide synthase: molecular cloning and characterization of a distinct constitutive molecular isoform. *Proc Natl Acad Sci USA* 89: 6348–6352

88 O'Brien AJ, Young HM, Povey JM, Furness JB (1995) Nitric oxide synthase is localized predominantly in the Golgi apparatus and cytoplasmatic vesicles of vascular endothelial cells. *Histochemistry* 103: 221–225

89 Garcia-Cardena G, Oh P, Liu J, Schnitzer JE, Sessa WC (1996) Targeting of nitric oxide synthase to endothelial cell caveolae via palmitoylation: implications for nitric oxide signaling. *Proc Natl Acad Sci USA* 93: 6448–6453

90 North AJ, Star RA, Brannon TS, Ujiie K, Wells LB, Lowenstein CJ et al (1994) Nitric oxide type I and type III gene expression are developmentally regulated in rat lung. *Am J Physiol* 266: L635–L641

91 Halbower AC, Tuder RM, Franklin WA, Pollock JS, Förstermann U, Abman SH (1994) Maturation-related changes in endothelial nitric oxide synthase immunolocalization in developing ovine lung. *Am J Physiol* 267: L585–L591

92 Kawai N, Bloch DB, Fillipov G, Rabkina D, Suen HC, Losty PD et al (1995) Constitutive endothelial nitric oxide synthase gene expression is regulated during lung development. *Am J Physiol* 268: L589–L595

93 Hislop AA, Springall DR, Buttery LD, Pollock JS, Haworth SG (1995) Abundance of endothelial nitric oxide synthase in newborn intrapulmonary arteries. *Arch Dis Child Fetal Neonatal* 73: F17–F21

94 Shaul PW, North AJ, Wu LC, Wells LB, Brannon TS, Lau KS et al (1994) Endothelial nitric oxide synthase is expressed in cultured human bronchiolar epithelium. *J Clin Invest* 94: 2231–2236

95 Xue C, Botkin SJ, Johns RA (1996) Localization of endothelial NOS at the basal microtubule membrane in ciliated epithelium of rat lung. *J Histochem Cytochem* 44: 463–471

96 Jain B, Rubinstein I, Robbins RA, Leise KL, Sisson JH (1993) Modulation of airway epithelial cell ciliary beat frequency by nitric oxide. *Biochem Biophys Res Commun* 191: 83–88

97 Asano K, Chee CB, Gaston B, Lilly CM, Gerard C, Drazen JM et al (1994) Constitutive and inducible nitric oxide gene expression, regulation and activity in human lung epithelial cells. *Proc Natl Acad Sci USA* 91: 10089–10093

98 Morrison KJ, Gao Y, Vanhoutte PM (1990) Epithelial modulation of airway smooth muscle. *Am J Physiol* 258: L254–L262

99 Nijkamp FP, van der Linde HJ, Folkerts G (1993) Nitric oxide synthase inhibitors induce airway hyperresponsiveness in the guinea-pig *in vivo* and *in vitro*. Role of the epithelium. *Am Rev Respir Dis* 148: 727–734

100 Rengasamy A, Xue C, Johns RA (1994) Immunohistochemical demonstration of a paracrine role of nitric oxide in bronchial function. *Am J Physiol* 267: L704–L711

101 Yan ZQ, Kramer K, Bast A, Timmerman H (1994) The involvement of nitric oxide synthase in the effect of histamine on guinea-pig airway smooth muscle tone *in vitro*. *Agents Actions* 41: c111–C112

102 Barnes PJ, Liew FY (1995) Nitric oxide and asthmatic inflammation. *Immunol Today* 16: 128–130

103 Kharitonov SA, Yates D, Robbins RA, Logan-Sinclair R, Shinebourne EA, Barnes PJ (1994) Increased nitric oxide in exhaled air of asthmatic patients. *Lancet* 343: 133–135

104 Kharitonov SA, Wells AU, O'Connor BJ, Cole PJ, Hansell DM, Logan-Sinclair RB et al (1995) Elevated levels of exhaled nitric oxide in bronchiectasis. *Am J Respir Crit Care Med* 151: 1889–1893

105 Hamid Q, Springall DR, Riveros-Moreno V, Chanez P, Howarth P, Redington A et al (1993) Induction of nitric oxide synthase in asthma. *Lancet* 342: 1510–1513

106 Belvisi MG, Barnes PJ, Larkin S, Yacoub M, Tadjarimi S, Williams TJ et al (1995) Nitric oxide synthase activity is elevated in humans. *Eur J Pharmacol* 283: 255–258

107 Geller DA, Lowenstein CJ, Shapiro RA, Nussler AK, Silvio M, Wang SC et al (1993) Molecular cloning and expression of inducible nitric oxide synthase from human hepatocytes. *Proc Natl Acad Sci USA* 90: 3491–3495

108 Oguchi S, Iida S, Adachi H, Oshima H, Esumi H (1992) Induction of Ca^{2+}/calmodulin-dependent NO synthase in various organs of rats by Proprionibacterium acnes and lipopolysaccharide treatment. *FEBS Lett* 308: 22–25

109 Liu SF, Adcock IM, Old RW, Barnes PJ, Evans TW (1996) Differential regulation of the constitutive and inducible nitric oxide synthase mRNA by lipopolysaccharide treatment *in vivo* in the rat. *Crit Care Med* 24: 1219–1225

110 Buttery LD, Springall DR, da Costa FA, Oliveira H, Hislop AA, Haworth SG et al (1995) Early abundance of nerves containing NO synthase in the the airways of newborn pigs and subsequent decrease with age. *Neurosci Lett* 201: 219–222

111 Fischer A, McGregor GP, Saria A, Philippin B, Kummer W (1996) Induction of tachykinin-gene and -peptide-expression in guinea-pig nodose primary afferent neurons by allergic airway inflammation. *J Clin Invest* 98: 2284–2291

112 Heppelmann B, Bscheidl C (1995) Proportion of NADPH-diaphorase reactive sympathetic efferents innervating the normal and inflamed knee joint of the cat. *Neurosci Lett* 185: 199–202

113 Hoheisel U, Reinert A, Mense S (1995) Changes in the NADPH-diaphorase activity in the rat dorsal horn following an acute experimental myositis. *Histochemistry* 103: 459–462

114 Fiallos-Estrada CE, Herdegen T, Kummer W, Mayer B, Bravo R, Zimmermann M (1993) Long-lasting increase of nitric oxide synthase immunoreactivity, NADPH-diaphorase reaction and c-JUN co-expression in rat dorsal root ganglion neurons following sciatic nerve transsection. *Neurosci Lett* 150: 169–173

115 Vizzard MA, Erdman SL, de Groat WC (1995) Increased expression of neuronal nitric oxide synthase (NOS) in visceral neurons after nerve injury. *J Neurosci* 15: 4033–4045

116 Giaid A, Saleh D (1995) Reduced expression of endothelial nitric oxide synthase in the lungs of patients with pulmonary hypertension. *N Engl J Med* 333: 214–221

117 Kane DW, Tesauro T, Koizumi T, Gupta R, Newman JH (1994) Exercise-induced pulmonary vasoconstriction during combined blockade of nitric oxide synthase and beta adrenergic receptors. *J Clin Invest* 93: 677–683

118 Cobbs CS, Brenman JE, Aldape KD, Bredt DS, Israel MA (1995) Expression of nitric oxide synthase in human central nervous system tumors. *Cancer Res* 55: 727–730

119 Edwards P, Cendan JC, Topping DB, Moldawer LL, McKay S, Copeland EMIII et al (1996) Tumor cell nitric oxide inhibits cell growth *in vitro*, but stimulates tumorigenesis and experimental lung metastasis *in vivo*. *J Surg Res* 63: 49–52

120 Dong Z, Staroselsky AH, Qi X, Xie K, Fidler IJ (1994) Inverse correlation between expression of inducible nitric oxide synthase activity and production of metastasis in K-1735 murine melanoma cells. *Cancer Res* 54: 789–793

121 Xie K, Dong Z, Fidler IJ (1996) Activation of nitric oxide synthase gene for inhibition of cancer metastasis. *J Leuk Biol* 59: 797–803

122 Xie K, Huang S, Dong Z, Juang SH, Gutman M, Xie QW et al (1995) Transfection with the inducible nitric oxide synthase gene suppresses tumorigenicity and abrogates metastasis by K-1735 murine melanoma cells. *J Exp Med* 181: 1333–1343

Nitric Oxide in Pulmonary Processes:
Role in Physiology and Pathophysiology of Lung Disease
ed. by M. G. Belvisi and J. A. Mitchell
© 2000 Birkhäuser Verlag Basel/Switzerland

CHAPTER 5
Role of Nitric Oxide in the Regulation of Pulmonary Vascular Tone

Shu F. Liu[1] and Timothy W. Evans[2]

[1] Long Island Jewish Medical Center, Albert Einstein College of Medicine,
270-5 76th Avenue, New Hyde Park, NY 11040, USA
[2] Unit of Critical Care, Royal Brompton Hospital, National Heart and Lung Institute,
Sidney Street, London SW3 6NP, UK

1   Introduction
2   Nitric Oxide (NO) Inhibits Adrenergic Contraction
2.1 Adrenergic Regulation of Pulmonary Vascular Tone
2.2 NO Inhibits Adrenergic Responses
3   NO Mediates Cholinergic Responses
3.1 Cholinergic Regulation of Pulmonary Vascular Tone
3.2 NO Mediates Cholinergic Responses
4   NO as an Inhibitory Non-Adrenergic, Non-Cholinergic (NANC) Neurotransmitter
4.1 NANC Nerves
4.2 NANC Neurotransmitters
4.3 NO as an Inhibitory NANC transmitter
4.4 NANC Regulation of Pulmonary Vascular Tone
5   NO and Humoral Regulation
5.1 Effects of Humoral Substances
5.2 Humoral Regulation of Pulmonary Vascular Tone
5.3 NO and Humoral Regulation
5.4 Role of Basal Release of NO
6   NO Modulates Hypoxic Pulmonary Vasoconstriction (HPV)
6.1 HPV
6.2 NO Modulates HPV
7   Summary
8   References

1. Introduction

The pulmonary circulation is a low pressure, low resistance, high flow system regulated through both active and passive factors [1–4]. Active factors alter pulmonary vascular resistance and tone by causing contraction or relaxation of vascular smooth muscle and include neural and humoral mechanisms, and gaseous regulators. Passive factors alter pulmonary vascular resistance and/or blood flow independently of changes in vascular tone and include variation in cardiac output, left atrial, airway and interstitial pressures, gravitational force, and vascular obstruction or recruitment. Although passive factors may be important, the pulmonary circulation is regulated overwhelmingly by active control mechanisms [1–4].

Nitric oxide (NO) plays an important role in the regulation of pulmonary vascular tone [5]. It modulates adrenergic contraction, mediates cholinergic pulmonary vasodilatation and acts as a novel neurotransmitter of inhibitory nonadrenergic, noncholinergic (iNANC) nerves. NO serves as a second messenger molecule in the pulmonary vascular response to many vasoactive substances and inhibits hypoxic pulmonary vasoconstriction. Pulmonary vascular endothelial cells generate NO continuously. This basal-release of NO acts as braking mechanism to avoid an "overreaction" of pulmonary smooth muscle to vasoconstrictors.

This chapter deals with the physiological regulatory mechanisms of pulmonary vascular tone with emphasis on the role of NO in this process.

2. NO Inhibits Adrenergic Contraction

2.1. Adrenergic Regulation of Pulmonary Vascular Tone

Sympathetic nerves supplying the pulmonary vessels arise from nerve cell bodies in the first five thoracic ganglia, the satellite ganglia, and middle and inferor cervical ganglia [1–4]. Post-ganglionic fibers from these sites intermingle with parasympathetic nerve fibers to form anterior and posterior plexi, at the tracheal bifurcation [1, 4]. Nerve fibers arising from these plexi enter the lungs to form a periarterial plexus innervating the pulmonary vascular tree, and a peribronchial plexus which innervates the bronchial tree. The distribution and density of catecholamine-containing nerve fibers vary across species [2, 4], but pulmonary arteries of many species, including humans, are densely innervated with these nerve fibers. These nerve fibers extend to pulmonary arteries with an outer diameter of < 60 μm [2, 4].

Stimulation of sympathetic nerves in a perfused canine lobe causes a frequency-related increase in pulmonary vascular resistance independent of changes in respiration, bronchomotor tone and bronchial blood flow [6]. Sympathetic nerve stimulation also increases pulmonary input impedance [4, 5]. Thus, sympathetic activation increases pulmonary vascular resistance and decreases pulmonary vascular compliance, thereby increasing pulmonary arterial pressure. Both effects are mediated by α-adrenoceptors [3, 4, 7], primarily of the α_1-subtype [3–5]. There appears also to be β-adrenoceptor-mediated pulmonary vasodilatation in response to sympathetic nerve stimulation which is observed in the presence of α-adrenoceptor blockade [3–5]. Further β-adrenoceptor blockade enhances the constrictor response to sympathetic nerve stimulation [3].

Sympathetic nerves also influence basal pulmonary vascular tone, for example α-adrenoceptor antagonists cause pulmonary vasodilatation and β-adrenoceptor antagonists induce pulmonary vasoconstriction, in conscious dogs [8]. After left lung autotransplantation in dogs there is an increased response to α-agonists, which may be a manifestation of denervation supersensitivity [4, 9]. Sympathetic nerves are likely to mediate pulmonary vasoconstrictor responses to cold exposure, reperfusion (hypoperfusion followed by hyperperfusion) and pulmonary embolism [4, 9].

2.2. NO Inhibits Adrenergic Responses

NO has an important modulatory role on the adrenergic response, exercised through complex NO-smooth muscle and NO-adrenergic nerve interactions [5]. In 1983, Cocks and Angus [10] observed a marked potentiation in the contractile response to noradrenaline (NA) following removal of the vascular endothelium in canine and pig coronary arteries. This phenomenon was later demonstrated in pulmonary vessels in response either to adrenergic agonists or to adrenergic nerve stimulation [4, 5]. Several mechanisms have been explored. Endothelium-derived vasodilator prostaglandins are unlikely to be involved [4, 5]. Reduction of NA degradation due to removal of endothelium may play a role, but is unlikely to be important [11].

The role of endogenous NO in the modulation of adrenergic neural contraction was demonstrated *in vitro* on pulmonary arteries from guinea-pig, rabbit and dog. Electrical field stimulation (EFS) of the intramural adrenergic nerves of these vessels caused a frequency-dependent contraction, which was markedly enhanced by the NO synthase (NOS) inhibitors N^G-monomethyl L-arginine (LNMMA) or N^G-L-arginine methylester (L-NAME) in a concentration-dependent and L-arginine reversible manner [4, 9]. D-NAME induced no such potentiation [9]. Further, exogenous NO applied as acid nitrite inhibited the adrenergic neural constriction in guinea-pig pulmonary arteries [12]. Whereas, NOS inhibition augments the pressor response to sympathetic nerve stimulation *in vivo* [4, 5].

Several mechanisms can explain NO-mediated inhibition of adrenergic contraction. An interaction between NO and adrenergic nerves has been suggested [9, 13, 14]. Immunohistochemical studies have localised neuronal NOS (nNOS) to both sympathetic and parasympathetic neurons [15, 16]. There are both immunohistochemical and pharmacological data indicating that NO is a neurotransmitter of NANC vasodilator nerves in the pulmonary vessels (see section 4.3). It is possible that NO released from these nerve endings can diffuse either to the adrenergic nerves inhibiting NA release or to smooth muscle cells antagonising adrenergic neural contraction. Supporting this possibility is the demonstration that the NOS inhibitor, L-NAME, markedly augmented EFS-induced adrenergic contraction, but had no effect on exogenous NA-induced contraction in endothelium-denuded pulmonary artery rings [17]. Endothelially-derived NO may also play an important role in this process. Activation of endothelial α_2-adrenergic receptors leading to the release of NO from endothelial cells has been reported to be responsible for the inhibition of adrenergic contraction in the vascular bed of skeletal muscle [5, 9]. Although endothelial α_2-adrenoceptors exist in pulmonary vessels, and NO does mediate α_2-adrenoceptor agonist-induced pulmonary vasodilatation [4, 5], their role in the modulation of adrenergic neural contraction is less important and appears to vary between species. This mechanism seems to contribute to the NO-mediated inhibition of adrenergic neural contraction in rabbit pulmonary arteries, but is unlikely to be important under physiological conditions in guinea-pig pulmonary arteries, since NA has little relaxant effect on these vessels, even when vascular tone is elevated [4, 5]. Pulmonary vascular endothelial cells release NO basally. Both endothelial shear stress, due to changes in perfusate velocity and viscosity, and mechanical deformation of the vessel wall have been demonstrated to release NO [18, 19], which also inhibits adrenergic contractions to EFS in systemic arteries [18]. This mechanism has not yet been confirmed in pulmonary vessels, but presumably should be operative.

NO can inhibit adrenergic contraction through either prejunctional or postjunctional actions, or both. Both endogenous and exogenous NO inhibit NA release from cardiac sympathetic nerves of rats and perivascular adrenergic nerves of dog mesenteric arteries [9, 13, 14]. In isolated dog intrapulmonary arteries and veins, removal of endothelium enhances, whilst effluent from endothelium-intact donor aorta inhibits, EFS-induced NA release. This suggests that that both neuronal and endothelial-derived NO can act pre-junctionally to inhibit NA release in these pulmonary vessels [5, 9, 11]. Similar mechanisms are unlikely to be operative in the pulmonary arteries of guinea-pigs and rabbits, however, since in vessels from these species, neither endothelial removal nor NO inhibition enhances NA release induced by EFS [4, 9, 12]. Moreover, in these studies exogenous NO did not inhibit EFS-induced NA release [4, 9, 12].

NO may modulate pulmonary vascular tone through central or reflex pathways. Inhibition of NO by L-NMMA increases NA release in the medial basal hypothalamus [14]. L-NMMA also increases central sympathetic outflow, which is abolished by spinal cord transection and reversed by L-arginine [9]. Exogenous L-arginine decreases renal sympathetic nerve activity [9]. The NOS inhibitor, L-NAME, enhances the gain of baroreceptor-cardiac reflex, which is reversed by the NO donor, sodium nitroprusside (SNP) [20]. NO and the NO donor, S-nitrosocycteine, suppress carotid sinus baroreceptor activity [9].

Although several factors contribute to the NO-mediated inhibition of adrenergic contraction, the basal and mechanically-stimulated release of NO from endothelial cells is likely to be mainly responsible for the inhibition. This could explain the uniform augmentation by NOS inhibitors of the contractile responses to vasoconstrictors with diverse mechanisms of action [4, 5].

3. NO Mediates Cholinergic Responses

3.1. Cholinergic Regulation of Pulmonary Vascular Tone

Intrapulmonary arteries of many species are innervated with cholinergic nerves arising from the vagal nuclei of the brain stem [1, 2, 4, 9]. The distribution of these post-ganglionic nerve fibers along the pulmonary vascular tree varies considerably between species [2, 4, 9]. The intrapulmonary arteries of rabbit, dog, monkey, sheep and cat are intensively innervated, as are those of human. However, cholinergic inervation of bovine, rat, mouse and guinea-pig intrapulmonary arteries is low or absent [2, 4, 9].

Although the pulmonary circulation of many species is innervated with cholinergic nerves, their functional significance is unclear. They do not appear to be important in the maintenance of low pulmonary vascular tone, since cholinergic blockade does not alter basal pulmonary arterial pressure or vascular resistance [4, 8, 9]. Earlier studies on the effects of vagal stimulation on the pulmonary circulation provided conflicting results. Vagal stimulation induces pulmonary vasoconstriction in perfused dog and guinea-pig lungs, but causes pulmonary vasodilatation in adult pig and fetal lamb lungs [4, 9]. Daly and Hebb observed increased, decreased, or biphasic changes in pulmonary artery pressure in response to vagal stimulation in the dog [21]. This is not surprising, since canine vagal nerves contain sympathetic nerve fibers [21]. Vagal stimulation is therefore likely to cause an adrenergic vasoconstriction as well as vasodilatation. Further, changes in cardiac output, airway pressure, and bronchial blood flow induced by vagal stimulation may also affect pulmonary arterial pressure. For example, vagally-induced increases in airway pressure would increase pulmonary vascular resistance and thereby confound any decrease in pulmonary arterial pressure induced by vagal stimulation [22]. In the perfused cat pulmonary vascular bed, vagal stimulation evokes an increase in pulmonary perfusion pressure under basal conditions, whereas perfusion pressure decreases under conditions of elevated vascular tone [23]. The pressor and depressor responses are blocked by phenoxybenzamine and atropine respectively, confirming that both adrenergic vasoconstriction and cholinergic vasodilatation are induced by vagal stimulation. After chemical sympathectomy with 6-hydroxydopamine, vagal stimulation induces a frequency-dependent decrease in lobar artery pressure under conditions of elevated vascular tone induced by the thromboxane mimetic U44169 or hypoxia. Exogenously-administered acetylcholine (ACh) mimics the response to vagal stimulation. The responses to both vagal stimulation and ACh are blocked by atropine and enhanced by physostigmine, a cholinesterase inhibitor. Moreover, this vagally-induced vasodilatation is not affected by elevating airway pressure, nor by reducing systemic blood pressure [23]. Vagally-released ACh acts on the vascular endothelium to induce NO release which then causes vasodilatation [24].

Vagal nerves also participate in reflex responses under both physiological and pathophysiological conditions. Stimulation of carotid chemoreceptors during local hypoxic pulmonary vasoconstriction blunts the response, an effect probably mediated via cholinergic nerves, although inconsistent results have been reported [4, 9]. Depending on the level of pre-existing tone, exogenous ACh induces either vasoconstrictor or vasodilator responses [4, 9]. ACh induces a pressor response under resting conditions, but causes a depressor response during elevated vascular tone [4, 9]. There also appears to be a species variation in the ACh response, as both the mechanism and characteristics of the vasoconstriction in the rabbit are different from those in the feline pulmonary circulation [4, 9]. In humans, ACh induces a clear vasodilator response both under resting conditions and during acute hypoxic pulmonary vasoconstriction [25]. Human isolated pulmonary arteries relax in response to ACh in an endothelium-dependent manner [4, 9]. Endothelial removal converts the relaxation to a small contractile response [4, 9]. Muscarinic receptors mediating the increase in pulmonary vascular resistance appear to be M_1-like receptors in rabbit, whereas both M_1- and M_2-receptors are involved in canine pulmonary vascular beds [4, 9]. In isolated rabbit large pulmonary arteries, both the contractile and relaxant responses are mediated via M_3-receptors [9]. ACh elicited relaxation of the rat precontracted pulmonary vascular bed is mediated through M_1-Receptors [26].

3.2. NO Mediates Cholinergic Responses

ACh was the first endothelium-depenent vasodilator to be described [27]. Studies using NOS inhibitors have revealed that NO mediates the vasodilator response to exogenous ACh in the pulmonary vascular beds of various species *in vivo* and *in situ*, although inconsistent results have been reported [5, 9]; and NO also mediates the vasodilator response to neurally-released ACh. In the precontracted cat pulmonary vascular bed, vagal stimulation elicits a frequency-dependent relaxation, which is blocked by atropine and greatly inhibited by the NOS inhibitor, L-NAME [24]. This neural relaxation is also markedly inhibited by the guanylyl cyclase inhibitor methylene blue [28]. By contrast, in the same preparation L-NAME has no inhibitory effects on the dilator response to drugs with diverse mechanisms of action, including adenosine, nicorandil, isoprenaline, sodium nitroprusside, prostaglandin E_1 (PGE_1), or 8-bromo-cGMP. How ACh released from cholinergic nerve terminals at the adventitio-medial border exerts its action on endothelial cells is unclear, since this presumably involves diffusion through the smooth muscle layer. Upon reaching endothelial cells, ACh stimulates the phosphoinositide cycle generating inositol 1,4,5-triphosphate to release calcium, which binds to calmodulin and activates NOS resulting in the release of NO. NO activates guanylyl cyclase and elevates the intracellular level of cyclic guanosine monophosphate (cGMP) in vascular smooth muscle cells, which reduces intracellular free calcium and thus initiates vasodilatation.

NO may modulate cholinergic responses via a prejunctional action. nNOS has been localised to cholinergic nerve endings [15, 16]. In myenteric neurons, NO donors stimulate basal [^{3}H]-ACh release, but inhibit EFS-induced [^{3}H]-ACh release [29]. The NOS inhibitors, L-NMMA and L-NAME, potentiate the EFS-induced [^{3}H]-ACh release [9]; implying that NO induces basal ACh release, but inhibits depolarisation-induced release from cholinergic nerves. This mechanism has not been explored in pulmonary vessels.

4. NO as an Inhibitory Non-Adrenergic, Non-Cholinergic (iNANC) Neurotransmitter

4.1. NANC Nerves

In addition to classic adrenergic and cholinergic innervation, there are neural mechanisms that are not inhibited by adrenergic and cholinergic blockade [4, 9]. NANC nerves may represent separate neural pathways, but are more likely to be manifestations of neural co-transmission in sympathetic, parasympathetic, and sensory nerves. NANC neural responses that are excitatory (eNANC, vasoconstrictor) and inhibitory (iNANC, vasodilator) have been demonstrated in pulmonary vessels of several species [5, 9, 30–32], including human intrapulmonary arteries [32]. In rat small pulmonary arteries, EFS evokes an excitatory junction potential, which is insensitive to adrenergic, cholinergic, histaminergic, and serotonergic blockade, and unaffected by catecholamine depletion or sympathetic denervation, but which is abolished by tetrodotoxin and inhibited by α-, β-methylene ATP [30], suggesting an adenosine triphosphate (ATP)-mediated eNANC transmission. In precontracted pulmonary artery rings of cat, guinea-pig and human, EFS induces frequency-dependent relaxation, which is abolished by tetrodotoxin, but largely unaffected by treatment with a combination of adrenergic and cholinergic antagonists, indicating that the main component of this relaxation is mediated via iNANC mechanism [5, 9, 30–32]. EFS also relaxes precontracted pulmonary arteries of dog, rabbit, and cow, but these responses are not of neural origin, since they are tetrodotoxin resistant [9].

4.2. NANC Neurotransmitters

As mentioned in a previous section, eNANC neurotransmitters may be ATP in small pulmonary arteries of rat [30]. Other mediators proposed as iNANC neurotransmitters include calcitonin gene-related peptide (CGRP), substance P (SP), a vasoactive intestinal polypeptide (VIP), ATP and NO [4, 9]. CGRP-like immunoreactive nerves are located around pulmonary arteries of several species [9]. CGRP-like immunoreactivity is released during stimulation of vagus nerve [33] and upon stimulation of the perivascular nerves of guinea-pig *main* pulmonary arteries [31]. CGRP is a potent vasodilator of guinea-pig *main* pulmonary arteries, mimicking the NANC vasodilator response [5, 9]. Pretreatment with capsaicin to deplete sensory neuropeptides including CGRP markedly inhibits the iNANC response in these vessels [4, 5, 9]. However, CGRP may not mediate the iNANC response in the *branch* pulmonary arteries of guinea-pig, as it does not mimic iNANC relaxation in these vessels. Further, the iNANC response in *branch* pulmonary arteries is partially endothelium-dependent, but CGRP is an endothelium-independent vasodilator in this vessel. Finally, capsaicin treatment *in vivo* and *in vitro* has no significant effect on the iNANC response in *branch* vessels [5, 9], but abolishes or greatly reduces the iNANC response in *main* pulmonary artery [4, 5, 9].

SP-like immunoreactive nerves have also been localised to pulmonary vessels of several species [2, 9]. SP is a potent vasodilator, and SP-like immunoreactivity is released during perivascular nerve stimulation by EFS in guinea-pig pulmonary artery [9, 31]. However, SP is unlikely to be important in mediating the iNANC vasodilator response, since the vasodilator response to SP is endothelium-dependent, whereas the iNANC response in this vessel is not [31]. Moreover, pretreatment with capsaicin to deplete SP from sensory nerves, or use of specific NK_1 receptor antagonist to block SP action has no effect on the iNANC vasodilator response [4, 9].

VIP-immunoreactive nerve fibers are localised to pulmonary arteries of several species [4, 9], including human [34]. VIP-immunoreactivity is released from perivascular nerves of cat extrapulmonary arteries in response to EFS [35]. VIP is a potent pulmonary vasodilator in several species, including human both *in vitro* and *in situ* [4, 5, 9]. However, VIP is unlikely to mediate the iNANC vasodilator response in guinea-pig pulmonary arteries. VIP has minimal relaxant effects on these vessels, and α-chymotrypsin, which degrades VIP, has no effect on the iNANC response [4, 9].

ATP may act as an iNANC transmitter in pulmonary vessels. ATP is released upon stimulation of perivascular nerves in rabbit pulmonary arteries by EFS [36]. The iNANC vasodilator response is significantly inhibited by the P_{2y}-purinoceptor antagonist, reactive blue 2, in guinea-pig *branch* pulmonary arteries [5, 9]. ATP mimics the iNANC vasodilator response in these vessels [4, 9]. P_{2y}-purinergic receptors that mediate the pulmonary vasodilator response to ATP have been identified on pulmonary vessels [4, 5, 9].

4.3. NO as an iNANC Transmitter

There is increasing evidence to support NO as an iNANC neurotransmitter in many organs [37]. Most of the direct evidence for the release of NO from iNANC nerve endings and for the increse in nNOS activity upon EFS comes from studies on enteric neuron and gastrointestinal tissues [37 – 39]. There are also immunocytochemical and pharmacological evidence supporting NO as an iNANC neurotransmitter in pulmonary arteries. Immuno-cytochemical staining for nNOS and NADPH-diaphorase, which is a marker of NOS, has demonstrated NOS-immunoreactive nerves distributing around extra- and intrapulmonary arteries [40, 41]. In precontracted, endothelium-denuded guinea-pig *branch* pulmonary arteries, the iNANC vasodilator response is markedly inhibited by the NOS inhibitors, L-NMMA or L-NAME, in an L-arginine reversible manner, D-arginine being inactive [4, 9, 17]. Pyrogallol, an agent known to inactivate NO through superoxide radical generation, also inhibits this iNANC relaxation, which is restored fully by adding superoxide dismutase at the point of peak inhibition. Inhibition of the formation of cGMP, the second messenger of NO action, by methylene blue (5 µM) causes >80% inhibition in iNANC relaxation. Additionally, iNANC-induced relaxation is significantly potentiated by zaprinast, a type V phosphodiesterase inhibitor which prevents cGMP degradation [17]. Further, iNANC relaxation is accompanied by a marked increase in tissue cGMP content, which is significantly inhibited by L-NMMA [17]. In endothelium-denuded pulmonary arteries, NOS inhibitors significantly augment adrenergic contraction, without any effect on basal vascular tone and contration evoked by exogenous NA, suggesting that there is neural release of NO, which acts as a functional antagonism to the adrenergic neural contraction [9, 17].

Both sympathetic and parasympathetic nerves contain NOS immuno-reactive neurons [15, 16]. Under *in vitro* conditions, application of EFS activates intramural adrenergic, cholinergic, and NANC nerves simultaneously. NO can be released from adrenergic and/or cholinergic nerves as a co-transmitter with NA or ACh. However, NO is unlikely to be released from adrenergic nerves, since chemical sympathetic denervation by 6-hydroxyl dopamine has no effect on EFS-induced relaxation in these vessels [9, 17]. It will be difficult to distinguish whether NO is released from cholinergic or NANC nerves until a method is developed to selectively destroy cholinergic nerves. Nevertheless, it is possible that NO can be released from separate NANC nerves. NOS immunoreactivity is co-localised with VIP-immunoreactive nerve fibers [15, 41], suggesting NO may be co-released with VIP. This further supports an iNANC transmitter role for NO.

The cellular source of NO has been a matter of debate, but recent evidence indicates that NO is released from intrinsic NANC nerves [38, 39]. The nNOS in nitrergic nerves is activated by calcium entry when the nerves are depolarized, thereby releasing NO. Endothelium-derived NO may also play a part. In guinea-pig pulmonary arteries, the iNANC vasodilator response is partially mediated by ATP-induced NO release from vascular endothelial cells [5, 9]. Earlier studies have suggested that VIP released from NANC nerves causes NO production from smooth muscle cells [42]. But more recent data indicate that NO is generated in nitrergic neurons on demand [39].

4.4. NANC Regulation of Pulmonary Vascular Tone

Although iNANC mediated pulmonary vasodilatation has bene demonstrated *in vitro* [4, 5, 17, 32], it has not been described *in vivo*. Therefore, the roles of this neural mechanism in the regulation of pulmonary vascular tone remain to be explored. Since the major part of the relaxant response of pulmonary vessels to EFS is mediated through an iNANC pathway, this neural mechanism may play a role in the regulation of pulmonary vascular tone and pulmonary blood flow. The role of NANC mechanisms in the maintenance of low basal pulmonary vascular tone is suggested by the demonstration that inhibition of NO production elevates pulmonary vascular blood pressure or pulmonary vascular resistance both in animals and humans [4, 5]. Although basal-release of NO from endothelial cells is mainly responsible in these circumstances, neuronally derived NO may also participate. The pulmonary circulation undergoes significant changes during the physiological adaptation to exercise, pregnancy, cold exposure and birth, to which NANC mechanisms may contribute. NO contributes to the pulmonary vasodilatation of exercise [4, 9], and to the low pulmonary arterial pressure and low pulmonary vascular resistance of pregnancy [4] and plays an important part in the transitional adaptation of the fetal pulmonary circulation to adult [43]. ATP participates in the O_2-induced pulmonary vasodilatation that occurs at birth [44]. NO, ATP, CGRP and SP inhibit the pulmonary vasoconstriction to hypoxia [4, 5], suggesting that these transmitters modulate hypoxic mvasoconstriction (HPV). CGRP counteracts the development of hypoxic pulmonary hypertension. CGRP-like immunoreactivity is increased in lung neuroendocirne cells of rats exposed to chronic hypoxia [4, 9]. Chronic infusion of CGRP prevents, and immunoneutralization with CGRP antibody, or infusion of CGRP receptor antagonist peptides, exacerbates hypoxic pulmonary hypertension in rats exposed to chronic hypoxia [4, 9]. A reduction in CGRP-containing NANC vasodilator nerves has been suggested to contribute to the development and maintenance of systemic hypertension in spontaneously hypertensive rats [4, 9]. Hypoxia inhibits NANC neuroeffector transmission in non-vascular tissues [4, 9]. It is possible that the normal vasodilator action of iNANC nerves is inhibited during hypoxia and may be impaired with repeated hypoxic episodes, thus promoting the development of hypoxic hypertension.

5. NO and Humoral Regulation

5.1. Effects of Humoral Substances

The pulmonary circulation is under continuous bombardment by a large body of vasoactive substances, including bioamines, kinins, peptides, purines and arachidonate metabolites [4, 5]. These substances influence pulmonary vascular tone by constricting or relaxing pulmonary vascular smooth muscle through the activation of specific receptors on smooth muscle and endothelial cells (Tab. 1 and 2). They can also increase or decrease pulmonary vascular resistance and/or compliance by changing cardiac output and bronchial tone, or closing or recruiting the pulmonary microvascular bed [4, 5]. The effects of these mediators and hormones on pulmonary vascular tone vary with species, age and pre-existing tone. In general, angiotensin II (A-II), neuropeptide Y (NPY), leucine-enkephalin, thrombin, thrombin receptor activation peptide, prostaglandins D_2, E_2 and F_{2a} are pulmonary vasoconstrictors, whereas atrial natriuretic peptide (ANP), VIP, CGRP, adenosine monophosphate (AMP), prostaglandins E_1 and I_2 are pulmonary vasodilators. There are exceptions in that PGD_2 and PGE_2 cause pulmonary vasodilatation in fetal lambs, and PGI_2 increases pulmonary vascular resistance in rabbits [4, 5]. Bradykinin (BK), arginine vasopressin (AVP), endothelins, pituitary adenylyl cyclase activating peptide (PACAP), SP, N-formal-methionyl-leucyl-phenylalanine (FMLP), histamine, 5-hydroxytryptamine (5-HT), platelet-activating factor (PAF), arachidonic acid, adenosine, ADP and ATP have dueal effects on pulmonary vascular tone, causing contraction when the vascular tone is low, but relaxation, when it is high [4, 5]. A detailed description of the effects of these humoral substances on pulmonary circulation is available elsewhere [4, 5].

5.2. Humoral Regulation of Pulmonary Vascular Tone

Although the pulmonary vasculature responds to these mediators and autocoids, the precise physiological and pathophysiological roles of most of them have not yet been defined. Inhibition of the production or blockade of the receptors of these substances has no effect on basal pulmonary vascular tone, suggesting that none in isolation is responsible for the maintenance of low pulmonary vascular tone, although they may be contributory if there is a synergistic interaction [45]. The maintenance of low pulmonary vascular tone seems to be the result of a balance between the vasoconstrictors and vasodilators, with the latter holding sway under normal physiological conditions [4, 5, 45]. Other factors such as recruitment and distention of the pulmonary vasculature, the meagerness of smooth muscle, low α-adrenergic activity and the ability of pulmonary endothelial cells to take up and remove both systematically or locally released vasoconstrictor substances may also contribute [4, 5, 45].

Humoral mediators may be important in some pathological conditions. 5-HT, histamine and thromboxane A_2 (TxA$_2$) mediate pulmonary hypertension during pulmonary embolism [4, 5, 45]. TxA$_2$ and leukotriene B$_4$ (LTB$_4$) may play a role in the early pulmonary hypertension seen in lung injury [4, 5, 45]. Many vasoactive substances, including A-II, ANP, AVP, ATP, ACh, BK, dopamine, endothelin (ET)-1, PAF, PGD$_2$, PGI$_2$ and SP have been reported to inhibit HPV, suggesting that these substances may modulate HPV. Some cyclooxygenase and lipoxygenase products may be involved in the etiology of hypoxic pulmonary hypertension [4, 5]. ET-1 and PAF may mediate and/or contribute to the development of hypoxic pulmonary hypertension, whereas ANP and cGMP may be important inhibitors of hypoxic pulmonary hypertension. ET-1 may play an important role in the occurrence and progression of other types of pulmonary hypertension. 5-HT is likely to be involved in the pathogenesis of monocrotaline-induced pulmonary hypertension [4, 5]. ET-1 and 5-HT have been reported to stimulate the proliferation of cultured pulmonary vascular smooth muscles [4, 5], which further supports their possible role in the development of pulmonary hypertension.

5.3. NO and Humoral Regulation

The importance of NO in the humoral regulation of pulmonary vascular tone is evidenced by the demonstration that many neural and humoral substances exert their pulmonary vasodilator actions via endothelium-dependent mechanisms and NO generation (Tabs. 1 and 2). Substances that have

Table 1. Autonomic receptors in pulmonary vessels

Receptors	Subtype	Response	Endothelium-dependency
Adrenergic	a_1	contraction	no
	a_2	contraction	no
		relaxation	yes
	β_2	relaxation	yes or no
Muscarinic	M_1	contraction	no
	M_3	relaxation	yes
Purinergic	P_{2x}	contraction	no
	P_{2y}	relaxation	yes
Tachykinin	NK_1	relaxation	yes
	NK_2	contraction	no
VIP	?	relaxation	yes or no
CGRP	?	relaxation	no

Table 2. Humoral receptors in pulmonary vessels

Receptors	Subtypes	Responses	Endothelium-dependency
Adenosine	A_1	contraction	no
	A_2	relaxation	no
Angiotensin	AT	contraction	no
ANP	ANP_A	relaxation	no
	ANP_B	relaxation	no
Bradykinin	B_1?	relaxation	yes
	B_2	relaxation	yes
Endothelin	ET_A	contraction	no
	ET_B	relaxation	yes
Histamine	H_1	relaxation	yes
	H_2	relaxation	no
5-HT	$5\text{-}HT_1$	contraction	no
	$5\text{-}HT_{1c}$	relaxation	yes
Thromboxane	TP	contraction	no
Vasopressin	V_1	relaxation	yes

been reported to induce pulmonary vasodilatation through endothelium-derived NO release include ACh, NA, BK, SP, ATP, ADP, histamine, 5-HT, ET-1, ET-3, thrombin and arachidonic acid [4, 5, 24, 31]. Further, both blood flow and mechanical deformation of the vascular wall impose shear stress on vascular endothelial cells and induce release of NO [4, 5, 18, 19]. Thus, an increase in pulmonary blood flow and possibly endothelium deformation due to pulmonary vasoconstriction causes NO release, which counteracts the increase in pulmonary blood pressure. Activation of calcium-activated K^+ channels appears to be involved in shear stress-induced NO release [46].

5.4. Role of Basal Release of NO

Accumulating evidence suggests that the basal-release of NO participates in the maintenance of pulmonary homeostasis, in the regulation of pulmonary vascular tone and in the modulation of pulmonary microvascular permeability. Infusion of L-NMMA acutely or administration of L-NAME orally for periods of 4 weeks causes a dose-dependent increase in systemic arterial blood pressure that is associated with a reduction in aortic cGMP content [4, 5, 47], indicating that basal release of NO plays an important role in the regulation of systemic blood pressure. The effects of basal NO released into the pulmonary circulation appears to vary between species. L-NMMA or N^G-nitro-L-arginine (L-NA) increase baseline pulmonary arterial pressure in guinea-pigs, rabbits, and lambs [4, 5]. L-NA reduces pulmonary vascular conductance with no change in pulmonary arterial pressure in pigs *in vivo*, suggesting an increase in pulmonary vascular resistance [4, 5]. Methylene blue also increases pulmonary arterial pressure in cats [4, 5]. By contrast, L-NA and L-NAME have no effect on pulmonary vascular resistance in dogs either under basal conditions or when the pulmonary venous pressure is slightly elevated to ensure that the circulation is under zone 3 conditions [48, 49]. L-NMMA and haemoglobin increase baseline vascular tone in isolated pulmonary artery rings from pigs, guinea-pigs and lambs, but not rats [4, 5]. L-NMMA and L-NA have no effect or slightly increse pulmonary perfusion pressure under basal conditions [4, 5], but increase pulmonary arterial pressure and vascular resistance under hypertensive conditions [50, 51] or when the venous pressure is slightly elevated in the rats [49]. Under the same conditions, the cyclooxygenase inhibitor, indomethacin, has no effect on baseline pulmonary vascular resistance in rats, but induces a rise in dogs [49]. Thus, vasodilator prostaglandins regulate basal canine pulmonary vascular tone, whereas NO performs this role in rats, cats, guinea-pigs, pigs, and sheep. Basal release of NO also plays an important role in the maintenance of low pulmonary vascular tone in humans [52, 53]. Infusion of L-NMMA into healthy volunteers or children with congenital heart disease; but with normal pulmonary blood flow, pressure, and resistance, causes a dose-dependent increase in pulmonary vascular resistance [53], or decrease in pulmonary blood flow, with no change in pulmonary arterial pressure [52]. Moreover, the increased pulmonary vascular resistance is associated with a reduced plasma NO_3^- level [53]. Together with the observation that basal release of NO inhibits the contractile response to adrenergic stimulation and other vasoconstrictors, such results indicate that NO plays an important part in the regulation of pulmonary vascular tone, both with or without elevated tone. Basal NO release increases when pulmonary arterial pressure or vascular resistance is increased, thus providing a tonic antagonism to the elevation in vascular tone. Basal NO release also plays an important role in the pulmonary vascular adaptation to exercise, pregnancy and during the transitional adaptation after birth [4, 5].

6. NO Modulates Hypoxic Pulmonary Vasoconstriction (HPV)

6.1. HPV

HPV is a physiological response whereby circulating blood is diverted away from hypoxic alveoli, thus optimizing the matching of perfusion and ventilation and maximizing arterial oxygenation. Because it is unique to the pulmonary circulation, HPV has been an area of intensive investigation and much debate since it was first described by von Euler and Liljestrand [54].

Despite over four decades of investigation, the mechanisms of HPV remain mysterious [4, 5]. Early work established that autonomic innervation does not appear to be necessary for the pressor response of the adult lung to hypoxia [4, 5], suggesting that the response is intrinsic to the lung. Two main hypotheses have been proposed. Firstly, the mediator hypothesis suggests that endogenous vasoconstrictors or vasodilators are released or suppressed by hypoxia. The other proposes a direct effect of hypoxia and the pulmonary vascular smooth muscle, inducing contraction.

Many vasoactive substances have been considered in the search for chemical mediators, including catecholamines, histamine, A-II, vasoconstrictor prostaglandins, 5-HT, PAF and ATP [4, 5]. None has proven essential for HPV, although a number of such substances may have a modulatory role or may establish the background conditions that are necessary for HPV to occur. LTC_4 and LTD_4 are still under investigation, but their definitive role in HPV still remains to be confirmed. ET-1 may play a role in the development of chronic hypoxic pulmonary hypertension, but is unlikely to mediate acute HPV response [4, 5].

Failure to identify conclusive mediator(s) promoted the alternative proposal that HPV represents a direct effect of hypoxia on pulmonary vascular smooth muscle cells. In support of this hypothesis, small pulmonary arteries of cat and human contract in response to hypoxia *in vitro* [4, 5], and hypoxia contracts pulmonary vascular smooth muscle cells in culture [55]. Several possible mechanisms have been proposed to explain how hypoxia directly causes pulmonary vasoconstriction. The K^+ channel hypothesis suggests that hypoxia closes oxygen-sensitive K^+ channels, leading to smooth muscle depolarisation and Ca^{2+} entry, thus inducing contraction. Hypoxia inhibits both voltage-gated and Ca^{2+}-activated K^+ channels, and induces depolarisation of pulmonary artery smooth muscle cells, but not renal nor mesenteric artery smooth muscle cells [4, 5, 56]. Hypoxia causes Ca^{2+} influx into pulmonary artery smooth muscle cells in adult rat and fetal lambs [4, 5, 56]. However, ATP-dependent K^+ channels have been shown to mediate secondary vasodilatation rather than the initial constriction to severe hypoxia [4]. The "energy-state" hypothesis suggests that HPV is initiated by decreased oxidative phosphorylation [4, 5, 57]. The cytochrome P_{450} hypothesis proposes that cytochrome P_{450} acts a sensor which initiates HPV [58]. The redox hypothesis states that oxygen tension regulates the production of reactive oxygen species or peroxide which control transmembrane Ca^{2+} flux and hence vascular tone through a direct action on sulfyldryl groups in the calcium channel protein of vascular smooth muscle [4, 5, 59]. All these hypotheses are still under exploration.

6.2. NO Modulates HPV

It has long been recognized that endothelium has an inhibitory role on HPV and hypoxic contractions [4, 5]. A role of endogenous NO in inhibiting

HPV was first suggested by Brashers et al. [60] who showed a marked potentiation of HPV by non-selective endothelium-derived relaxing factor (EDRF) inhibitors in the rat perfused pulmonary vascular bed. Subsequently, several groups have reported a marked augmentation of HPV by inhibiting the NO pathway, either by the use of selective NOS inhibitors [4, 5, 61, 62] or by use of guanylyl cyclase inhibitors [63]. The precursor of NO, L-arginine, has no effect on baseline pulmonary hemodynamics, but inhibits HPV [62, 64]. The effect of L-arginine on HPV is inhibited by methylene blue and potentiated by zaprinast, a type V phosphodiesterase inhibitor that inhibits cGMP degradation [64]. Moreover, exogenous NO and cGMP inhibit HPV (4, 5). Hypoxic contraction of pulmonary vessel rings *in vitro* is also potentiated by the removal of endothelium and by inhibition of NO using L-NMMA, haemoglobin, and methylene blue [4, 5, 65]. These results indicate that endogenous NO acts to attenuate HPV. Loss of this feedback mechanism would therefore potentiate hypoxia-induced contraction. The marked augmentation in HPV induced by NOS inhibitors in perfused pulmonary vascular beds can be explained through the inhibition of either basal or stimulated NO release, or both. This contention is not necessarily contradictory to the demonstration that hypoxia inhibits endothelial NOS (eNOS) expression and activity in cultured pulmonary artery endothelial cells [66], since the inhibition of eNOS activity requires several hours hypoxic incubation [66]. By contrast, HPV is a rapid on/off response. Alternatively, even though enzymatic activity is inhibited to some extent, it may still increase in response to stimuli. For example, hypoxia inhibits cyclooxygenase activity in rat pulmonary arteries *in vitro*, whereas *in vivo* hypoxia results in a marked increase in tissue PGI_2 production [4, 5]. During HPV, several factors, including endothelial shear stress resulting from changes in blood flow profile and endothelial deformation induced by smooth muscle contraction could stimulate NO release [19].

Whether acute hypoxia itself stimulates or inhibits NO production, and/ or NO activity still remains open to speculation. Earlier studies have provided conflicting results [4, 5]. Moderate ($PO_2 = 40$ mmHg) or severe ($PO_2 = 4-17$ mmHg) hypoxia inhibit endothelium-dependent relaxation to methacholine, ACh, ATP, and A23187 and the associated cGMP accumula tion in rabbit and rat extrapulmonary arteries and in small pulmonary artery rings of sheep [4, 5, 67, 68]. In porcine small pulmonary artery rings, hypoxia inhibits the relaxant response to ACh, reduces basal cGMP content, and augments the contractile response to phenylephrine, an effect abolished by endothelium removal [65]. By contrast, hypoxia does not inhibit endothelium-dependent relaxation to ACh and BK in isolated canine intrapulmonary arteries [69]. In the isolated extrapulmonary artery rings of rats, moderate hypoxia (48 mmHg) inhibits basal, but not ACh-, A23187- or SNP-induces tissue cGMP accumulation [70]. In cultured bovine pulmonary artery endothelial cells, moderate hypoxia (40 mmHg) increases basal, and potentiates BK-induced NO release, but severe hypoxia

(15 mmHg) inhibits BK-induced NO generation [4, 5, 71]. In isolated perfused bovine pulmonary artery and vein, both the activity and half-life of EDRF increase by reduction in oxygen tension in the perfusate [4, 5]. In isolated neonatal pig lung perfused with physiological salt solution, moderate hypoxia reduces both NO (the NO decomposition product) accumulation in perfusate and NO content in exhaled air, whereas in the isolated adult rat lung preparation, hypoxia (23 mmHg) reduces NO content in exhaled air, but has no effect on perfusate NO [72, 73]. Hypoxia can affect NO production and/or action at multiple steps; including NOS expression and activity, substrate and enzyme cofactor availability, NO half-life and signaling pathways, and the whole signal transduction cascade from receptor occupation to NO action in the case of agonist-induced NO-release. Consequently, more studies are required before firm conclusions can be drawn. Further, NOS activity and endothelial response may vary with species, maturity or the severity of hypoxia.

The effects of *chronic* hypoxia on NO production and/or activity are equally controversial. Both reduced and enhanced NO production and/or activity have been reported [4, 5]. Evidence supporting reduced NO production and/or activity include: a reduced or diminished endothelium-dependent relaxant responses to ACh, ATP or A-23187 observed in isolated pulmonary artery rings and perfused pulmonary vascular beds of rats with hypoxic pulmonary hypertension [4, 5], and in intrapulmonary artery rings from patients with chronic obstructive pulmonary disease [74]. Hypoxia reduces eNOS mRNA, protein and enzyme activity in bovine pulmonary artery endothelial cells [66]. Hypoxia inhibits pulmonary artery endothelial L-arginine uptake [75] and L-arginine synthesis from citrulline [76], and patients with pulmonary hypertension display reduced eNOS mRNA and protein expression in pulmonary vessels [77]. The pulmonary circulation undergoes rapid adaptational changes during the transitional period from fetal to neonatal life. Changing from a hypoxic to normoxic environment results in marked pulmonary vasodilatation [4, 5]. There is evidence that NO mediates this oxygen-dependent pulmonary vasodilatation [4, 5]. Moreover, eNOS gene and protein expression and activity are upregulated by increasing oxygen tension in fetal pulmonary artery endothelial cells [78]. This may represent another piece of evidence for hypoxic inhibition of eNOS expression and activity. There are also data suggesting increased NO production and activity after chronic exposure to hypoxia. Chronic hypoxia augments endothelium-dependent vasodilator responses to ACh, BK, SP, ET-1 or A-23187 in rat and calf pulmonary vascular beds [4, 5, 50, 51, 79, 80]. Chronic hypoxia also enhances the pulmonary vasoconstrictor response to L-NAME, suggesting an enhanced basal NO production [50, 51, 79]. Isolated lungs from rats with hypoxic pulmonary hypertension releases more NO [79]. Moreover, chronic hypoxia increases eNOS mRNA, protein expression and NOS activity in rat lung homogenates [81, 82]. Chronic hypoxia also increases inducible NOS expression both at mRNA and protein level [81]. Chronic hypoxia does not appear to change the smooth muscle sensitivity to NO nor for function of the smooth muscle contractile/relaxant machinery in perfused pulmonary vascular beds, the relaxant response to NO donors, sodium nitroprusside, 3-morpholinosydnonimine (SIN-1) or S-nitroso-N-acetylpenicillamine (SNAP) being unchanged by chronic hypoxia [4, 5, 80]. However, in extra-pulmonary arterial rings, chronic hypoxia diminishes the smooth muscle sensitivity to NO donors, probably through desensitization at guanylyl cyclase level [4, 5]. Again, this difference could be explained in several ways, and further research is needed to clarify this discrepancy.

7. Summary

Pulmonary vascular tone is under the regulation of adrenergic, cholinergic, and NANC vasodilator nerves and humoral mechanisms. Hypoxic pulmonary vasoconstriction also plays an important role in the active regulation of pulmonary vascular tone. Adrenergic nerves, HPV and vasoconstrictor humoral substances represent the vasoconstricting forces; whereas cholinergic, NANC mechanisms, vasodilator humoral substances, and basal and stimulated release of NO represent dilating forces. A balance between

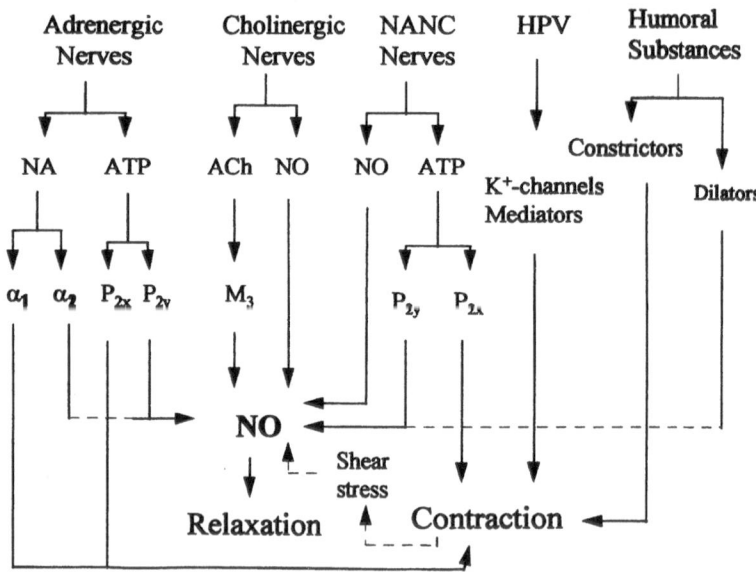

Figure 1. A schematic diagram summarizing the roles of nitric oxide in the regulation of pulmonary vascular tone. NA, noradrenaline; ATP, adenosine triphosphate; ACh, acetylcholine; α_1, α_1-adrenoceptor; α_2, α_2-adrenoceptor; P_{2x}, P_{2x}-purinoceptor; P_{2y}, P_{2y}-purinoceptor; M_3, M_3-muscarinic receptor.

these opposing forces influences normal resting pulmonary vascular tone. Disturbance of this balance may result in and/or contribute to the development of some disease such as pulmonary hypertension. NO plays an important role in regulating pulmonary vascular tone (Fig. 1). It inhibits adrenergic contraction, modulates hypoxic pulmonary vasoconstriction and counteracts the contractile response to many pulmonary vasoconstrictors. NO mediates the pulmonary vasodilator response to cholinergic stimulation and to a variety of vasodilator substances, and acts as an novel iNANC neurotransmitter.

8. References

1 Daly IDB, Hebb C (1986) Innervation of the lungs. In: Daly IDB, Hebb C (eds). Pulmonary and bronchial vascular systems. Baltimore: William & Wilkins, 89–117
2 McLean JR (1986) Pulmonary vascular innervation. In: Bergofsky EH (ed) Abnormal pulmonary circulation. London: Churchill Livingstone, 27–81
3 Hyman AL, Lippton Hl, Dempesy CW, Fontana CJ, Richardson D, Rieck R et al (1989) Autonomic control of the pulmonary circulation. In: Weir EK, Reeves JT (eds). Pulmonary vascular physiology and pathophysiology. New York: Marcel Dekker, 291–324
4 Barnes PJ, Liu SF (1995) Regulation of pulmonary vascular tone. *Pharmacol Rev* 47: 87–131
5 Liu SF, Barnes PJ (1994) Role of endothelium in the control of pulmonary vascular tone. *Endothelium* 2: 11–33
6 Kadowitz PJ, Hyman AL (1973) Effect of sympathetic nerve stimulation on pulmonary vascular resistance in the dogs. *Circ Res* 32: 221–227
7 Kadowitz PJ, Knight DS, Hibbs RG, Ellison JP, Joiner PD, Brody MJ et al (1976) Influence of 5- and 6-hydroxydopamine on adrenergic transmission and nerve terminal morphology in the canine pulmonary vascular bed. *Cir Res* 39: 191–199
8 Murray PA, Lodato RF, Michael JR (1986) Neural antagonists modulate pulmonary vascular pressure-flow plots in conscious dogs. *J Appl Physiol* 60: 1900–1907
9 Liu SF, Barnes PJ (1997) Neural control of pulmonary vascular tone. In: Crystal RG, West JB, Barnes PJ, Weibel ER (eds) The Lung, Scientific Foundations. Philadelphia: Lippincott-Raven Publisher, 1457–1472
10 Cocks TM, Angus JA (1983) Endothelium-dependent relaxation of coronary arteries by noradrenaline and serotonin. *Nature* 305: 627–630
11 Greenberg S, Diecke FPJ, Peevy K, Tanaka TP (1989) Endothelium modulates adrenergic neurotransmission to canine pulmonary arteries and veins. *Eur J Pharmacol* 162: 67–80
12 Cederqvist B, Gustafsson LE (1994) Modulation of neuroeffector transmission in guinea-pig pulmonary artery and vas deferens by endogenous nitric oxide. *Acta Physiol Scand* 150: 75–81
13 Schwarz P, Diem R, Dun NJ, Förstermann U (1995) Endogenous and exogenous nitric oxide inhibits norepinephrine release from rat heart sympathetic nerves. *Cir Res* 77: 841–848
14 Seilicovich A, Lasaga M, Befumo M, Duvilanski BH, del Carmen Diaz M et al (1995) Nitric oxide inhibits the release of norepinephrine and dopamine from the medial basal hypothalamus of the rat. *Proc Natl Acad Sci USA* 92: 11299–11302
15 Ceccatelli S, Lundberg JM, Zhang X, Åman K, Hökfelt T (1994) Immunohistochemical demonstration of nitric oxide synthase in the peripheral nervous system. *Brain Res* 656: 381–395
16 Fischer A, Hoffman B, Mayer B, Kummer W (1993) Nitric oxide synthase in the innervation of the human respiratory tract. *Am Rev Respir Dis* 147: A662
17 Liu SF, Crawley DE, Rohde JAL, Evans TW, Barnes PJ (1992) Role of nitric oxide and guanosine 3'-,5'-cyclic monophosphate in mediating nonadrenergic noncholinergic neural relaxation in guinea-pig pulmonary arteries. *Br J Pharmacol* 107: 861–866

18 Tesfamariam B, Cohen RA (1988) Inhibition of adrenergic vasoconstriction by endothelial cell shear stress. *Circ Res* 63: 720–725
19 Lamontagne D, Pohl U, Busse R (1992) Mechanical deformation of vessel wall and shear stress determine the basal release of endothelium-derived relaxing factor in the intact rabbit coronary vascular bed. *Circ Res* 70: 123–130
20 Minami N, Imai Y, Hashimoto J, Abe K (1995) The role of nitric oxide in the baroreceptor-cardiac reflex in conscious Wistar rats. *Am J Physiol* 269: H851–H855
21 Daly IDB, Hebb C (1952) Pulmonary vasomotor fibbers in the cervical vagosympathetic nerve of dog. *Q J Exp Physiol* 37: 19–43
22 Colebatch HJH, Halmagyi DFJ (1963) Effect of vagotomy and vagal stimulation on lung mechanics and circulation. *J Appl Physiol* 18: 871–878
23 Nandiwad PA, Hyman AL, Kadowitz PJ (1983) Pulmonary vasodilator responses to vagal stimulation and acetylcholine in the cat. *Circ Res* 53: 86–95
24 McMahon TJ, Hood JS, Kadowitz PJ (1992) Pulmonary vasodilator response to vagal stimulation is blocked by N-omega-nitro-L-arginine methyl ester in the cat. *Circ Res* 70: 364–369
25 Fritts J, Harris P, Clauss RH, Odell JE, Cournand A (1958) The effect of acetylcholine on the human pulmonary circulation under normal and hypoxic conditions. *J Clin Invest* 37: 99–110
26 Wilson PS, Khimenko PL, Barnard JW, Moore TM, Taylor AE (1995) Muscarinic agonists and antagonists cause vasodilation in isolated rat lung. *J Appl Physiol* 78: 1404–1411
27 Furchgott RF, Zawadzki JV (1980) The obligatory role of endothelial cells in the relaxation of arterial smooth muscle by acetylcholine. *Nature* 288: 373–376
28 McMahon TJ, Kadowitz PJ (1992) Methylene blue inhibits neurogenic cholinergic vaso-dilator responses in the pulmonary vascular bed of the cat. *Am J Physiol* 263: L575–L584
29 Hebeiß K, Kilbinger H (1996) Differential effects of nitric oxide donors on basal and electrically evoked release of acetylcholine from guinea-pig myenteric neurons. *Br J Pharmacol* 118: 2073–2076
30 Inoue T, Kannan MS (1988) Nonadrenergic and noncholinergic excitatory neurotransmission in rat intrapulmonary artery. *Am J Physiol* 254: H1142–H1148
31 Maggi CA, Patachini R, Perretti F, Tramontana M, Manzini S, Geppetti P et al (1990) Sensory nerves, vascular endothelium and neurogenic relaxation of the guinea-pig isolated pulmonary artery. *Naunyn-Schmied Arch Pharmacol* 342: 78–84
32 Scott JA, Craig I, McCormack DG (1996) Nonadrenergic noncholinergic relaxation of human pulmonary arteries is partially mediated by nitric oxide. *Am J Respir Crit Care Med* 154: 629–632
33 Marting CR (1987) Sensory nerves containing tachykinins and CGRP in the lower airways. Functional implications for bronchoconstriction, vasodilatation and protein extravasation. *Acta Physiol Scand* 563 (Suppl): 1–57
34 Dey RD, Shannon WA, Said JR (1981) Localization of VIP-immunoreactive nerves in airways and pulmonary vessels of dogs, cat, and human subjects. *Cell Tissue Res* 220: 231–238
35 Kubota E, Sata T, Soas AH, Paul S, Said SI (1985) Vasoactive intestinal peptide as a possible transmitter of nonadrenergic, noncholinergic relaxation of pulmonary artery. *Trans Assoc Am Physicians* 98: 233–242
36 Mohri K, Takeuchi K, Shinozuka K, Bjur RA, Westfall DP (1993) Simultaneous determination of nerve-induced adenine nucleotides and nucleosides released from rabbit pulmonary artery. *Anal Biochem* 210: 262–267
37 Rand MJ, Li CG (1995) Nitric oxide as a neurotransmitter in peripheral nerves: nature of transmitter and mechanism of transmission. *Annu Rev Physiol* 57: 659–682
38 Chakder S, Rattan S (1996) Evidence for VIP-induced increase in NO production in myenteric neurons of opossum internal and sphincter. *Am J Physiol* 270: G492–G497
39 Mashimo H, He XD, Huang PL, Fishman MC, Goyal RK (1996) Neuronal constitutive nitric oxide synthase is involved in murine enteric inhibitory neurotransmission. *J Clin Invest* 98: 8–13
40 Klimaschewki L, Kummer W, Mayer B, Couraud JY, Preissler U, Philippin B et al (1992) Nitric oxide synthase in cardiac nerve fibers and neurons of rat and guinea-pig heart. *Cir Res* 71: 1533–1537
41 Shimosegawa T, Toyota T (1994) NADPH-diaphorase activity as a marker for nitric oxide synthase in neurons of the guinea-pig respiratory tract. *Am J Respir Crit Care Med* 150: 1402–1410

42 Grider JR, Murthy KS, Kin J, Makhlouf GM (1992) Stimulation of nitric oxide from muscle cells by VIP: prejunctional enhancement of VIP release. *Am J Physiol* 262: 774–778

43 Abman SH, Chatfield BA, Hall SL, McMurtry IF (1990) Role of endothelium-derived relaxing factor during transition of pulmonary circulation at birth. *Am J Physiol* 259: H1921–H1927

44 Konduri GG, Gervasio CT, Theodorou AA (1993) Role of adenosine triphosphate and adenosine in oxygen-induced pulmonary vasodilatation in fetal lambs. *Pediatr Res* 33: 533–539

45 McMurtry I (1986) Humoral control. In: Bergosfky EH (ed) Abnormal Pulmonary Circulation. London: Churchill Livingstone, 83–125

46 Cooke JP, Rossitch EJr, Andon NA, Loscalzo J, Dzau VJ (1991) Flow activates an endothelial potassium channel to release an endogenous nitrovasodilator. *J Clin Invest* 88: 1663–1671

47 Arnal J-F, Warin L, Michel J-B (1992) Determinants of aortic guanosine monophosphate in hypertension induced by chronic inhibition of nitric oxide synthase. *J Clin Invest* 90: 647–652

48 Nishiwaki K, Nyhan DP, Rock P, Desai PM, Peterson WP, Pribble CG et al (1992) N omega-nitro-L-arginine and pulmonary vascular pressure-flow relationship in conscious dogs. *Am J Physiol* 262: H1331–H1337

49 Barnard JW, Wilson PS, Moore TM, Thompson JW, Taylor AE (1993) Effect of nitric oxide and cyclooxygenase products on vascular resistance in dog and rat lungs. *J Appl Physiol* 74: 2940–2949

50 Oka M, Hasunuma K, Webb SA, Stelzner TJ, Rodman DM, McMurtry IF (1993) EDRF suppresses an unidentified vasoconstritor mechanism in hypertensive rat lungs. *Am J Physiol* 264: L587–L597

51 Barer G, Emergy C, Stewart A, Bee D, Howard P (1993) Endothelial control of the pulmonary circulation in normal and chronic hypoxic rats. *J Physiol* 463: 1–16

52 Celermajer DS, Dollery C, Burch M, Deanfield JE (1994) Role of endothelium in the maintenance of low pulmonary vascular tone in normal children. *Circulation* 89: 2041–2044

53 Stamler JS, Loh E, Roddy M, Currie KE, Creager MA (1994) Nitric oxide regulates basal systemic and pulmonary vascular resistance in healthy humans. *Circulation* 89: 2035–2040

54 Von Euler US, Liljestrand G (1947) Observations on the pulmonary arterial pressure in the cat. *Acta Physiol Scand* 12: 301–320

55 Murray TR, Chen L, Marshall BE, Macarak EJ (1990) Hypoxic contraction of cultured pulmonary vascular smooth muscle cells. *Am J Respir Cell Mol Biol* 3: 457–465

56 Cornfield DN, Stevens T, McMurtry IF, Abman SH, Rodman DM (1994) Acute hypoxia causes membrane depolarization and calcium influx in fetal pulmonary artery smooth muscle cells. *Am J* 266: L469–L475

57 Rounds S, McMurtry IF (1981) Inhibitors of oxidative ATP production cause transient vasoconstriction and block subsequent pressor responses in rat lungs. *Circ Res* 48: 393–400

58 Miller MA, Hales CA (1979) Role of cytochrome P-450 in alveolar hypoxic pulmonary vasoconstriction in dogs. *J Clin Invest* 64: 666–673

59 Archer SL, Will JA, Weir EK (1986) Redox status in the control of pulmonary vascular tone. *Herz* 11: 127–141

60 Brashers VL, Peach MJ, Rose CEJ (1988) Augmentation of hypoxic pulmonary vasoconstriction in the isolated perfused rat lung by *in vitro* antagonists on endothelium-dependent relaxation. *J Clin Invest* 82: 1495–1502

61 Sprauge RS, Tjiemermann C, Vane JR (1992) Endogenous endothelium-derived relaxing factor opposes hypoxic pulmonary vasoconstriction and supports blood to hypoxic alveoli in anesthetized rabbits. *Proc Natl Acad Sci USA* 89: 8711–8715

62 Liu SF, Crawley DE, Barnes PJ, Evans TW (1991) Endothelium derived nitric oxide inhibits hypoxic pulmonary vasoconstriction in isolated blood perfused rat lungs. *Am Rev Respir Dis* 143: 32–37

63 Mazmanian GM, Baudet B, Brink C, Cerrina J, Kirkiachrian S, Weiss M (1989) Methylene blue potentiates vascular reactivity in isolated rat lungs. *J Appl Physiol* 66: 1040–1045

64 Fineman JR, Chang R, Soifer S (1991) L-arginine, a precursor of EDRF *in vitro*, produces pulmonary vasodilation in the lambs. *Am J Physiol* 261: H1563–H1569

65 Ogata M, Ohe M, Katayose D, Takishima T (1992) Modulatory role of EDRF in hypoxic contraction of isolated porcine pulmonary arteries. *Am J Physiol* 262: H691–H697

66 Liao JK, Zulueta JJ, Yu FS, Peng HB, Cote CG, Hassoun PM (1995) Regulation of bovine endothelial constitutive nitric oxide synthase by oxygen. *J Clin Invest* 96: 2661–2666

67 Johns RA, Linden JM, Reach MJ (1989) Endothelium-dependent relaxation and cyclic GMP accumulation in rabbit martery are selectively impaired by moderate hypoxia. *Cir Res* 65: 1508–1515

68 Rodman DM, Yamaguchi T, Hasunuma K, O'Brien RF, McMurtry IF (1990) Effects of hypoxia on endothelium-dependent relaxation of rat pulmonary artery. *Am J Physiol* 258: L207–L214

69 Chand N, Altura BM (1981) Acetylcholine and bradykinin relax intrapulmonary arteries by acting on endothelial cells: role in lung vascular diseases. *Science* 213: 1376–1379

70 Shaul PW, Wells LB, Horning KM (1993) Acute and prolonged hypoxia attenuate endothelial nitric oxide production in rat pulmonary arteries by different mechanisms. *J Cardiovasc Pharmacol* 22: 819–827

71 Hampl V, Cornfield DN, Cowan NJ, Archer SL (1995) Hypoxia potentiates nitric oxide synthesis and transiently increases cytosilic calcium levels in pulmonary artery endothelial cells. *Eur Respir J* 8: 515–522

72 Nelin LD, Thomas CJ, Dawson CA (1996) Effect of hypoxia on nitric oxide production in neonatal pig lung. *Am J Physiol* 271: H8–14

73 Grimminger F, Spriestersbach R, Weissmann N, Walmrath D, Seeger W (1995) Nitric oxide generation and hypoxic vasoconstriction in buffer-perfused rabbit lungs. *J Appl Physiol* 78: 1509–1515

74 Dinh-Xuan AT, Higenbottam TW, Clelland CA, Pepke-Zaba J, Cremona G, Butt AY et al (1991) Impairment of endothelium-dependent pulmonary artery relaxation in chronic obstructive lung disease. *N Engl J Med* 324: 1539–1547

75 Block ER, Herrera H, Couch M (1995) Hypoxia inhibits L-arginine uptake by pulmonary artery endothelial cells. *Am J Physiol* 269: L574–80

76 Su Y, Block ER (1995) Hypoxia inhibits L-arginine synthesis from L-citrulline in procine pulmonary artery endothelial cells. *Am J Physiol* 269: L581–7

77 Giaid A, Saleh D (1995) Reduced expression of endothelial nitric oxide synthase in the lungs of patients with pulmonary hypertension. *N Engl J Med* 333: 214–221

78 North AJ, Lau KS, Brannon TS, Wu LC, Wells LB, German Z, Shaul PW (1996) Oxygen upregulates nitric oxide synthase gene expression in ovine fetal pulmonary artery endothelial cells. *Am J Physiol* 270: L643–L649

79 Isaacson TC, Hampl V, Weir EK, Nelson DP, Archer SL (1994) Increased endothelium-derived NO in hypertensive pulmonary circulation of chronically hypoxic rats. *J Appl Physiol* 76: 933–940

80 Resta TC, Walker BR (1996) Chronic hypoxia selectively augments endothelium-dependent pulmonary arterial vasodilation. *Am J Physiol* 270: H888–H896

81 Xue C, Rengasamy A, Le Cras TD, Koberna PA, Dailey GC, Johns RA (1994) Distribution of NOS in normoxic vs. hypoxic rat lung: upregulation of NOS by chronic hypoxia. *Am J Physiol* 267: L667–78

82 Shaul PW, North AJ, Brannon TS, Ujiie K, Wells LB, Nisen PA, Lowenstein CJ, Snyder SH, Star RA (1995) Prolonged *in vivo* hypoxia enhances nitric oxide synthase type I and type III gene expression in adult rat lung. *Am J Respir Cell Mol Biol* 13: 167–174

Nitric Oxide in Pulmonary Processes:
Role in Physiology and Pathophysiology of Lung Disease
ed. by M. G. Belvisi and J. A. Mitchell
© 2000 Birkhäuser Verlag Basel/Switzerland

CHAPTER 6
Nitric Oxide and Bronchial Hyperresponsiveness

Frans P. Nijkamp and Gert Folkerts

Department of Pharmacology and Pathophysiology, Faculty of Pharmacy, Utrecht University, The Netherlands

1 Introduction
2 Nitric Oxide (NO) and Asthma
3 Airway Inflammation and Peroxynitrite Production
4 NO and Airway Hyperresponsiveness
5 NO and Virus-Induced Hyperresponsivenes
6 References

1. Introduction

Increasing evidence points to an important role for nitric oxide (NO) in the regulation of pulmonary functions and in pulmonary disease [1–4]. NO is present in exhaled air of animals and humans [1, 5]. The respiratory tract, nerves endothelial cells, vascular and airway smooth muscle cells, inflammatory cells (macrophages, neutrophils, mast cells) and the airway epithelium are sources for NO production [2]. The different effects of NO are mediated by the activation of soluble guanylyl cyclase, with as a consequence, an increase of cyclic guanosine monophosphate (cGMP) in the target cell.

NO synthases (NOSs) catalyse the conversion of L-arginine to L-citrulline and during this reaction NO is produced. NO is the product of the five-electron oxidation of one of the chemically equivalent guanidino nitrogens of L-arginine. NO can occur in biological systems in different forms, as NO^- (nitroxyl anion) or NO^+ (nitrosium) [4, 6]. In particular, the aqueous environment in the lung with an acidic pH can influence the type of NO metabolite produced [4, 6]. However, in most physiological systems NO has a short half-life (0.1–5 sec) [7, 8]. Different NOS isoforms have been isolated, cloned and sequenced [9–11]. Immunohistological studies have identified the presence of endothelial cell, neuronal and inducible NOS (eNOS, nNOS, iNOS) in human lung [12, 13]. Functionally, there are constitutive and inducible forms of NOS. The constitutive forms (eNOS and nNOS9 are normally expressed in endothelial and neuronal cells, but also in platelets, mast cells and neutrophils [2, 14]. These forms are calcium and calmodulin-dependent and produce picomoles of NO in response to cellular stimulation [15]. The inducible form of NOS is not dependent on intracellular calcium or calmodulin and requires a number of co-factors. The enzyme is regulated at the level of transcription and can be induced by certain cytokines, for example interferon-γ (IFN-γ), interleukin-1β (IL-1β) and tumor necrosis factor-α (TNF-α), and endotoxin lipopolysaccharides (LPSs) which probably act through the release of cytokines. The amounts of NO produced by the iNOS are much larger (nanomoles) than after activation of the constitutive enzymes. These high amounts of NO may contribute to the pathophysiological effects. Interestingly, glucocorticoids inhibit the induction of inducible, but not the activity of constitutive NOS. Furthermore, a number of cytokines, for example transforming growth factors [16], IL-4 [17] and IL-10 [18] have been shown to inhibit the expression of inducible NOS.

Research on the role of NO has been particularly facilitated by the discovery of analogues of L-arginine, which appeared to act as false substrates for the enzyme, thereby preventing the formation of endogenous NO. Examples of these analogues are N^G-monomethyl-L-arginine (L-NMMA), N^G-nitro-L-arginine (L-NA), N^G-nitro-L-arginine methylester (L-NAME) [19].

2. NO and Asthma

Expression of iNOS has been found in the epithelium of asthmatic patients but not in healthy subjects [12, 20]. Glucocorticoids inhibit the expression of iNOS [21, 22]. From animal studies it appeared that NO is produced in upper and lower airways [24]. Alving et al. (1993) [25] compared the production of NO in exhaled air between breathing through the nose or the mouth. They suggested that in normal human airways the production of NO is restricted to the nasal mucosa. However, in mild asthmatics, the level of exhaled NO during oral breathing increased 2–3 fold, indicating the involvement of the lower airways [25]. These data may point to the involvement of macrophages, which produce high amounts of NO [26]. These cells are found in much higher number in the bronchial, compared to the nasal airways [27]. NO can have proinflammatory effects. In particular, the high amounts of NO formed by the iNOS in asthmatic patients may be deleterious. The increased release of NO from epithelial cells could increase airway blood flow and cause hyperaemia and further airway oedema by plasma exudation. The level of exhaled NO is elevated in patients with asthma who are not receiving glucocorticoid therapy [25, 28, 29]. Glucocorticoids reduce exhaled NO levels in asthmatic patients [28, 30], suggesting that the increase in exhaled NO reflects iNOS activity. Kharitonov et al. [31] showed an increase in exhaled NO during the late asthmatic reaction after allergen challenge. This increase was absent during the early bronchoconstrictor response, suggesting that iNOS had been induced after allergen challenge. The cellular source of iNOS is not clear. Structural cells, such as epithelial cells, smooth muscle cells and endothelial cells [32–34] or alternatively, macrophages, mast cells, neutrophils and other inflammatory cells may contribute [34].

Inhibition of endogenous NO production reduces plasma exudation in the airways, possibly by inhibition of its potent vasodilator activity. Also, neurogenic airway oedema can be prevented by inhibitors of NOS [35]. Interestingly, in ovalbumin sensitised guinea-pigs insufflation pressure and NO in exhaled air immediately increased in a dose-dependent manner, in response to challenge with nebulised allergen [5]. An immediate increase in NO levels paralleled the degree of bronchoconstriction. NO acts as a feedback against bronchoconstriction since inhibition of endogenous NO production leads to a substandial potentiation of the allergen-induced bronchoconstriction [23, 36].

3. Airway Inflammation and Peroxynitrite Production

It has now been generally accepted that asthma is an inflammatory disease [37, 38]. The number of inflammatory cells is increased in the broncho-alveolar lavage (BAL) fluid of asthmatic patients. One of the major products that can be released by inflammatory cells is superoxide anion. Calhoun et al. [39] measured the superoxide production by bronchoalveolar cells obtained 12 min and 48 h after segmental antigen challenge. It was demonstrated that the superoxide anion production was significantly enhanced after the early and late phase. In addition to these *in vitro* observations superoxide production *in vivo* during asthma might also be increased [40, 41]. Therefore, during asthmatic reactions the pro inflammatory mediators NO and superoxide are likely to be formed. In inflamed tissue NO can react very quickly with superoxide anions, leading to the formation of peroxynitrite [42].

$$NO^{\cdot} + O_2^{\cdot -} \rightarrow OONO^- \tag{1}$$

The rate constant for the reaction of $NO^{\cdot}$ with $O_2^{\cdot -}$ is 6.7×10^9 l/mol/s which is close to the rate constant for diffusion of NO [43]. Peroxynitrite is a potent and relatively long lived oxidant with a half-live ≤ 1 sec at pH 7.4 [44].

$$ONOO^- + H^+ \leftrightarrow ONOOH \tag{2}$$

Since peroxynitrite is a highly reactive anion, it reacts and oxidises many cellular components such as lipids and proteins, thereby disturbing their function, and thus cellular homeostasis [42]. Peroxynitrite oxidises membrane lipids [45], tissue sulfhydryls [46] and is believed to damage membrane sodium channels in colon [47] and lung [48] and calcium channels in the myocardium [49]. Peroxynitrite is a potent oxidant that has bactericidal activity [50].

Are there reasons to assume that peroxynitrite is formed under (patho)-physiological conditions? NO is a hydrophobic gas, it will accumulate in higher concentrations within the hydrophobic core of the membrane near the site of superoxide formation. McCall et al. [51] demonstrated in a bioassay that stimulated rat peritoneal neutrophils release the platelet in-hibitory factor, NO. As the degree of stimulation increased, the inhibitory action was progressively inhibited by concomitant release of superoxide anions, pointing to an interaction between NO and superoxide. Moreover, it has been reported that peroxynitrite is formed by macrophage-derived NO [52]. The peroxynitrite production was as high as 0.11 nmol/10^6 cells/min. Rat lung contains approximately 10^7 macrophages (lining fluid = 1 µl), the average rate of peroxynitrite formation would be 1 µM/min within the whole lung and 1 mM/min in the epithelial lining fluid. Furthermore, immediate peroxynitrite production was detectable by luminol-enhanced chemiluminescence from cultured bovine aortic endothelial cells exposed to bradykinin or the calcium ionophore A23187 [53].

Overproduction or uncontrolled formation of peroxynitrite, is an impor-tant factor in the tissue damaging mechanisms during pathological situa-tions such as chronic inflammation. There are several reports suggesting the formation of peroxynitrite during the inflammatory process. The nitra-tion of tyrosine residues in proteins by peroxynitrite to 3-nitrotyrosine is an indication of the presence of peroxynitrite [42]. Immunoreactivity to nitrotyrosine residues and iNOS are colocalised in guinea-pig ileitis, suggesting that peroxynitrite is formed following iNOS induction [54]. Moreover, an increased immunofluorescence to nitrotyrosine residues was detected at the sites of inflammation in acute lung injury in rats and humans [55, 56], acute endotoxemia in rats [57], influenza-induced pneumonia in mice [58] and in rheumatoid patients [59]. Inhalation of silica produces a dramatic inflammatory and toxic response within the lungs of humans and laboratory animals. Interestingly, 24 h after silica inhalation, lung tissue and BAL cells from the rat produce significantly more peroxynitrite than controls [60]. The luminol-dependent chemiluminescence was markedly decreased by either superoxide dismutase or the NOS inhibitor (L-NAME). When the animals were pretreated with the steroid dexamethasone, there was a complete protection against the biochemical, cellular, and chemilu-minescence indices of damage caused by silica. The above mentioned data provided evidence that peroxynitrite can be formed by a number of cells in the lung after receptor or non-receptor stimulation. Peroxynitrite, unlike its precursor NO, is probably not an intercellular messenger molecule because of its limited stability and diffusion range, but from the presently available evidence one cannot exclude the possibility that peroxynitrite serves as an intra- or pericellular messenger [42]. Since the rate of peroxynitrite formation depends upon the production of superoxide and NO, it will increase 100-fold for every 10-fold increase in superoxide and NO. Thus relatively small increases in the rats of superoxide and NO production may greatly increase rates of peroxynitrite formation to potentially cyto-toxic levels.

At different levels in this cascade there are opportunities for therapeutic intervention. Steroids or aminoguanidine, drugs which inhibit the expression/activity of iNOS, can be used to prevent NO production. The production of superoxide can be inhibited by apocynin or the inactivation of superoxide may be enhanced by superoxide dismutase. This will lead finally to a diminished peroxynitrite production. Further, there are a number of drugs that can scavenge peroxynitrite e.g. urate, cysteine and penicillamine.

It has also been reported that exogenously administered peroxynitrite mimics some inflammatory conditions. Indeed, intrarectally administered peroxynitrite in the rat induces transmucosal necrosis, acute inflammation, and exudative oedema 24 h later [61]. Resolution of oedema, mucin repletion, thickening of the muscularis mucosa and propria, and fibrosis were observed at 3 weeks. In guinea-pigs, peroxynitrite caused airway epithelial damage and hyperresponsiveness *in vitro* and *in vivo* [62]. Sadeghi-Hashjin et al. [62] showed that incubation of peroxynitrite on the mucosal side of the guinea-pig trachea caused a significant hyperresponsiveness, the maximal contractions in response to histamine and methacholine were enhanced 30% and 40% respectively. In the peroxynitrite-treated group, clear epithelial damage as well as eosinophil destruction were detected. Moreover, 3, 5, and 10 days after intratracheal instillation of peroxynitrite (100 nmol), a significant rise in airway resistance to histamine of anesthetised animals was observed. It is suggested that the generation of peroxynitrite from NO and superoxide radicals during inflammatory processes induces epithelial damage, mediator release, and hence airway hyperresponsiveness.

4. NO and Airway Hyperresponsiveness

Evidence points to an important role for the airway epithelium in modulating the responsiveness of the underlying smooth muscle. Hyperresponsiveness of the airways, which is a feature of asthma, is associated with damage or loss of the airway epithelium in bronchial asthma [37, 63]. Removal of the epithelial layer from isolated airways of several mammalian species enhanced the contractile response to various bronchoconstrictor agents, including histamine, acetylcholine, 5-hydroxytryptamine and leukotrienes C_4 and D_4 [64, 65]. In addition, arachidonic acid induces a relaxation in intact tracheae and a contraction in epithelium-denuded tissues [66]. These findings led to the concept that intact epithelium may act as a protective barrier between constrictors and airway smooth muscle [67–69] or it may modulate the airway tone through the release of relaxant bustances, which may include prostanoids and epithelium-derived relaxing factor(s). Major differences in contractile responses or perfusion pressures to agents applied from the serosal and the luminal side of intact guinea-pig trachea have been detected [67, 69, 70]. The sensitivity was much less on the inside than on the outside and this difference disappeared when the epithelium was removed. It has been proposed that the epithelial layer produces an "epithelial derived relaxing factor", which is similar to EDRF [65, 68]. Whether this EDRF is similar to NO and whether any other relaxing substances are involved is as yet not certain. Gao and Vanhoutte [71] demonstrated an inhibitory role for an endogenous NO-like substance during contractions of canine bronchi evoked by acetylcholine. However the epithelial layer did not seem to play a major role in this effect. A cultured human epithelial cell line produces nitrite spontaneously, which can be suppressed by an NO synthesis inhibitor and restored by L-arginine, suggesting the constitutive production of NO [72]. cNOS and iNOS are present in rat and human epithelial cells [12, 20, 73]. A number of contractile agents, including histamine, stimulate cNOS [2]. Immunoreactivity for NOS has been demonstrated in epithelium of both large and small airways [73, 74]. Rengasamy et al. [75] showed NOS immunoreactivity within rat respiratory epithelium but not in the bronchial smooth muscle. In contrast, guanylyl cyclase activity was shown in respiratory smooth muscle but not in the epithelium pointing to a paracrine role of NO in bronchial function. Robbins et al. [76] clearly substantiated the role of iNOS in a murine epithelial cell line. Stimulation with a mixture of cytokines (IL-1β, TNF-α and IFN-γ), elevated nitrite levels by 873%, increased iNOS activity and the expression of iNOS mRNA. Dexamethasone decreased these cytokine induced increases. Also in primary cultured human airway epithelial cells the same mixture of cytokines increased iNOS expression [76]. Human type II alveolar epithelial cells also express iNOS after exposure to LPS [12] or cytokines [77]. Cytokines released by mononuclear cells can therefore stimulate airway epithelial cells to express iNOS and to release NO. On the other hand, Guo et al. [78] demonstrated that NO synthesis in normal human airways is due to a continuous expression of the iNOS in airway epithelial cells.

We have provided pharmacological evidence that one of the epithelium-derived relaxing factors might be NO [79]. In a perfused tracheal tube set up according to Pavlovic et al. [70], in which selectively the serosal (out)side or the mucosal (in)side of the trachea can be stimulated with drugs, it was demonstrated that luminal perfusion of guinea-pig tracheal tubes *in vitro* with NO synthesis inhibitors shifted the maximum effect of the histamine concentration-response curve upwards by 335%. This effect was mimicked by removal of airway epithelium, suggesting that the airway epithelial layer releases NO which counteracts the bronchoconstrictor effect of spasmogens [79]. Furthermore the effect of L-NAME was concentration-dependently inhibited by co-incubation with L-arginine. In accordance with the findings of Fedan et al. [80] and Sparrow and Mitchell [69], the intact preparations did not reach a clear plateau after a complete histamine concentration-response curve (up to 10^{-3} M). This is comparable with the observations in healthy humans in which a decrease in the forced expiratory volume in one second (FEV$_1$) greater than 20% is not obtained, even when very high concentrations of histamine are nebulised. In further experiments we investigated whether these effects were species specific. When 4th and 5th generation airways of the horse were incubated with L-NAME, the maximal contraction in response to histamine was increased by 250%. Similar findings have been observed in human bronchi [81]. This means that the effect with the NO synthesis inhibitors is not species specific.

Interestingly the hyperresponsiveness after NOS inhibition is mediated by leukotrienes [82]. Preincubation of isolated trachea with a 5-lipoxygenase inhibitor (AA-861) or a leukotriene C$_4$, D$_4$, E$_4$ receptor antagonist (FPL 55712) totally blocked the L-NAME induced tracheal hyperresponsiveness. These data are in line with the findings of Adcock and Garland [83] who demonstrated that guinea-pig tracheal hyperresponsiveness to histamine after cyclooxygenase inhibition was attributable to an augmenting effect of lipoxygenase products. Now, abundant evidence has been obtained that leukotrienes are involved in airway hyperresponsiveness [84]. Recently, it became clear that NO can stimulate cyclooxygenase, an enzyme responsible for the synthesis of prostaglandins. Indeed, in previous studies we demonstrated that the histamine-induced contractions of the guinea-pig trachea were associated with the release of both prostaglandin E$_2$ and NO [64, 85]. Also, enhanced tracheal contractions in animal models of airway hyperresponsiveness coincide with a decreased prostaglandin E$_2$ and NO production [64, 85]. The L-NAME induced airway hyperresponsiveness was associated with a decrease in prostaglandin E$_2$ production [82]. Therefore, inhibition of NO synthesis decreases cyclooxygenase activity and, maybe as a consequence, increases lipoxygenase activity. Alternatively, NO may have a tonic inhibition on the lipoxygenase pathway. The effects of inhibitors of NOS can also be observed *in vivo*. The administration by aerosol of NO synthesis inhibitors to spontaneously breathing anesthetised guinea-pigs resulted in a significant enhancement of lung resistance after increasing intravenous doses of histamine [126–282%) [79]. Differences in endogenous NO production also contributes to strain-related differences in airway responsiveness in rats [86]. The Fischer strain is hyperresponsive to inhaled agonists in comparison to other strains such as the Lewis rat. Jia et al. [86] further showed that inhibition of NOS induced airway hyperresponsiveness to cholinergic receptor stimulation *in vivo* and *in vitro* in Lewis rats, but had almost no effect in Fischer rats. The effect of the NOS inhibitor was abolished by removal of the epithelium. Carbachol induced a NO dependent increase in cGMP levels in tracheal tissue but to a lesser extent in Fischer than in Lewis rats. Jia et al. [86] thus demonstrated the involvement of an endogenous NO-cGMP pathway in the regulation of airway responsiveness in Lewis rats.

The role of cGMP in airway responsiveness was further substantiated by Sadeghi-Hashjin et al. [87]. We demonstrated that drugs that prevented the increase of cGMP after histamine stimulation of perfused isolated guinea-pig trachea, such as cystamine and methylene blue (guanylyl cyclase inhibitors) or pyrogallol (a generator of superoxide that may inactivate NO) increased the contractile response to histamine. A functional role for endogenous NO in the modulation of airway contractile responses has further been suggested by a number of different research groups [23, 88]. Interestingly, endogenous NO also has an inhibitory effect on bronchial obstruction in a model of antigen-induced bronchoconstriction [23, 36]. The increased NO release during allergen challenge was likely to be due to actions of histamine and leukotrienes since the increase in exhaled NO concentration was abolished by histamine and leukotriene receptor antagonists [23]. Inhalation of NOS inhibitors in asthmatic patients does not increase airway obstruction or increase the bronchoconstrictor responses to histamine [30]. However in asthmatic patients the level of exhaled NO is markedly elevated probably by enhanced iNOS activity [25, 28, 29]. Large amounts of NO downregulate cNOS [89–91], which may explain the absence of effect of NOS inhibitors in human. In the lung vasculature, NO has been implicated in the modulation of the pulmonary circulation [92] and in the vasoconstriction which follows hypoxia [93]. It is unlikely that the pulmonary vasculature contributes to the airway hyperresponsiveness since the effects observed *in vivo* were confirmed *in vitro* using a perfused tracheal tube in which the role of the vasculature can be excluded.

Besides NO, the epithelium probably releases other factors that modify the level of intracellular cGMP. Hay and colleagues demonstrated in a coaxial bioassay system, that the guinea-pig tracheal epithelium releases a factor that can relax the rat aorta and increase the level of cGMP. However, both phenomena were not inhibited by methylene blue [94]. A comparable observation was found in the perfused guinea-pig trachea. The osmotic-induced release of an epithelium-derived relaxing factor by mannitol was suppressed by haemoglobin and methylene blue, but not by L-NMMA [68]. Thus, other (NO-related-)products that can modify cGMP levels in smooth muscle are released by the epithelial layer. A diminished production of epithelium-derived relaxing factors caused by destruction of the epithelial layer may contribute to the increased airway responses in asthmatic patients. In addition, we demonstrated that histamine stimulates NO synthesis [85] and the release of histamine has been implicated in the bronchoconstriction after exercise, viral infections [95] and allergen exposure [96]. In asthmatic patients with an enhanced bronchial responsiveness, an increased spontaneous histamine release by bronchoalveolar mast cells is found. Moreover, the concentration of histamine in bronchoalveolar lavage fluid in asthmatics is related to the level of airway responsiveness [37]. The histamine-induced increase in cGMP production in the cardiovascular [97] and respiratory system [98] has been shown to be an L-arginine dependent process. It is tempting to speculate that the epithelial layer by releasing NO, acts as a negative feedback system to histamine-induced contractions and that the combination of increased histamine levels and epithelial damage induces airway hyperresponsiveness in asthamtic patients. A number of substances have been shown to induce tracheal relaxation after intraluminal perfusion in precontracted tissues, e.g. endothelin [99] and bradykinin [100, 101]. These relaxations are inhibited or reversed into contractions by inhibitors of NO synthesis, indicating that the relaxations are mediated by the release of NO.

In standard organ bath experiments potassium induces an initial contraction followed by a relaxation and a sustained contraction of intact tracheae [102]. We showed [103] that potassium induces a monophasic contraction when it was added on the serosal side. In contrast, potassium induced a relaxation when added on the inside. From these results it may be concluded that depolarisation of smooth muscle cells leads to a contraction, whereas depolarisation of epithelial cells results in a relaxation of tracheal tubes. This effect is mediated by NO since L-NAME prevents the relaxation. Epithelium removal caused a reversal of the relaxation into a potent contractile response. Addition of potassium on the inside of intact trachea does not stimulate the smooth muscle cells because incubation with L-NAME on the inside only prevented the relaxation. The relaxation did not reverse into a contraction as seen in epithelium-denuded tissues. From the present results it is likely that the epithelial layer acts as a firm barrier, since even a relative simple molecule as potassium is not able to penetrate through the epithelial layer [103].

5. NO and Virus-Induced Hyperresponsiveness

Epidemiological studies have demonstrated a close temporal association between respiratory viral infections and exacerbations of asthma [104–107]. In addition, in otherwise healthy people, respiratory infections induce airway hyperresponsiveness. Viruses have been identified in up to 50% of wheezing illnesses and asthma exacerbations occurring in childhood and in up to 20% of those in adults. Moreover, viral infections have been shown to develop into late asthmatic reactions [108]. Epithelial damage, airway inflammation and an enhanced release of reactive oxygen species by inflammatory cells are observed both during viral respiratory infections and asthma [37–39, 63]. We showed that intra-tracheal inoculation of parainfluenza type 3 virus to guinea-pigs induces a marked increase in airway responsiveness to histamine *in vivo* and *in vitro* [109–112]. After inhalation of low doses of L-arginine this hyperresponsiveness is completely blocked [85]. Moreover, the histamine-induced release of NO from virus-inoculated tracheal tubes was diminished by 75%. Therefore, it is likely that the deficiency in endogenous NO after a viral infection is due to a dysfunction of cNOS. Interestingly, Saiboku-to, a traditional Chinese herbal medicine that has been widely used in the treatment of asthma in Asian countries stimulates epithelial NO generation [113].

There are at least three possible mechanisms which may account for the NO deficiency in virally infected airways. Firstly, the decreased NO production can be explained by substrate limitation, e.g. a decreased concentration of L-arginine in virus-treated animals. However, intracellular levels of arginine are already high and the supply of arginine is normally not rate-limiting for the constitutive enzyme [114]. On the other hand, it cannot be excluded that the activity of arginase, the enzyme that breaks down arginine, is increased. Arginase is widely distributed in the body including the lungs [115] and is elevated during growth of tissues and tumors [116]. Whether, the arginase activity is increased in the lungs during viral respiratory infections needs to be investigated.

Secondly, the epithelial layer is damaged in virus-infected animals [109, 117]. Therefore, a likely explanation for the lack of NO in virus-treated animals, is a diminished activity or availability of the cNOS which might be due to epithelial damage. In biopsies of human airways, immunoreactivity to iNOS was seen in the epithelium in 22 of 23 asthmatic cases, but only 2 of 14 non-asthmatic controls [118]. Although, in normal subjects during symptomatic upper respiratory tract infections the concentration of NO in exhaled air is markedly increased [119], it cannot be excluded that the NO released by the activity of the constitutive enzyme is diminished during bronchoconstriction. Although eNOS has been described as constitutive, its expression can be regulated. MacNaul and Hutchinson [120] demonstrated that concurrent treatment of human aortic endothelial cells with IL-1β, TNF-α, IFN-γ, and LPS decreased the eNOS mRNA level [121–124] and eNOS protein [121]. In bovine cultured coronary venular endothelial cells LPS alone already causes down regulation of eNOS [91]. Interestingly, during viral infections IFN-γ is produced. This might stimulate iNOS and the high amount of NO could subsequently inactivate cNOS [89–91].

A third mechanism by which the concentration of NO can be decreased is the following. NO is inactivated by products released from inflammatory cells, i.e. superoxide anions [2, 125]. Parainfluenza type 3 virus activates inflammatory cells [40, 117] and the number of inflammatory cells is increased in lungs of virus-infected guinea-pigs [40, 110]. Naive guinea-pig tracheas incubated with inflammatory cells obtained from lungs of virus-treated animals become hyperresponsive to histamine [126]. Besides decreasing the NO concentration, the reactive peroxynitrite (ONOO$^-$) is produced by the interaction of superoxide anions with NO [2, 127], which accordingly may lead to "additional" epithelial damage. Interestingly, Akaike et al. [58] recently demonstrated a role for peroxynitrite in the pathogenesis of influenza virus-induced pneumonia in mice. They showed by means of an immunohistochemical study formation of peroxynitrite by inflammatory cells, including macrophages and neutrophils, and of intra-alveolar exudate. There results suggest formation of peroxynitrite in the lung through the reaction of NO with superoxide, which is generated by alveolar phagocytic cells and xanthine oxidase. Moreover, isolated guinea-pig epithelial cells themselves can release reactive oxygen species [128]. Therefore, a number of processes may act additively or synergistically during the development of virus-induced airway hyperresponsiveness.

6. References

1 Gustafsson LE, Leone AM, Persson MG, Wiklund NP, Moncada S (1991) Endogenous nitric oxide is present in the exhaled air of rabbits, guinea-pigs and humans. *Biochem Biophys Res Commun* 181: 852–857
2 Barnes PJ, Belvisi MG (1993) Nitric oxide and lung disease. *Thorax* 48: 1034–1043
3 Jorens PG, Vermeire PA, Herman AG (1993) L-arginine-dependent nitric oxide synthase: a new metabolic pathway in the lung and airways. *Eur Respir J* 6: 258–266
4 Gaston B, Drazen JM, Loscalzo J, Stamler JS (1994) The biology of nitric oxides in the airways. *Am J Respir Crit Care Med* 149: 538–551
5 Persson MG, Gustafsson LE (1993) Allergen-induced airway obstruction in guinea-pigs is associated with changes in nitric oxide levels in exhaled air. *Acta Physiol Scand* 149: 461–466
6 Stamler JS, Singel DJ, Loscalzo J (1992) Biochemistry of nitric oxide and its redox-activated forms. *Science* 258: 1898–1902
7 Palmer RMJ, Ferrige AG, Moncade S (1987) Nitric oxide release accounts for the biological activity of endothelium-derived relaxing factor. *Nature* 327: 524–526
8 Kelm M, Schrader J (1990) Control of coronary vascular tone by nitric oxide. *Circ Res* 66: 1561–1575
9 Bredt DS, Hwang PM, Glatt CE, Lowenstein C, Reed RR, Snyder SH (1991) Cloned and expressed nitric oxide synthase structurally resembles cytochrome P-450 reductase. *Nature* 351: 714–718
10 Janssens SP, Shimouchi A, Qertermous T, Bloch DB, Bloch KD (1992) Cloning and expression of cDNA encoding human endothelium-derived relaxing factor/nitric oxide synthase. *J Biol Chem* 267: 14519–14522
11 Lyons CR, Orloff GJ, Gunningham JM (1992) Molecular cloning and functional expression of an inducible nitric oxide synthase from a murine macrophage cell line. *J Biol Chem* 267: 6370–6374
12 Kobzik L, Bredt DS, Lowenstein CJ, Drazen J, Gaston B, Sugarbaker D et al (1993) Nitric oxide synthase in human and rat lung: Immunocytochemical and histochemical localization. *Am J Respir Cell Mol Biol* 9: 371–377
13 Tracey WR, Xue C, Klinghoffer V, Barlow J, pollock JS, Forstermann U et al (1994) Immunocytochemical detection of inducible NO synthase in human lung. *Am J Physiol* 266: 722–727
14 Nathan C (1992) Nitric oxide as a secretory product of mammalian cells. *FASEB* 6: 3051–3064
15 Moncada S (1992) L-arginine: nitric oxide pathway. *Acta Physiol Scand* 145: 201–227
16 Ding A, Nathan CF, Graycar J, Derynck R, Stuehr DJ, Srimal S (1990) Macrophage deactivating factor and transforming growth factors-β1, β2 and β3 inhibit induction of macrophage nitrogen oxide synthesis by IFN-γ. *J Immunol* 145: 940–944
17 Liew FY, Li Y, Severn A, Millott S, Schmidt J, Salter M et al (1991) A possible novel pathway of regulation by murine T helper type-2 (Th$_2$) cells of a Th$_1$ cell activity via the modulation of the induction of nitric oxide synthase on macrophages. *Eur J Immunol* 21: 2489–2494
18 Cunha FQ, Moncada S, Liew FY (1992) Interleukin-10 (IL-10) inhibits the induction of nitric oxide synthase by interferon-γ in murine macrophages. *Biochem Biophys Res Commun* 186: 1155–1159
19 Rees DD, Cellek S, Palmer RMJ, Moncada S (1990) Dexamethasone prevents the induction by endotoxin of a nitric oxide synthase and the associated effects on vascular tone: an insight into endotoxin shock. *Biochem Biophys Res Commun* 173: 541–547

20 Hamid Q, Springall DR, Riveros-Moreno V, Chanez P, Howarth P, Redington A et al (1993) Induction of nitric oxide synthase in asthma. *Lancet* 342: 1510–1513
21 Radomski MW, Palmer RMJ, Moncada S (1990) An L-arginine/nitric oxide pathway present in human platelets regulates aggregation. *Proc Natl Acad Sci* 87: 5193–5197
22 Liu SF, Adcock IM, Old RW, Barnes PJ, Evans T (1993) lipopolysaccharide treatment *in vivo* induces widespread expression of inducible oxide synthase mRNA. *Biochem Biophys Res Commun* 196: 1208–1213
23 Persson MG, Friberg SG, Gustafsson LE, Hudqvist P (1995) The promotion of patent airways and inhibition of antigen induced bronchial obstruction by endogenous nitric oxide. *Brit J Pharmacol* 116: 2957–2962
24 Persson MG, Midtvedt T, Leone AM, Gustafsson LE (1994) Ca^{2+}-dependent and Ca^{2+}-independent exhaled nitric oxide; presence in germ-free animals and inhibition by arginine analogues. *Eur J Pharmacol* 264: 13–20
25 Alving K, Weitzberg E, Lundberg JM (1993) Increased amount of nitric oxide in exhaled air of asthmatics. *Eur Respir J* 6: 1368–1370
26 Juliusson S, Bachert C, Klementsson H (1991) Macrophages on the nasal mucosal surface in provoked and naturally ocurring allergic rhinitis. *Acta Otolaryngol* 111: 946–953
27 Marletta MA, Yoon PS, Iyengar R, Leaf CD, Wishnok JS (1988) Macrophage oxidation of L-arginine to nitrite and nitrate: nitric oxide is an intermediate. *Biochemistry* 27: 8706–8711
28 Kharitonov SA, Yates D, Robbins RA, Logan-Sinclair R, Shinebourne EA, Barnes PJ (1994) Increased nitric oxide in exhaled air of asthmatic patients. *Lancet* 343: 133–135
29 Persson MG, Zetterstrom O, Argenius V, Ihre E, Gustafsson LE (1994) Single-breath oxide measurements in asthmatic patients and smokers. *Lancet* 343: 146–147
30 Yates DH, Kharitonov SA, Robbins RA, Thomas PS, Barnes PJ (1995) Effect of nitric oxide synthase inhibitor and a glucocorticosteroid on exhaled nitric oxide. *Am J Respir Crit Care Med* 152: 892–896
31 Kharitonov SA, O'Connor BJ, Evans DJ, Barnes PJ (1995) Allergen-induced late asthmatic reactions are associated with elevation of exhaled nitric oxide. *Am J Respir Crit Care Med* 151: 1894–1995
32 Geng Y, Hansson GK, Holme E (1992) Interferon-β and tumor necrosis factor synergize to induce nitric oxide production and inhibit mitochondrial respiration in vascular smooth muscle. *Cir Res* 71: 1268–1276
33 Hansson GK, Geng YJ, Holm J, Hardhammar P, Wennalm A, Jennische E (1994) Arterial smooth muscle cells express nitric oxide synthase in response to endothelial injury. *J Exp Med* 180: 733–738
34 Moncada S, Higgs A (1993) The L-arginine-nitric oxide pathway. *N Engl J Med* 329: 2002–2012
35 Kuo H-P, Liu S, Barnes PJ (1992) The effect of endogenous nitric oxide on neurogenic plasma exudation in guinea-pig airways. *Eur J Pharmacol* 221: 385–388
36 Persson MG, Friberg SG, Hedqvist P, Gustafsson LE (1993) Endogenous nitric oxide counteracts antigen-induced bronchoconstriction. *Eur J Pharmacol* 249: R7
37 Djukanovic R, Roche WR, Wilson JW, Beasley CRW, Twentyman OP, Howarth PH et al (1990) Mucosal inflammation in asthma. *Am Rev Resp Dis* 142: 434–457
38 Folkerts G, Nijkamp FP (1993) Cells and mediators involved in airway hyperresponsiveness. In: Tarayre JP, Vergaftig B, Carilla E (eds). New concepts in asthma. London: Macmillan 224–244
39 Calhoun WJ, Reed HE, Moest DR, Stevens CA (1992) Enhanced superoxide production by alveolar macrophages and air-space cells, airway inflammation, and alveolar macrophage density changes after segmental antigen bronchoprovocation in allergic subjects. *Am Rev Resp Dis* 145: 317–325
40 Folkerts G, Esch B van, Janssen M, Nijkamp FP (1992) Virus-induced airway hyperresponsiveness in guinea-pigs *in vivo*: study of broncho-alveolar cell number and activity. *Eur J Pharmacol* 228: 219–227
41 Henricks PAJ, Van Esch B, Engels F, Nijkamp FP (1993) Effects of parainfluenza type 3 virus on guinea-pig pulmonary alveolar macrophage functions *in vitro*. *Inflammation* 17: 663–675
42 Muijsers RBR, Folkerts G, Henricks PAJ, Sadeghi-Hashjin G, Nijkamp FP (1997) Peroxynitrite: a two faced metabolite of nitric oxide. *Life Sci* 60: 1833–1845

43 Huie RE, Padmaja S (1993) The reaction of NO with superoxide. *Free Rad Res Comm* 18: 195–199
44 Crow JP, Spruell C, Chen J, Gunn C, Ischiropoulos H, Tsai M et al (1994) On the pH-dependent yield of hydroxyl radical products from peroxynitrite. *Free Rad Biol Med* 16: 331–338
45 Radi R, Beckman JS, Bush KM, Freeman BA (1991) Peroxynitrite-induced membrane lipid peroxidation: the cytotoxic potential of superoxide and nitric oxide. *Arch Biochem Biophys* 288: 481–487
46 Radi R, Beckman JS, Bush KM, Freeman BA (1991) Peroxynitrite oxidation of sulfhydryls. The cytotoxic potential of superoxide and nitric oxide. *J Biol Chem* 266: 4244–4250
47 Bauer ML, Beckman JS, Bridges RJ, Fuller CM, Matalon S (1992) Peroxynitrite inhibits sodium uptake in rat colonic membrane vesicles. *Biochim Biophys Acta* 1104: 87–94
48 Hu P, Ischiropoulos H, Beckman JS, Matalon S (1994) Peroxynitrite inhibition of oxygen consumption and sodium transport in alveolar type II cells. *Am J Physiol* 266: L628–L634
49 Ishida H, Ichimori K, Hirota Y, Fukahori M, Nakazawa H (1996) Peroxynitrite-induced cardiac myocyte injury. *Free Rad Biol Med* 20: 343–350
50 Zhu L, Gunn C, Beckman JS (1992) Bactericidal activity of peroxynitrite. *Arch Biochem Biophys* 298: 452–457
51 McCall TB, Boughton-Smith NK, Palmer RMJ, Whittle BJR, Moncada S (1989) Synthesis of nitric oxide from L-arginine by neutrophils. Release and interaction with superoxide anion. *Biochem J* 261: 293–296
52 Ischiropoulos H, Zhu L, Beckman JS (1992) Peroxynitrite formation from macrophage-derived nitric oxide. *Arch Biochem Biophys* 298: 446–451
53 Kooy NW, Royall JA (1994) Agonist-induced peroxynitrite production from endothelial cells. *Arch Biochem Biophys* 310: 352–359
54 Miller MJS, Thompson JH, Zhang XJ, Sadowska-Krowicka H, Kakkis JL, Munshi UK et al (1995) Role of inducible nitric oxide synthase expression and peroxynitrite formation in guinea-pig ileitis. *Gastroenterology* 109: 1475–1483
55 Royall JA, Kooy NW, Beckman JS (1995) Nitric oxide-related oxidants in acute lung injury. *New Horiz* 3: 113–122
56 Haddad IY, Pataki G, Hu P, Galliani C, Beckman JS, Matalon S (1994) Quantitation of nitrotyrosine levels in lung sections of patients and animals with acute lung injury. *J Clin Invest* 94: 2407–2413
57 Wizemann TM, Gardner CR, Laskin JD, Quinones S, Durham SK, Goller NL et al (1994) Production of nitric oxide and peroxynitrite in the lung during acute endotoxemia. *J Leukocyte Biol* 56: 759–768
58 Akaike T, Noguchi Y, Ijiri S, Setoguchi K, Suga M, Zheng YM et al (1996) Pathogenesis of influenza virus-induced pneumonia: involvement of both nitric oxide and oxygen radicals. *Proc Natl Acad Sci* 93: 2448–2453
59 Kaur H, Haliwell B (1994) Evidence for nitric-oxide-mediated oxidative damage in chronic inflammation, nitrotyrosine in serum and synovial fluid from rheumatoid patients. *FEBS Lett* 350: 9–12
60 Van Dyke K, Antonini JM, Wu L, Ye Z, Reasor MJ (1994) The inhibition of silica-induced lung inflammation by dexamethosone as measured by bronchoalveolar lavage fluid parameters and peroxynitrite-dependent chemiluminescence. *Agents and Actions* 41: 44–49
61 Rachmilewitz D, Stamler JS, Karmelli F, Mullins ME, Singel DJ, Loscalzo J et al (1993) Peroxynitrite-induced rat colitis-a new model of colonic inflammation. *Gastroenterology* 105: 1681–1688
62 Sadeghi-Hashjin G, Folkerts G, Henricks PAJ, Verheyen AKCP, Van der Linde HJ, Van Ark I et al (1996) Peroxynitrite induces airway hyperresponsivenes in guinea-pigs *in vitro* an *in vivo*. *Am J Respir Crit Care Med* 153: 1697–1701
63 Laitinen LA, Heino M, Laitinen A, Kava T, Haahtela T (1985) Damage of the airway epithelium and bronchial reactivity in patients with asthma. *Am Rev Resp Dis* 131: 599–606
64 Folkerts G, Engels F, Nijkamp FP (1989) Endotoxin-induced hyperreactivity of the guinea-pig isolated trachea coincides with decreased prostaglandin E_2 production by the epithelial layer. *Br J Pharmacol* 96: 388–394
65 Folkerts G, Nijkamp FP (1998) Airway epithelium: more than just a barrier! *TiPS* 19: 334–341

66 Nijkamp FP, Folkerts G (1986) Reversal of arachidonic acid-induced tracheal relaxation into contraction after epithelium removal. *Eur J Pharmacol* 131: 315–316

67 Munakata M, Huang I, Mitzner W, Menkes H (1989) Protective role of the epithelium in the guinea-pig airway. *J Appl Physiol* 66: 1547–1552

68 Munakata M, Masaki Y, Sakuma I, Ukita H, Otsuka Y, Homma Y et al (1990) Pharmacological differentiation of epithelium-derived relaxing factor from nitric oxide. *J Appl Physiol* 69: 665–670

69 Sparrow MP, Mitchell HW (1991) Modulation by the epithelium of the extent of bronchial narrowing produced by substances perfused through the lumen. *Br J Pharmacol* 103: 1160–1164

70 Pavlovic D, Fournier M, Aubier M, Pariente R (1989) Epithelial vs. serosal stimulation of tracheal muscle: role of epithelium. *J Appl Physiol* 67: 2522–2526

71 Gao Y, Vanhoutte PM (1993) Attenuation of contractions to acetylcholine in canine bronchi by an endogenous nitric oxide-like substance. *Br J Pharmacol* 109: 887–891

72 Chee C, Gaston B, Gerard C, Loscalzo J, Kobzik L, Drazen JM et al (1993) Nitric oxide is produced by human epithelial cell line. *Am Rev Resp Dis* 147: A433

73 Schmidt HHHW, Gagne GD, Nakane M, Pollock JS, Miller MF, Murad F (1992) Mapping of neural nitric oxide synthase in the rat suggests frequent co-localization with NADPH diaphorase but not with soluble guanylyl cyclase, and novel paraneural functions for nitrinergic signal transduction. *J Histochem Cytochem* 40: 1439–1456

74 Fischer A, Mundel P, Mayer B, Preissler U, Phillipin B, Kummer W (1992) Nitric oxide synthase in guinea-pig lower airway innervation. *Neurosci Lett* 149: 157–160

75 Rengasamy A, Xue C, Johns RA (1994) Immunohistochemical demonstration of a paracine role of nitric oxide in bronchial function. *Am J Physiol* 267: L704–L711

76 Robbins RA, Springall DR, Warren JB, Kwon OJ, Buttery LDK, Wilson AJ et al (1994) Inducible nitric oxide synthase is increased in murine lung epithelial cells by cytokine stimulation. *Biochem Biophys Res Commun* 198: 835–843

77 Punjabi CJ, Laskin JD, Pendino KJ, Goller NL, Durham SK, Laskin L (1994) Production of nitric oxide by rat type II pneumocytes: increased expression of inducible nitric oxide synthase following inhalation of a pulmonary irritant. *Am J Respir Cell Mol Biol* 11: 165–172

78 Guo FH, De Raeve HR, Rice TW, Stuehr DJ, Thunissen FBJM, Erzurum SC (1995) Continuous nitric oxide synthesis by inducible nitric oxide synthase in normal human airway epithelium *in vivo*. *Proc Natl Acad Sci* 92: 7809–7813

79 Nijkamp FP, Van der Linde HJ, Folkerts G (1993) Nitric oxide synthesis inhibitors induce airway hyperresponsiveness in the guinea-pig *in vivo* and *in vitro*. *Am Rev Resp Dis* 148: 727–734

80 Fedan FS, Nutt ME, Frazer DG (1990) Reactivity of guinea-pig isolated trachea to methacholine, histamine and isoproterenol applied serosally versus mucosally. *Eur J Pharmacol* 190: 337–345

81 Folkerts G, Van der Linde H, Schreurs AJM, Verheyen FKCP, Blomjous FJ, Nijkamp FP (1995) Hyperresponsiveness of human bronchi after nitric oxide synthesis inhibition. *Am J Respir Crit Care Med* 151: A832

82 Folkerts G, Van der Linde H, Van de Loo PGF, Engels F, Nijkamp FP (1995) Leukotrienes mediate tracheal hyperresponsiveness after nitric oxide synthesis inhibition. *Eur J Pharmacol* 285: R1–2

83 Adcock JJ, Garland LG (1980) A possible role for lipoxygenase products as regulators of airway smooth muscle reactivity. *Br J Pharmacol* 69: 167–169

84 O'Byrne PM (1994) Eicosanoids and Asthma. *Ann NY Acad Sci* 744: 251–261

85 Folkerts, Linde van der HJ, Nijkamp FP (1995) Virus-induced airway hyperresponsiveness in guinea-pigs is related to a deficiency in nitric oxide. *J Clin Invest* 95: 26–30

86 Jia YL, Xu LJ, Turner DJ, Martin JG (1996) Endogenous nitric oxide contributes to strain-related differences in airway responsiveness in rats. *J Appl Physiol* 80: 404–410

87 Sadeghi-Hashjin G, Folkerts G, Henricks PAJ, Van de Loo PGF, Van der Linde HJ, Dik IEM (1996) Induction of guinea-pig airway hyperresponsiveness by inactivation of guanylate cyclase. *Eur J Pharmacol* 302: 109–115

88 Lach E, Daeffler L, Waeldele F, Gies J-P (1995) Bombesin-induced contractions of guinea-pig lungstrips are modulated by endogenous nitric oxide. *Naunyn-Schmiedeberg's Arch Pharmacol* 352: 419–423

89 Rengasamy A, Johns RA (1993) Regulation of nitric oxide synthase by nitric oxide. *Molecular Pharmacology* 44: 124–128

90 De Kimpe SJ, Tielemans W, Van Heuven-Nolsen D, Nijkamp FP (1994) Reversal of bradykinin-induced relaxation to contraction after interferon-γ bovine isolated mesenteric arteries. *Eur J Pharmacol* 261: 111–120

91 Lu J-L, Schmiege LM, Kuo L, Liao JC (1996) Downregulation of endothelial constitutive nitric oxide synthase expression by lipopolysaccharide. *Biochem Biophys Res Commun* 225: 1–5

92 Persson MG, Gustafsson LE, Wiklund NP, Moncada S, Heqvist P (1990) Endogenous nitric oxide as a probable modulator of pulmonary circulation and hypoxic pressor response *in vivo*. *Acta Physiol Scand* 140: 449–457

93 Archer SL, Tolins JP, Raij L, Weir EK (1989) Hypoxic pulmonary vasoconstriction is enhanced by inhibition of the synthesis of an endothelium derived relaxing factor. *Biochem Biophys Res Commun* 164: 1198–1205

94 Hay DPW, Muccitelli RM, Page CP, Spina D (1992) Correlation betwen airway epithelium-induced relaxation of rat aorta in the co-axial bioassay and cyclic nucleotide levels. *Br J Pharmacol* 105: 954–958

95 Welliver RC, Wong DT, Sun M, Middelton EJ, Vaugan RS, Ogra PL (1981) The development of respiratory syncytial virus-specific IgE and the release of histamine in nasopharyngeal secretions after infection. *N Engl J Med* 305: 841–846

96 Jarjour NN, Calhoun WJ, Schwartz LB, Busse WW (1991) Elevated bronchoalveolar lavage fluid histamine levels in allergic asthmatics are associated with increased airway obstruction. *Am Rev Resp Dis* 144: 83–87

97 Moncada S, Palmer RMJ, Higgs EA (1991) Nitric oxide: physiology, pathophysiology, and pharmacology. *Pharmacol Rev* 43: 109–141

98 Leurs R, Brozium MM, Jansen W, Bast A, Timmerman H (1991) Histamine H_1-receptor-mediated cyclic GMP production in guinea-pig lung tissue is an L-arginine-dependent process. *Biochem Pharmacol* 42: 271–277

99 Filep JG, Battistini B, Sirois P (1993) Induction by endothelin-1 of epithelium-dependent relaxation of guinea-pig trachea *in vitro*: role for nitric oxide. *Br J Pharmacol* 109: 637–644

100 Schemper V, Calixto JB (1994) Nitric oxide pathway-mediated relaxant effect of bradykinin in the guinea-pig isolated trachea. *Br J Pharmacol* 111: 83–88

101 Figini M, Ricciardolo FLM, Javdan P, Nijkamp FP, Emanueli C, Pradelles P et al (1996) Evidence that epithelium-derived relaxing factor released by braykinin in the guinea-pig trachea is nitric oxide. *Am J Respir Crit Care Med* 153: 918–923

102 Nielsen-Kudsk JE, Karlsson J-A, Persson CGA (1986) Relaxant effects of xanthines, a β_2-receptor agonists and Ca^{2+} antagonists in guinea-pig tracheal preparations contracted by potassium or carbachol. *Eur J Pharmacol* 128: 33–40

103 Folkerts G, Linde van der H, Verheyen AKCP, Nijkamp FP (1995) Endogenous nitric oxide modulation of potassium-induced changes in guinea-pig airway tone. *Br J Pharmacol* 115: 1194–1198

104 Folkerts G, Busse WW, Nijkamp FP, Sorkness R, Gern JE (1998) Virus-induced airway hyperresponsiveness and asthma. *Am J Respir Crit Care Med* 157: 1708–1720

105 Bardin PG, Johnston SL, Pattemore PK (1992) Viruses as precipitants of asthma symptoms. II. Physiology and mechanisms. *Clin Exp Allergy* 22: 809–822

106 Sterk PJ (1993) Virus-induced airway hyperresponsiveness in man. *Eur Respir J* 6: 894–902

107 Folkerts G, Nijkamp FP (1995) Virus-induced airway hyperresponsiveness: Role of inflammatory cells and mediators. *Am J Resp Crit Care Med* 151: 1666–1674

108 Gern JE, Busse WW (1995) The effects of rhinovirus infections on allergic airway responses. *Am J Respir Crit Care Med* 152: S40–S45

109 Folkerts G, Verheyen AKCP, Geuens GMA, Folkerts HF, Nijkamp FP (1993) Virus-induced changes in airway responsiveness, morphology, and histamine levels in guinea-pigs. *Am Rev Resp Dis* 147: 1569–1577

110 Folkerts G, De Clerck F, Reijnart I, Span P, Nijkamp FP (1993) Virus-induced airway hyperresponsiveness in the guinea-pig: possible involvement of histamine and inflammatory cells. *Br J Pharmacol* 108: 1083–1093

111 Oosterhout AJM, Ark van I, Folkerts G, Linde van der HJ, Savelkoul HFJ, Verheyen AKCP et al (1995) Antibody to interleukin-5 inhibits virus-induced airway hyperresponsiveness to histamine in guinea-pigs. *Am J Respir Crit Care Med* 151: 177–183

112 Ladenius ARC, Folkerts G, Linde van der HJ, Nijkamp FP (1995) Potentiation by viral respiratory infection of ovalbumin-induced guinea-pig tracheal hyperresponsiveness: role for tachykinins. *Br J Pharmacol* 115: 1048–1052

113 Tamaoki J, Kondo M, Ciyotani A, Takemura H, Konno K (1995) Effect of Saiboku-to, an antiasthamtic herbal medicine, on nitric oxide generation from cultured canine airway epithelial cells. *Jpn J Pharmacol* 69: 29–35

114 McCall T, Vallance P (1992) Nitric oxide takes centre-stage with newly defined roles. *TIPS* 13: 1–6

115 Aminlari M, Vaseghi T (1992) Arginase distribution in tissues of domestic animals. *Comp Biochem Physiol* 103B: 385–389

116 Taylor AA, Stewart GR (1981) Tissue and subcellular localization of enzymes of arginine metabolism in pisum sativum. *Biochem Biophys Res Commun* 101: 1281–1289

117 Folkerts G, Verheyen A, Nijkamp FP (1992) Viral infection in guinea-pigs induces a sustained non-specific airway hyperresponsiveness and morphological changes of the respiratory tract. *Eur J Pharmacol* 228: 121–130

118 Springall DR, Hamid OA, Buttery LKD, Chanez P, Howarth P, Bousquet J et al (1993) Nitric oxide synthase induction in airways of asthmatic subjects. *Am Rev Resp Dis* 147: A515

119 Kharitonov SA, Yates D, Barnes PJ (1995) Increased nitric oxide in exhaled air of normal human subjects with upper respiratory tract infections. *Eur Respir J* 8: 295–297

120 MacNaul KL, Hutchinson NI (1993) Differential expression of iNOS and cNOS mRNA in human vascular smooth muscle cells and endothelial cells under normal and inflammatory conditions. *Biochem Biophys Res Commun* 196: 1330–1334

121 Mohamed F, Monge JC, Gordon A, Cernacek P, Blais D, Stewart DJ (1995) Lack of role for nitric oxide (NO) in the selective destabilization of endothelial NO synthase mRNA by tumor necrosis factor-α. *Arterioscler Thromb Vasc Biol* 15: 52–57

122 Nishida K, Harrison DG, Navas JP, Fischer AA, Dockery SP, Uematsu M et al (1992) Molecular cloning and characterization of the constitutive bovine aortic endothelial call nitric oxide synthase. *J Clin Invest* 90: 2092–2096

123 Yoshizumi M, Perella MA, Burnett JC, Lee ME (1993) Tumor necrosis factor down regulates an endothelial nitric oxide synthase mRNA by shorting its half-life. *Circ Res* 73: 205–209

124 Marsden PA, Schappert KT, Chen HS, Flowers M, Sundell CL, Wilcox JN et al (1992) Molecular cloning and characterization of human endothelial nitric oxide synthase. *FEBS Lett* 307: 287–293

125 Nijkamp FP, Folkerts G (1994) Nitric oxide and bronchial reactivity. *Clin Exp Allergy* 24: 905–914

126 Folkerts G, Verheyen A, Janssen M, Nijkamp FP (1992) Virus-induced airway hyper-responsiveness in the guinea-pig can be transferred by bronchoalveolar cells. *J Allergy Clin Immunol* 90: 364–372

127 Nijkamp FP, Folkerts G (1995) Nitric oxide and bronchial hyperresponsiveness. Archives internationales de Pharmacodynamie et de Therapie 329: 81–96

128 Kinnula VL, Adler KB, Ackley NJ, Crapo JD (1992) Release of reactive oxygen species by guinea-pig tracheal epithelial cells *in vitro. Am J Physiol* 262: L708–L712

Nitric Oxide in Pulmonary Processes:
Role in Physiology and Pathophysiology of Lung Disease
ed. by M. G. Belvisi and J. A. Mitchell
© 2000 Birkhäuser Verlag Basel/Switzerland

CHAPTER 7
Bronchodilator Actions of Nitric Oxide and Related Compounds

Sanjay Mehta[1] and Jeffrey M. Drazen[2]

[1] *Pulmonary Division, Departments of Medicine and Pharmacology/Toxicology, London Health Sciences Center, University of Western Ontario, London, Ontario, Canada NGA 4G5*
[2] *Pulmonary and Critical Care Division, Department of Medicine, Brigham and Women's Hospital, Harvard Medical School, Boston, MA 02115, USA*

1   Introduction
2   Bronchodilator Actions of Endogenous Nitric Oxide (NO)
2.1   Neural Inhibitory Non-Adrenergic Non-Cholinergic (iNANC) Bronchodilation
2.2   Paracrine Mediation of Airway Responses
2.2.1 Role of NO in Airway Responses to Vasoactive Intestinal Peptide (VIP)
2.2.2 Role of NO in Airway Responses to Other Agents
3   Modulation of Neural Constrictor Responses
4   Modulation of Bronchoconstriction in Response to Exogenous Contractile Agents
4.1   Role of NO in Bronchial Responsiveness of Normal Airways
4.2   Role of NO in Enhanced Bronchial Responsiveness Associated with Airway Inflammation
5   Modulation of Airway Responses to Antigen Exposure in Sensitised Animals
6   Bronchodilator Actions of Exogenous NO and NO-Related Compounds
6.1   Inhaled NO in Animals
6.2   Inhaled NO in Humans
6.3   Bronchodilator Actions of Exogenous NO-Related Compounds
7   Possible Mechanisms Involved in the Bronchodilator Response to NO and Sources of Endogenous NO
8   References

1. Introduction

Among its many roles in mammalian cells and organisms, nitric oxide (NO) has a multitude of physiological and pathophysiological roles in the lungs and airways. In the airways, NO and NO-related compounds modulate airway tone and microvascular leak from the airway circulation, mediate enhanced ciliary motility in response to various agents, and likely contribute to epithelial injury and denudation the setting of airway inflammation. NO is synthesized by a family of NO synthases (NOSs) which are found in a variety of cell types in the lungs and airways, including bronchial epithelial cells, endothelial cells and intrinsic airway postganglionic neurons [1, 4, 7, 8, 14, 22, 24, 27, 32, 45–47, 50].

An increasing amount of evidence supports the idea that endogenously-produced NO is an important modulator of airway function both in the basal state [2, 3, 34, 41, 54, 55] and in the setting of airway inflammation [15, 40]. For example, endogenously-produced NO can modulate airway responses to endogenous contractile stimuli, including vagal stimulation-induced contractile responses [2, 55]. Furthermore, in the setting of airway inflammation induced by viral infection or repeated antigen exposure, this endogenous NO-related bronchodilator mechanism may be dysregulated. In this review, the direct and indirect bronchodilator effects of endogenously-produced NO and the airway effects of exogenous (inhaled) NO and related compounds will be examined.

2. Bronchodilator Actions of Endogenous NO

2.1. Neural Inhibitory Non-Adrenergic Non-Cholinergic (iNANC) Bronchodilation

The first evidence of a role for endogenously-produced NO in the modulation of airway tone was derived from descriptions of neural, non-adrenergic, non-cholinergic (iNANC) airway smooth muscle relaxation in response to vagal activation. In these experiments it was shown that inhibition of NOS with various analogues of L-arginine attenuated the smooth muscle relaxant response which occurred after iNANC stimulation in guinea-pig and human airway tissue [3, 34, 54]. In the guinea-pig, the iNANC response was only partially, 40–60%, blunted by NOS inhibition, suggesting an important role for another mediator; which is thought to be vasoactive intestinal peptide (VIP) [34, 54]. In contrast, in human tracheal strips, iNANC responses were found to be solely NO-dependent and were almost completely inhibited by pre-incubation with N^G-nitro-L-arginine methyl ester (L-NAME), an L-arginine-analogue NOS inhibitor [3].

2.2. Paracrine Mediation of Airway Responses

2.2.1. Role of NO in Airway Responses to VIP: In addition to directly mediating neural bronchodilator responses, it has been shown that NO also has an important paracrine role in mediating the effects of agents such as VIP, bradykinin, and endothelin. For example, the bronchodilator response of isolated, tracheally-perfused guinea-pig lungs to geometrically-increasing concentrations of VIP is blunted by approximately 100-fold in the presence of 200 mM N^G-nitro-L-arginine (L-NA) in the perfusate (IC_{50} 32 nmol/kg *vs* 0.39 nmol/kg in control lungs) (Fig. 1) [35]. This inhibitory effect of L-NA could be overcome and VIP responses restored by addition of excess L-arginine to the perfusate, which restores endogenous

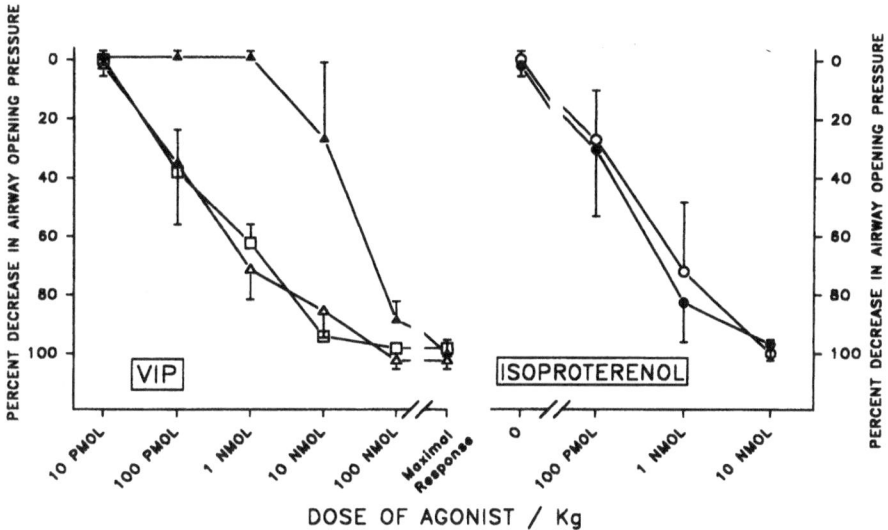

Figure 1. *Left*: dose-response relationship for vasoactive intestinal peptide (VIP) with N^G-nitro-L-arginine (L-NA), with L-NA and L-arginine, and with no additives present in perfusion buffer. *Right*: dose-response relationship for isoproterenol with and without L-NA present in perfusion buffer. Closed circles, isoproterenol with L-NA; open circles, isoproterenol without L-NA; closed triangles, VIP with L-NA; open squares, VIP with L-NA and L-arginine; open triangles, VIP without L-NA. Results are expressed as group mean with 95% confidence intervals (CI).

NO production. The role of NO as a paracrine mediator of VIP's effects was confirmed by the measurement of NO-equivalents by the Griess reagent method in the effluent from isolated, perfused lungs: VIP administration was associated, in a time course that immediately preceded the onset of bronchorelaxation, with an increase in the local pulmonary elaboration of NO-equivalents from 0.11 ± 0.04 to 0.78 ± 0.15 µM (p < 0.05).

2.2.2. Role of NO in airway responses to other agents: NO also appears to be critical in determining the bronchodilator response of airways to endothelin-1 (ET-1), which has been reported to exert both bronchoconstrictor and bronchodilator effects [13, 37]. In isolated guinea-pig trachea at low resting tone, ET-1 produces a dose-dependent constriction that is enhanced by removal of the epithelium, but not by pre-incubation with N^G-monomethyl-L-arginine (L-NMMA) or methylene blue. In contrast, at high resting tone, ET-1 induces a concentration-dependent slow tracheal relaxation which can be markedly blunted by pre-incubation with 100 µM L-NMMA or 10 µM methylene blue; removal of the epithelium changes this relaxant response to a more sustained constrictor response [13]. Similarly, it has been shown that bradykinin's relaxant effects on airway tone are partially NO-dependent [49].

3. Modulation of Neural Constrictor Responses

Besides its direct neural and paracrine bronchodilator effects, neurally released NO also modulates bronchoconstriction in response to neural
stimulation-induced acetylcholine release. In both guinea-pig and human
tissues, inhibition of NOS by pre-incubation of tracheal strips with
L-NMMA or L-NAME results in exaggerated constrictor responses to vagal
stimulation [2, 55]. Since the enhanced constrictor response following NOS
inhibition was not associated with any measurable increase in acetylcholine
release per se, NO's modulatory effects do not appear to be mediated
through interference with acetylcholine release. It is likely that NO modulates neural stimulation-induced bronchial responses at the level of the
acetylcholine receptor or postreceptor subcellular signaling systems [55].

4. Modulation of Bronchoconstriction in Response to Exogenous Contractile Agonists

Based on the above-described roles for endogenous NO in neural dilator
and constrictor responses, and on the established responses of vascular
smooth muscle to NO and NO-related compounds, subsequent studies on
the bronchodilator role of NO in the airways focused on NO-mediated
modulation of bronchoconstriction induced by exogenous agents. For
example, Gao et al. described an important role for an endogenous NO-like
substance in the attenuation of contractions in canine bronchial smooth
muscle induced by exogenous acetylcholine *in vitro* [16].

4.1. Role of NO in Bronchial Responsiveness of Normal Airways

Similar to its homeostatic role in airway responses to endogenous contractile mechanisms, endogenously-produced pulmonary NO also has an important modulatory action in bronchoconstriction induced by administration of contractile agonists, such as histamine [38, 41]. In isolated guinea-
pig tracheal tubes *in vitro*, luminal perfusion with 120 µM L-NAME and
L-NMMA enhanced maximal histamine responsiveness by 335% and
250%, respectively ($p < 0.01$ for each *vs* control), and these effects were
reversed in the presence of excess L-arginine (Fig. 2) [41]. This finding
indicates that endogenously-produced pulmonary NO has a significant role
in attenuating basal responsiveness to exogenous histamine. Moreover,
removal of the tracheal epithelium was associated with increased basal responsiveness to histamine and with loss of L-NAME's enhancing effect on
histamine-responsiveness. Thus, the airway epithelium was critical in this
endogenous NO-dependent homeostatic mechanism, presumably as the
source of NO.

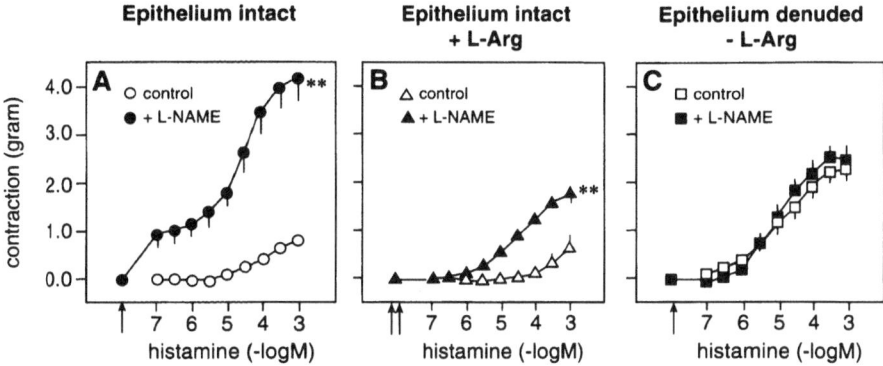

Figure 2. Effect of L-NAME (120 µM) and L-Arg (200 µM) incubation on isolated perfused guinea-pig tracheal tubes with or without epithelium. L-NAME (*arrow*) incubation for 30 min increased the basal tone of the tracheae. The histamine concentration-response curve was shifted upwards after L-NAME incubation (*closed circles*) compared with tissues incubated with the solvent solution (*open circles*) **p < 0.01, two-way ANOVA. L-Arg incubation together with L-NAME (*double arrows*) for 30 min prevented the increase in basal tone (*closed triangles*) and suppressed the histamine concentration-response curve compared with the L-NAME group (A, *closed circles*), but the concentration-response curve was increased compared with tissues incubated with the solvent solution (A, *open circles*) or with L-Arg (*open triangles*). **p < 0.01, two-way ANOVA. (C) Epithelium removed resulted in an upward shift in the histamine concentration-response curve compared with tissues with epithelium (A, *open circles*). L-NAME incubation (*arrow*) for 30 min did not influence basal tone (*closed squares*) and did not result in an additional upward shift in the histamine concentration-response curve compared with epithelium-denuded tissues incubated with solvent solution (*open squares*). Each data point is the mean ± SEM.

This homeostatic effect of NO has also been demonstrated in spontaneously breathing guinea-pigs using measurement of lung resistance (R_{lung}) as an outcome index [41]. In these experiments, treatment with aerosolized L-NAME and L-NMMA was associated with markedly enhanced airway constrictor responses: The peak R_{lung} response to intravenous histamine was increased by 126% and 282% (p < 0.01 for each *vs* control), respectively. Furthermore, in animals rendered hyperresponsive by competitive NOS inhibition, administration of aerosolized L-arginine, the substrate of NOS, was associated with return of airway histamine-responsiveness to pre-L-NAME levels.

We have confirmed a significant endogenous pulmonary NO-related modulatory effect on bronchoconstriction induced by both exogenous histamine and capsaicin in tracheotomised, mechanically ventilated guinea-pigs [38, unpublished observations]. Respiratory resistance (R_{resp}) responses to histamine were enhanced by 30 ± 8% after intravenous treatment with L-NAME (10 mg/kg) over control responses (Fig. 3). Our data agree in a broad sense with those previously reported by Nijkamp et al., although the magnitude of enhancement of the bronchoconstrictor response we observed was substantially less than that previously reported [41]. Indeed, others have been unable to replicate the findings reported by Nijkamp et al.

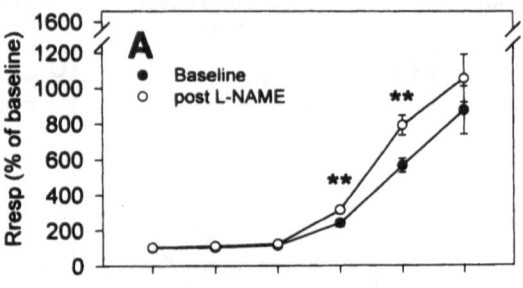

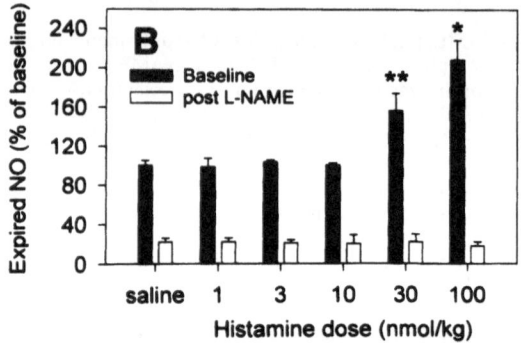

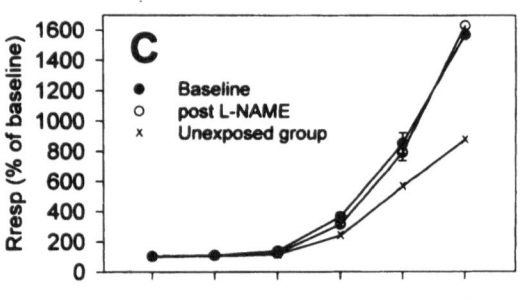

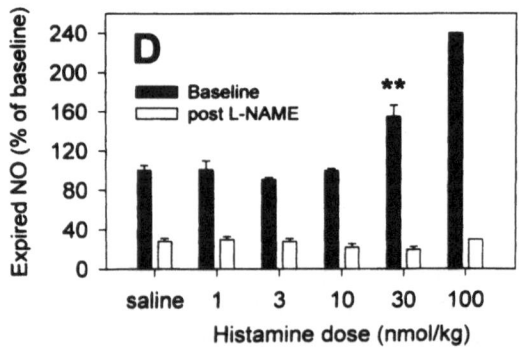

[12]. Although the differences in these various sets of observations are likely due to differences in the physiological parameter measured, i.e. R_{resp} vs R_{lung}, differing contributions of upper airway resistance in tracheotomised vs spontaneously-breathing animals, or differences in animal strains, no investigative group has clearly resolved these conflicting issues.

Besides demonstration of this endogenous, pulmonary, NO-related homeostatic mechanism, in our experiments we also observed significant transient elevations in the level of NO in mixed expired gas that were cotemporal with the increase in R_{resp} after administration of histamine (Fig. 4). Inhibition of endogenous pulmonary NO production with L-NAME, administered as an intravenous infusion, was associated with markedly reduced baseline expired NO levels and loss of the increase in expired NO during bronchoconstriction. Thus, the decrease in mixed expired NO levels after NOS inhibition and the loss of endogenous NO-related homeostatic bronchodilator effect are closely linked. We have documented significant, transient elevations of mixed expired NO levels with bronchoconstriction induced by histamine, methacholine, capsaicin, substance P and leukotriene-C_4 (unpublished observations). As with histamine, an increase in expired NO occurs during capsaicin-induced bronchoconstriction; NOS inhibition results in loss of the transient increase in expired NO levels that occurs with constriction as well as enhanced constrictor responses to capsaicin.

4.2. Role of NO in Enhanced Bronchial Responsiveness Associated with Airway Inflammation

The importance of an endogenous pulmonary NO-related homeostatic mechanism has been further demonstrated by studies in which this mechanism is altered by airway inflammation. *In vivo* bronchial responsiveness to histamine and the sensitivity of tracheal tubes *in vitro* to histamine were both enhanced by infection with parainfluenza type 3 virus in guinea-pigs

---

Figure 3. Bronchial responsiveness to histamine (panels A, C) and peak nitric oxide (NO) levels in mixed expired gas (panels B, D) during histamine-induced bronchoconstriction before (baseline) and after N^G-nitro-L-arginine methyl ester (L-NAME) administration in unexposed control guinea-pigs (n = 6) and antigen-exposed guinea-pigs 24 h after antigen exposure (n = 7). Histamine-induced bronchoconstriction was associated with significant increases in expired NO at higher doses of histamine (30 and 100 nmol/kg) in both unexposed (panel B) and antigen-exposed animals (panel D). Only two unexposed animals and one antigen-exposed animal received the 100 nmol/kg dose of histamine. In both unexposed and antigen-exposed animals, administration of L-NAME reduced basal expired NO and eliminated the increase in expired NO during bronchoconstriction. However, bronchial responsiveness to histamine was enhanced after L-NAME treatment in unexposed control animals (panel A), but not in antigen-exposed animals, 24 h after antigen exposure (panel C). Note that histamine responsiveness data from the unexposed control group (panel A) are reproduced in panel C for the sake of comparison. Rresp, respiratory resistance. *, p < 0.05 and **, p < 0.01, baseline vs post-L-NAME.

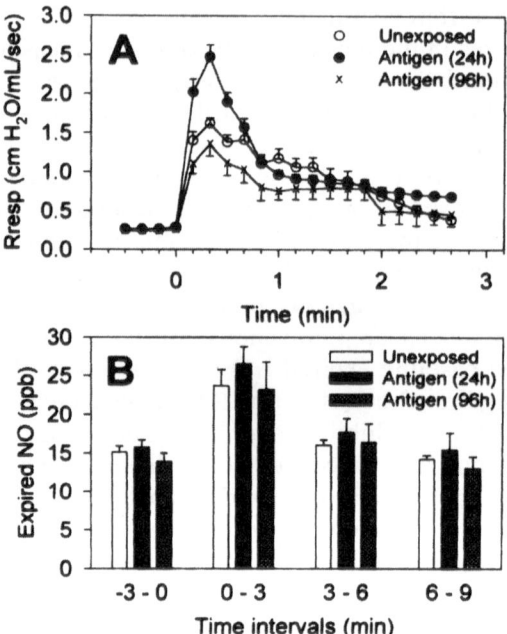

Figure 4. Time course of changes in respiratory resistance (Rresp, panel A) and expired nitric oxide (NO, panel B) following intravenous administration of 30 nmol/kg of histamine in unexposed and antigen-exposed guinea-pigs either 24 h or 96 h after antigen exposure. Following histamine administration at time = 0, the increase in Rresp ($p < 0.01$, peak vs baseline) was associated with a cotemporal increase in expired gas NO levels ($p < 0.01$, peak vs baseline); both Rresp and expired NO returned to baseline levels after 2–3 min. Histamine responsiveness was significantly enhanced 24 h $p < 0.01$, antigen-exposed vs unexposed), but not 96 h, after antigen exposure, but the increase in expired NO with histamine-induced bronchoconstriction was unaffected by antigen exposure.

[15]. In these studies, L-arginine exposure completely prevented the virus-induced airway hyperresponsiveness, whereas aerosolized L-NAME had no effect on histamine-responsiveness in virus-infected animals. Furthermore, using an NO-sensitive electrochemical probe, these authors were able to measure increased NO production *in vitro* after histamine-exposure of isolated tracheal strips from animals not infected by virus. In contrast, the histamine-stimulated liberation of NO into the tissue perfusate was markedly diminished when tracheas from virus-infected guinea-pigs were studied, but could be restored by incubation with excess L-arginine (Fig. 5). Thus, virus infection-induced airway inflammation results in enhanced bronchial hyperresponsiveness to histamine; this occurs with both a loss of endogenous NO-related modulatory activity and a decrease in directly measured histamine-induced local airway NO production *in vitro*.

We have reported a similar defect in the endogenous NO-related homeostatic mechanism in the setting of airway inflammation induced by repeated pulmonary exposure to antigen in guinea-pigs [38, 40]. Signifi-

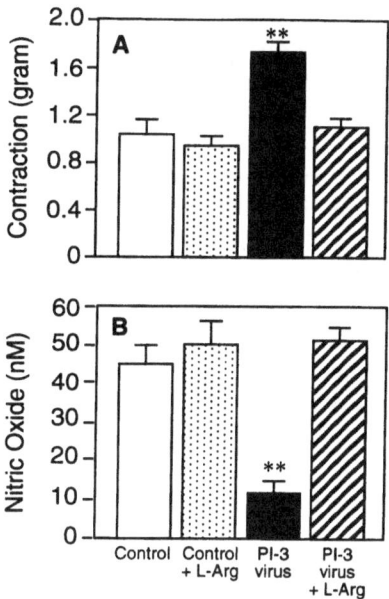

Figure 5. Histamine (10^{-3} M)-induced contraction and NO release, in the absence and presence of L-arginine (200 μM), of perfused isolated tracheal tubes obtained from control and virus-infected guinea-pigs. In control tissues the histamine-induced contraction was associated with a simultaneous release of NO (*open bars*, *A* and *B*, *n* = 4). L-Arginine incubation had no effect on the contraction or NO release (*stippled bars*, *A* and *B*, *n* = 4). The histamine-induced contraction in the virus-infected group was significantly enhanced (*black bar*, *A*, **p < 0.01, Student's unpaired *t* test, *n* = 5) and was associated with a significant decrease in NO production (*black bar*, *B*, ** p < 0.01, Student's unpaired *t* test, *n* = 5). Incubation of L-arginine completely prevented the enhanced contraction and the decreased NO production (*hatched bars*, *A* and *B*, *n* = 5).

cant bronchial hyperresponsiveness to histamine was induced, at 24 h after antigen exposure, in sensitized guinea-pigs and had largely resolved by 96 h after antigen exposure. Histamine-induced bronchoconstriction in antigen-exposed guinea-pigs was associated with significant increases in NO levels in expired gas which were proportional to the histamine dose and of similar magnitude to that observed in control, unsensitised guinea-pigs (Fig. 3). We assessed the modulatory role of endogenous pulmonary NO production through performance of two successive histamine dose-response curves, i.e. before and after an intervention. Intravenous administration of L-NAME (10 mg/kg), but not D-NAME, enhanced bronchial responsiveness to histamine on the second dose-response curve in unsensitised guinea-pigs. In contrast, in antigen-exposed animals 24 h after antigen exposure, at a time when hyperresponsiveness to histamine was present following antigen exposure, L-NAME administration had no further enhancing effect on bronchial responsiveness to histamine (Fig. 3). Furthermore, 96 h after antigen exposure, i.e. when antigen-induced histamine hyperresponsiveness had resolved, inhibition of endogenous NO production with L-NAME was again associated with enhanced responsiveness to histamine. Thus, an endogenous pulmonary NO-dependent modulatory activity, as reflected by enhanced responsiveness to histamine after L-NAME, is transiently lost cotemporally with the induction of airway inflammation-associated bronchial hyperresponsiveness. Furthermore, baseline expired NO levels and the dose-dependent increase in expired NO levels with histamine administration are similar between control and antigen-exposed animals (Fig. 4), indicating that a simple deficiency of NO production does not fully explain this transient absence of an NO-related homeostatic mechanism. It remains undetermined whether this defect is related to a loss of NO's relaxant effect at the level of the bronchial smooth muscle, or a problem of access of endogenously-produced NO to its site of action, possibly due to airway edema and inflammation.

5. Modulation of Airway Responses to Antigen Exposure in Sensitized Animals

The above-described endogenous pulmonary NO-related homeostatic mechanism also appears to be important in modulating acute airway responses to antigen challenge in sensitized guinea-pigs [40, 42]. Persson et al. first reported dose-dependent increases in expired gas NO and airway opening pressure following antigen (ovalbumin) challenge in sensitized guinea-pigs [42]. We have also reported that intratracheal antigen exposure in sensitized guinea-pigs produced an acute allergic bronchoconstrictor response that was associated with a marked, transient elevation of mixed expired gas NO levels from 17 ± 1 to a peak of 56 ± 8 part per billion (ppb) ($p < 0.01$, figure 6). The increase in expired NO was cotemporal with the increase in R_{resp} and correlated significantly with the magnitude of the acute bronchoconstrictor response, with a correlation coefficient of $r = 0.77$ ($n = 12$, $p < 0.01$). Inhibition of endogenous NO production by treatment with 30 mg/kg/day of L-NAME infused over $48-72$ h by a subcutaneously-implanted osmotic pump, reduced basal expired NO levels by 67% (6 ± 1 ppb vs 18 ± 1 ppb in non-L-NAME treated animals, $p < 0.01$) and eliminated the increase in expired NO during the acute allergic bronchoconstrictor response (Fig. 6). Furthermore, inhibition of endogenous NO production was associated with an exaggerated acute increase in R_{resp} following antigen challenge (660 ± 60 vs $497 \pm 42\%$ of baseline in non-L-NAME treated animals, $p < 0.05$). Thus, the increased expired NO during the acute allergic bronchoconstrictor response is not simply a marker of the severity of physiological airway obstruction, but reflects this important endogenous NO-related modulatory activity. Interestingly, the modulatory effect of endogenous NO may be more important in the larger airways, given the lack of effect of NOS inhibition on the decline in dynamic respiratory compliance (C_{dyn}) following antigen challenge.

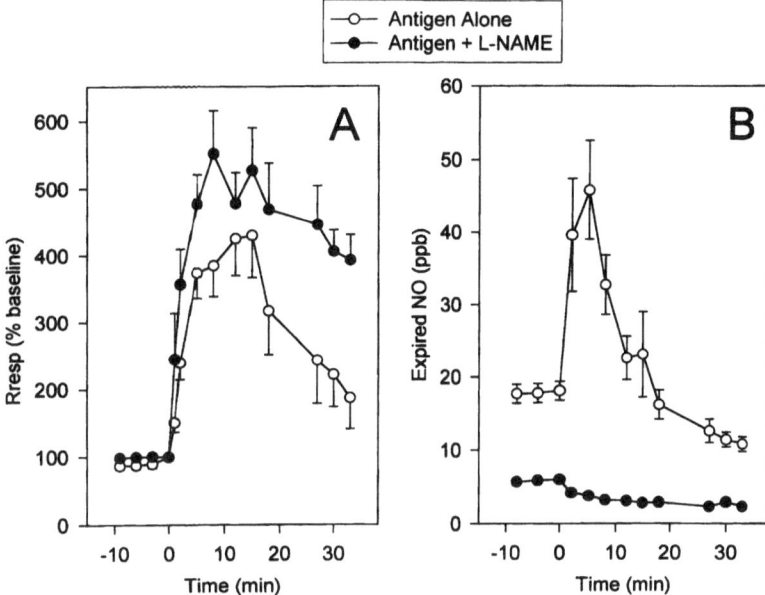

Figure 6. The effect of N^G-nitro-L-arginine methylester (L-NAME, a competitive inhibitor of NO synthase) on the increase in respiratory resistance (Rresp, panel A) and expired nitric oxide (NO, panel B) following antigen (ovalbumin) challenge in guinea-pigs. Treatment with L-NAME reduced basal expired NO by 67% ($p < 0.01$), eliminated the increase in expired NO following antigen challenge and resulted in an enhanced Rresp response to antigen challenge ($p < 0.05$). Note that error bars for expired NO in L-NAME treated animals are present (panel B, filled circles), but are hidden by the data points.

6. Bronchodilator Actions of Exogenous NO and NO-Related Compounds

In addition to the sensitivity of airway tissue to the modulatory effects of endogenous NO, exposure of bronchial smooth muscle *in vitro* to exogenous NO and NO-related compounds also produces relaxation [6, 10]. Furthermore, the administration of exogenous NO produces important bronchodilatory effects in intact animals and humans. Exogenous NO may be administered in either the gaseous form, i.e. inhaled NO, or as metabolically active adducts of NO and thiol-containing peptides and amino acids, such as the S-nitrosothiols, e.g. S-NO-glutathione.

6.1. Inhaled NO in Animals

The first evidence of a bronchodilatory effect of exogenous inhaled NO was reported in guinea-pigs by our group [9]. In mechanically ventilated, anesthetised guinea-pigs, C_{dyn} and R_{lung} were measured by plethysmography. In the absence of induced airway constriction, the inhalation of 300 parts per million (ppm) of NO had a slight bronchodilatory effect as it reduced R_{lung} from 0.138 ± 0.004 to 0.125 ± 0.002 cmH$_2$O/mL/sec ($p < 0.05$) (Fig. 7). In contrast to this slight bronchodilator effect in unconstricted airways, inhalation of 5–300 ppm of NO produced a rapid, dose-dependent, reversible decrease in R_{lung} in guinea-pigs receiving a continuous infusion of methacholine to induce airway obstruction (Fig. 8). Furthermore, over 1 h of treatment, there was no tolerance to the bronchorelaxant action of inhalation of 100 ppm NO nor was any substantial methemoglobinemia observed, as blood levels remained < 2%. Inhaled NO reversed changes in R_{lung} at concentrations that had no effect on C_{dyn}, indicating that the predominant site of action of NO was in the larger, central airways. Finally, with respect to the combined effects of inhaled NO and other bronchodilators, the actions of 100 ppm of inhaled NO and inhaled terbutaline were additive regardless of the sequence of administration.

A similar bronchorelaxant action of inhaled NO was reported by Hogman et al. in a crossover trial of methacholine-induced bronchoconstriction with and without NO in mechanically ventilated, intubated rabbits [23]. The inhalation of 80 ppm of NO had no effect on basal respiratory compliance and resistance, measured using the technique of rapid airway occlusion during constant-flow inflation. However, the bronchoconstrictor effect of exposure to nebulised methacholine (4 mg/mL) was significantly blunted, as resistance only increased to 72 ± 26 cmH$_2$O/L/sec (mean $\pm$ 95% CI) in the presence of inhaled NO vs 107 ± 52 cmH$_2$O/L/sec with methacholine alone ($p < 0.01$). Consistent with the above-described findings of Mehta et al. [40] and Dupuy et al. [9], the predominant action of NO appeared to be

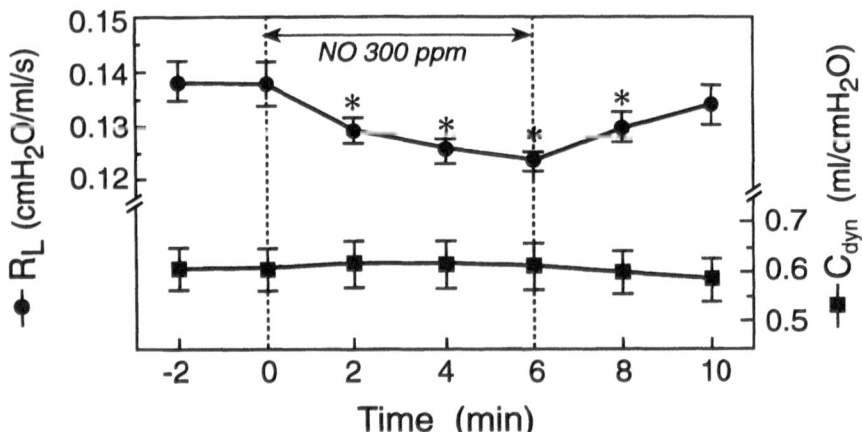

Figure 7. Effects of inhaling 300 ppm NO for 6 min on the baseline pulmonary resistance (R_L) and dynamic compliance (C_{dyn}) of anesthetized guinea-pigs ($n = 8$, mean $\pm$ SE). * $p < 0.05$ differs from time 0.

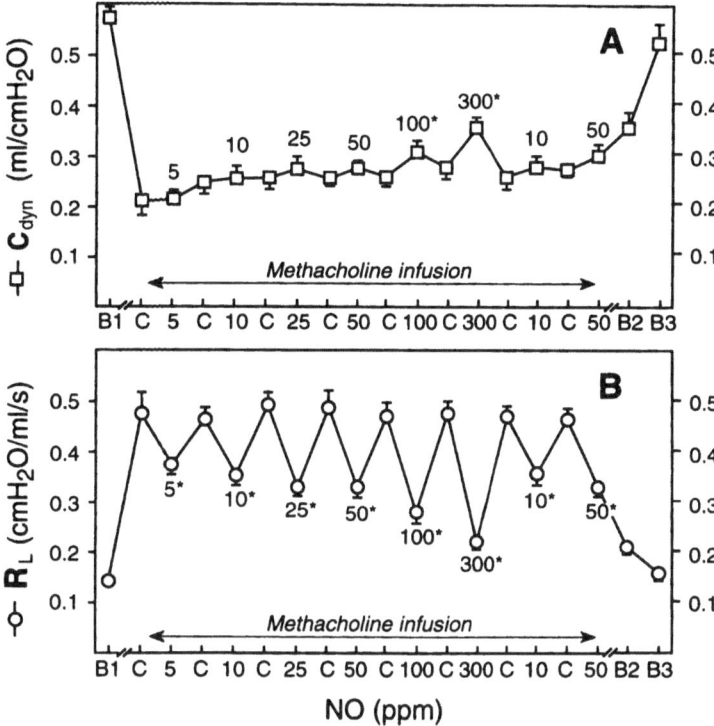

Figure 8. (*A*) Dynamic compliance and (*B*) pulmonary resistance during a continuous infusion of methacholine interspaced with inhalation of varying concentrations of NO (5–300 ppm) at FIO₂ 0.30–0.32. "C" indicates the mean value of R_L and C_{dyn} during the control period before each level of NO inhalation. "B" indicates baseline R_L and C_{dyn} before (*B1*) and after (*B2*) methacholine infusion, and after lung inflation with there times the tidal volume (*B3*) ($n = 8$, mean ± SE). *$p < 0.05$ differs from "C" value at that level of NO inhalation.

at the level of large airways, as inhaled NO had no significant effect on the methacholine-induced fall in respiratory compliance.

Brown et al. used high-resolution computed tomography to assess the effects of inhaled NO on the caliber of airways larger than 1 mm in diameter during exposure of anesthetised, mechanically ventilated dogs to histamine and methacholine [5]. After preconstriction of airways to approximately 60% of control airway area, 100–400 ppm of inhaled NO had a significant dose-dependent relaxant effect in the conducting airways (Fig. 9). At all concentrations, inhaled NO was more effective in reversing bronchoconstriction induced by histamine than by methacholine. Inhaled NO increased airway area to 110±10% of control airway area following histamine-induced constriction, but only to 75±2% of control airway area following methacholine-induced constriction. Attenuation of histamine-induced bronchoconstriction by inhaled NO was significantly blunted by a continuous infusion of 10 mg/min of methylene blue, confirming a cGMP-

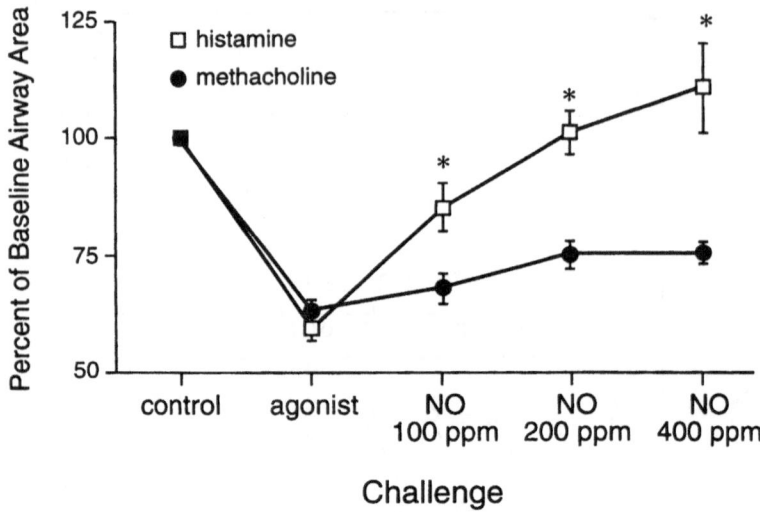

Figure 9. Dose-response attenuation by NO to histamine-induced (*open boxes*) and methacholine-induced (*closed diamonds*) airway constriction. The attenuation by NO of the histamine-induced constriction was significantly greater than the methacholine-induced constriction (*p < 0.01). NO at 200 and 400 ppm completely reversed the histamine-induced constriction (*p < 0.01).

dependent mechanism of NO's action. In this model, histamine's broncho-constrictor action appeared to be primarily mediated through central, vagal reflexes with little or no direct smooth muscle effect, as bronchoconstriction was completely blocked with atropine. Based on these findings, the authors suggest that the selectivity of NO's bronchodilator effects were due to a central, functional antagonism of the effects of histamine and were mediated through stimulation of vagal reflexes, as well as possibly due to a direct relaxant action of NO at the level of the smooth muscle. Moreover, this central action of inhaled NO is consistent with the well-described actions of NO in neural dilator and constrictor airway responses (*vide supra*).

Although several groups have suggested a greater action of both endogenous and inhaled NO in the larger, central airways, Gwyn et al. have demonstrated a bronchodilatory effect of inhaled NO in the peripheral airways of anesthetised dogs, as assessed by the measurement of peripheral airway resistance (R_{periph}) by a wedged bronchoscope technique [20]. These authors studied constrictor responses to acetylcholine, which acts directly on bronchial smooth muscle via muscarinic receptors, and hypocapnia, which does not appear to depend on activation of cholinergic reflexes. NO delivered directly to the peripheral airways via a bronchoscope, in concentrations of 14.5 to 250 ppm, had no effect on baseline R_{periph}, but it attenuated the constrictor responses to hypocapnia, aerosolized acetylcholine, and aerosolized histamine by up to $74 \pm 0\%$, $52 \pm 0\%$, and $83 \pm 6\%$, respectively. Thus, these investigators proposed that the peripheral airways, at least in dogs, respond to levels of inhaled NO that are within the clinically useful range of less than 100 ppm. Given that they had previously reported only a small bronchodilator effect of 250 ppm of inhaled NO in canine peripheral airways preconstricted with intravenous histamine [36], these data suggest that direct airway smooth muscle effects of NO are not the basis for the observed attenuation of hypocapnic and acetylcholine-induced bronchoconstriction. Furthermore, these investigators suggest that inhibition of cholinergic reflexes is also unlikely to be the mechanism of NO's peripheral airway action given that cholinergic reflex activity is limited in the lung periphery. Thus, Gwyn et al. hypothesize that the attenuation of peripheral bronchoconstriction by inhaled NO is mediated through relaxant actions on vascular smooth muscle, known to be sensitive to these relatively low concentrations of NO, and a resulting increase in blood flow to constricted segments, resulting in either washout of acetylcholine or attenuation of the degree of hypocapnia as a result of increased CO_2 delivery.

Consistent with these proposed mechanisms are the findings of Putensen et al. [44], who described the effects of inhaled NO on ventilation-perfusion (V/Q) distributions, as assessed by the multiple inert gas technique, during methacholine-induced bronchoconstriction in mechanically ventilated pigs. The inhalation of 20 and 80 ppm NO significantly reduced R_{lung} and increased lung compliance, and was associated with dose-dependent reductions in pulmonary vascular pressure (38 ± 2 to 31 ± 2 and 30 ± 2 mmHg, with 20 and 80 ppm of NO, respectively, $p < 0.05$ for each vs control) and pulmonary vascular resistance (510 ± 55 to 332 ± 22 and 329 ± 41 dyn sec/cm5, $p < 0.05$ for each vs control), as well as improvements in arterial oxygenation (PaO_2: 65 ± 4 to 90 ± 5 and 104 ± 6 mmHg, $p < 0.05$ for each vs control), oxygen delivery, and shunt fraction (31 ± 2 to 15 ± 2 and $11 \pm 2\%$, $p < 0.05$ for each vs control). In addition, inhalation of 20 and 80 ppm NO reduced blood flow to shunt units by 14 and 19% ($p < 0.05$) and increased perfusion of normal V/Q units by 12 ± 1 and $18 \pm 1\%$ ($p < 0.05$). Although nebulised terbutaline produced a similar reduction in airflow resistance as inhaled NO, it had no effect on pulmonary vascular hemodynamics, blood oxygenation of V/Q matching. Thus, the effects of inhaled NO on airway function may be due, in part, to the significant alterations of pulmonary hemodynamics and blood flow distribution induced by NO.

6.2. Inhaled NO in Humans

Hogman et al. first described the effects of inhaled NO on airway function in humans using plethysmographically-measured specific lung conductance (sGaw) [23 b]. The inhalation of 80 ppm NO had no effect on sGaw in healthy control subjects or in patients with a diagnosis of chronic obstructive pulmonary disease (COPD) whose when FEV_1 was $46 \pm 14\%$

of predicted normal. In nonsmoking subjects with normal spirometry but hyperresponsive airways, the inhalation of NO reduced the dose-normalised effect of methacholine on sGaw to $45 \pm 16\%$ of that observed without NO inhalation. Furthermore, inhaled NO had a significant bronchodilator action in stable, moderate-to-severe asthmatics with a mean FEV_1 of $52 \pm 13\%$. However, in these subjects, the increase in sGaw from 0.4 ± 0.1 to 0.6 ± 0.2 (kPa/sec) ($p < 0.05$) following NO inhalation was small relative to the marked increase to 1.2 ± 0.3 (kPa/sec) with inhaled isoprenaline (Fig. 10). Although it may have no effect on basal airway tone in normal subjects, a slight bronchodilator effect of 80 ppm of inhaled NO was found in normal humans with induced bronchoconstriction [48]. After the induction of long-lasting bronchoconstriction with aerosolized methacholine, sGaw values at specific time points were 23% greater in the presence of inhaled NO than without NO (0.085 ± 0.037 vs 0.069 ± 0.028 (cmH_2O/sec), $p < 0.05$). However, these authors also reported that the bronchodilator action of NO was much less than that usually observed after inhalation of β-sympathomimetic drugs.

Similarly, a minor but significant airway relaxant action of the inhalation of 100 ppm NO was reported after methacholine-induced bronchoconstriction in mild asthmatics not requiring regular steroid medication [28]. After preconstriction with methacholine to an $FEV_1 < 80\%$ of baseline, the inhalation of NO for 9 min produced significant increases in FEV_1 (2.33 ± 0.18 to 2.66 ± 0.18, $p < 0.01$) and FVC, although FEF25 and PEF were un-

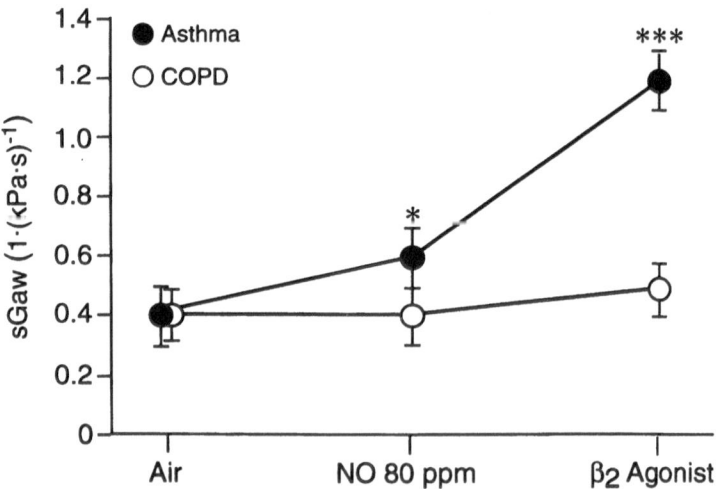

Figure 10. Specific airway conductance (SGaw) in two groups of adult patients with airflow limitations: bronchial asthma (*closed circles*) and chronic obstructive pulmonary disease (*open circles*). Mean values $\pm$ SEM are given for 10 min of air breathing through the system, after 10 min of nitric oxide (NO) at 80 ppm, and after inhalation of a β_2-agonist. *$p < 0.05$, ***$p < 0.0001$.

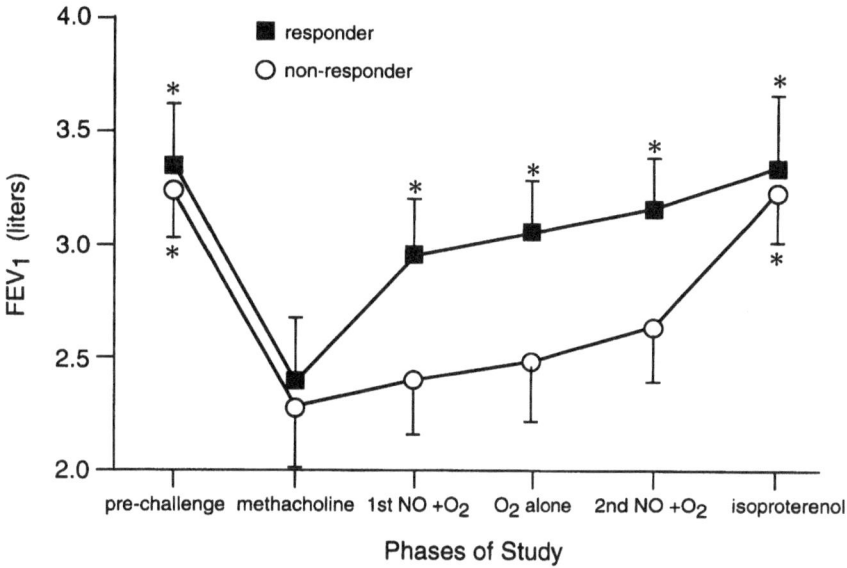

Figure 11. Test subjects were assigned to responder (n = 6) and nonresponder (n = 7) groups. Responders' FEV_1 increased by > 350 ml from the level achieved after methacholine challenge to the level achieved during the first NO inhalation. For all subjects the largest FEV_1, vital capacity (VC), and PEF from each phase was selected, and FEF_{25} was recorded from the breath with the largest VC. *p < 0.01 ANOVA for repeated measure versus methacholine challenge. All values mean ± SEM.

affected (Fig. 11). The improvement in spirometry was maintained after cessation of NO and was not enhanced by readministration of inhaled NO; the spirometric indices did, however, improve markedly and returned to baseline levels following administration of inhaled isoprenaline. In a post hoc subgroup analysis, subjects defined as NO-responders (increase in FEV_1 by $\geq 15\%$ or ≥ 350 mL) were found to have significantly lower levels of bronchial responsiveness to methacholine as evidenced by a higher provoking concentration for a $\geq 20\%$ fall in FEV_1 (PC_{20}, 6.8 ± 2.8 vs 0.46 ± 0.16 mg/mL, p < 0.05) than non-responders, although baseline spirometry was similar between the two groups.

Finally, in a study of pediatric subjects with mild asthma, all of whom were on regular antiinflammatory medication including inhaled steroids in the majority, there was no spirometric improvement after the inhalation of 40 ppm NO [43]; in contrast, inhaled albuterol produced significant improvement in all subjects.

6.3. Bronchodilator Actions of Exogenous NO-Related Compounds

Katsuki and colleagues first described the *in vitro* airway relaxant effects of the NO-releasing agents nitroprusside and nitroglycerin, on bovine and guinea-pig trachea and the concomitant elevation in tissue cyclic guanosine monophosphate (cGMP) levels [29, 30]. These findings have since been confirmed by many others [10, 19, 25, 31, 53]. Although bronchial smooth muscle relaxes in response to the administration of NO and NO-containing and liberating agents, it is generally far less sensitive to these agents than is vascular smooth muscle [52]. The first *in vivo* evidence for NO-congener-related airway relaxation came from Wright et al. who reported that the infusion of nitroprusside in anesthetised, endotoxemic sheep produced bronchodilation, presumably mediated by the liberation of NO [56].

Subsequently, several groups assessed the airway effects of other NO-containing compounds, the S-nitrosothiols (RSNO). Jansen et al. reported significant smooth muscle relaxant properties of RSNO on guinea-pig trachea *in vitro* [26]. Isolated tracheal rings were preconstricted (methacholine, histamine, leukotriene-D_4 (LTD_4)) and the dose of the RSNO required to produce a 50% relaxation (IC_{50}) estimated by linear interpolation. All of the RSNO species studied were effective smooth muscle relaxants with the rank of effectiveness being S-NO-glutathione > S-NO-penicillamine > S-N-acetylcysteine = S-NO-homocysteine > S-NO-cysteine ≫ S-NO-captopril. The effect of RSNO on airway tissue was partially mediated by activation of guanylyl cyclase and cGMP, as the relaxant effect was significantly, but not completely, inhibited by methylene blue ($p < 0.05$), and RSNO-induced, methylene blue-inhibitable increases in tissue cGMP could be measured ($p < 0.0005$). The RSNO species were most active against LTD_4-induced constriction, and progressively less so against contractions induced by histamine and methacholine. The authors suggested that the relaxant properties of the various RSNO species (IC_{50} 0.99–20 µM) were likely of physiological significance in airway homeostasis and potentially of pharmacological relevance as bronchodilators given their potency was intermediate between that of two classical airway smooth muscle relaxants, isoprenaline (IC_{50} 0.016 µM) and theophylline (IC_{50} 74 µM) (Fig. 12).

The observation that significant (nM – µM) levels of RSNO species, predominantly the adduct of NO with glutathione, were present in the airway lining fluid of healthy human subjects provided insight into a potential physiological role of these biologically active, metabolically stable adducts of NO [18]. At physiological concentrations, exogenous S-NO-glutathione induced significant relaxation of preconstricted human bronchial tissue *in vitro*. These initial observations on the relaxant actions of RSNO species on human bronchial tissue *in vitro* were extended by Gaston et al. [17]. As in guinea-pig trachea [26], various RSNO species produced significant relaxation of human bronchi; the order of potency as relaxant agonists in human bronchial tissue was S-NO-glutathione > S-NO-cysteine > S-NO-acetylcysteine ≫ S-NO-BSA. Thus, these agents had a relaxant potency (IC_{50} 3.3–36 µM) intermediate between that of isoprenaline (IC_{50} 0.020 µM) and theophylline (IC_{50} 263 µM). The bronchoconstrictor specificity of the relaxant action of RSNO species in human bronchi was different from

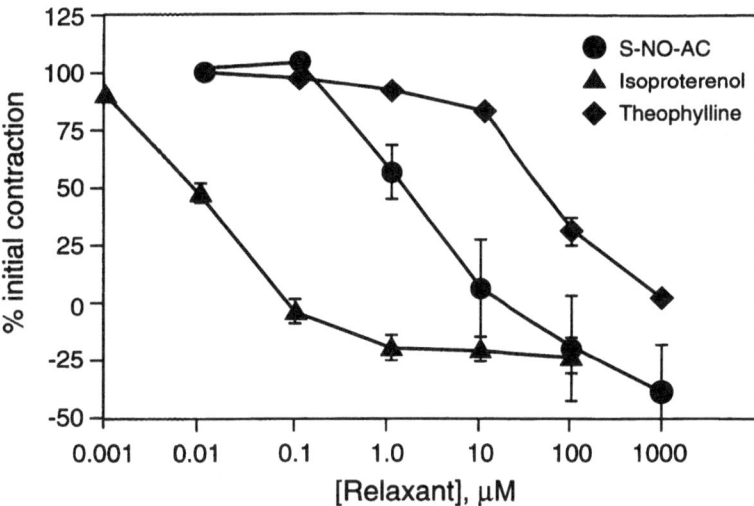

Figure 12. Tracheal relaxant effects of (S-NO-AC), isoproterenol and theophylline. The relaxant activity of S-NO-AC was compared against isoproterenol and theophylline in airways constricted with 3 μM histamine. Concentration-effect relationships reveal an order of potency: isoproterenol (▲) > S-NO-AC(●) > theophylline (◆). The concentration-response curves for these agents are each significantly different from each other by twoway analysis of variance to p < .01. Results are expressed as mean ± SEM (n = 3–5).

that described above in guinea-pig trachea; the relaxant effect was more marked after histamine-induced constriction than after constriction with either methacholine or LTD_4. As in guinea-pig airways, RSNO-induced human airway relaxation was associated with a four-fold increase in tissue cGMP levels; this increase could be significantly inhibited in the presence of methylene blue, but not haemoglobin (Fig. 13). In contrast, the relaxant action of the RSNO species in human bronchi was unaffected by either methylene blue or haemoglobin. These observations suggest that RSNO have a dilator mechanism of action other than simple NO release, as this latter mechanism would have been efficiently inactivated by hemoglobin binding of NO, and other than guanylyl cyclase activation, given the decline in cGMP levels without attenuation of the airway relaxant effect in the presence of methylene blue. Furthermore, the relatively similar potencies of RSNO species of markedly different physical size suggested that RSNO-dependent effects were relatively independent of translocation into the cell. Alternate mechanisms that have been proposed include cGMP-independent pathways such as ADP-ribosylation and nitrosylation of iron-heme centers and sulfhydryl groups of proteins [21, 51].

Of note, only one study has compared the relative potencies of inhaled NO and other NO-containing species: in guinea-pigs, the bronchodilator effect of 100 ppm of inhaled NO was similar to that of aerosolized S-nitroso-N-acetylpenicillamine (SNAP) [9].

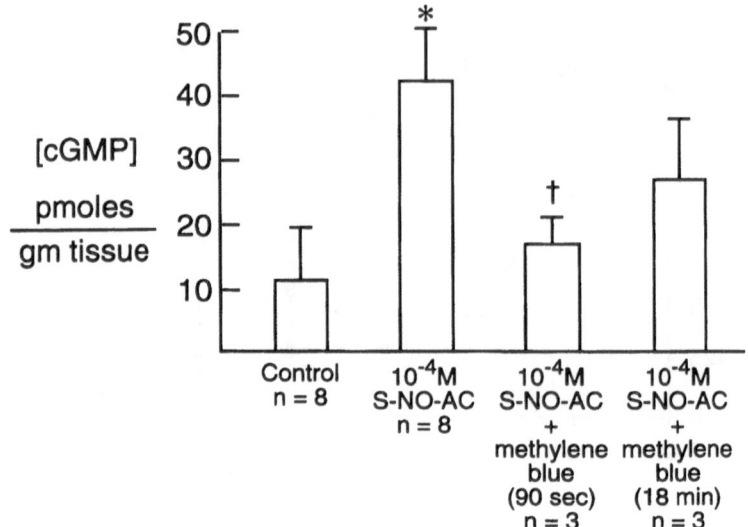

Figure 13. cGMP determinations after exposure to S-NO-AC. Bronchial rings incubated with S-NO-AC (100 µM) for 90 sec (shown) or 18 min (not shown) exhibited 4-fold increases in cGMP over basal levels. Increases in cGMP were attenuated significantly at 90 sec by pretreatment of the tissues with methylene blue (100 µM) for 30 min; the effects of methylene blue at 18 min did not reach statistical significance. Results are presented as mean ± SEM *p < 0.01 with respect to control; *p < 0.05 with respect to S-NO-AC alone.

7. Possible Mechanisms Involved in the Bronchodilator Response to NO and Sources of Endogenous NO

A large body of evidence, collected by many different groups, in different species, in different preparations, *in vitro* and *in vivo*, supports a physiologically and pathophysiologically significant bronchodilatory role of endogenously produced NO in the lungs and airways, and an important effect on airway tone of exogenous NO. Although some of the airway relaxant effects of inhaled NO may be due to a direct smooth muscle action, it is highly likely that the significant physiological effects of inhaled NO at levels between 15 and 100 ppm, especially in the preconstricted airways in animals and in the preconstricted or inflamed airways in humans, are mediated by mechanisms other than direct bronchodilation. Possible mechanisms include alterations of pulmonary vascular hemodynamics thus modifying ventilation-perfusion matching in the lung, and modulation of central, neurogenic reflexes. Similarly, the effects of exogenous NO-containing adducts, such as the RSNO, are clearly not simply due to release of NO or to guanylyl cyclase activation. Regardless of these unsettled questions, NO and the NO-containing compounds are important endogenous bronchodilators and have a lesser role as exogenous bronchodilators. Although they are not as potent as other agents in common clinical use, their limited side-effect profile is quite distinct.

Although a direct muscle effect remains possible for the actions of endogenous NO, other potential mechanisms of its homeostatic role include the modulation of airway microvascular leak [11, 33, 39], interaction with other effector mechanisms, such as neural cholinergic reflexes, the lipoxygenase-leukotriene and neuropeptide systems. Even though the majority of cell types normally present in the airway and lung have been found to have the synthetic capacity to produce and release NO, the most likely sources of endogenous NO are intrinsic airway neurons, bronchial epithelial cells, and vascular endothelial cells.

Finally, currently ongoing and future studies are likely to continue to focus on anatomic sources of the endogenous NO-dependent homeostatic mechanism, the mechanisms of NO's modulatory and bronchodilatory effects, the importance and utility of various measures of NO and NO-equivalents, for example, mixed expired gas NO levels, and on the role of NO in the unique environment of the lung, where the interaction of airway and vasculature is being increasingly appreciated.

8. References

1 Asano K, Chee CBE, Gaston B, Lilly CM, Gerard C, Drazen JM et al (1994) Constitutive and inducible nitric oxide synthase gene expression, regulation, and activity in human lung epithelial cells. *Proc Natl Acad Sci USA* 91: 10089–10093

2 Belvisi MG, Miura M, Stretton D, Barnes PJ (1993) Endogenous vasoactive intestinal peptide and nitric oxide modulate cholinergic neurotransmission in guinea-pig trachea. *Eur J Pharmacol* 231: 97–102

3 Belvisi MG, Stretton CD, Yacoub MH, Barnes PJ (1992) Nitric oxide is the endogenous neurotransmitter of bronchodilator nerves in humans. *Eur J Pharmacol* 210: 221–222

4 Bissonette EY, Hogaboam CM, Wallace JL, Befus AD (1991) Potentiation of tumor necrosis factor mediated cytotoxicity of mast cells by their production of nitric oxide. *J Immunology* 147: 3060–3065

5 Brown RH, Zerhouni EA, Hirshman CA (1994) Reversal of bronchoconstriction by inhaled nitric oxide: Histamine vs. methacholine. *Am J Respir Crit Care Med* 150: 233–237

6 Buga GM, Gold ME, Wood KS, Chaudhuri G, Ignarro JL (1989) Endothelium-derived nitric oxide relaxes nonvascular smooth muscle. *Eur J Pharmacol* 161: 61–72

7 Busse R, Mulsch A (1990) Induction of nitric oxide synthase by cytokines in vascular smooth muscle cells. *FEBS Lett* 275: 87–90

8 Dey RD, Mayer B, Said SI (1993) Colocalization of vasoactive intestinal peptide and nitric oxide synthase in neurons of the ferret trachea. *Neuroscience* 54: 839–843

9 Dupuy PM, Shore SA, Drazen JM, Frostell C, Hill WA, Zapol WM (1992) Bronchodilator action of inhaled nitric oxide in guinea-pigs. *J Clin Invest* 90: 421–428

10 Dusting GJ, Read MA, Stewart AG (1988) Endothelium-derived relaxing factor released from cultured cells: Differentiation from nitric oxide. *Clin Exp Pharmacol Physiol* 15: 83–92

11 Erjefält JS, Erjefält I, Sundler F, Persson CGA (1994) Mucosal nitric oxide may tonically suppress airways plasma exudation. *Am J Respir Crit Care Med* 150: 227–232

12 Fedan JS, Warner TE, Yuan LX, Robinson VA, Frazer DG (1995) Nitric oxide synthase inhibitor and lipopolysaccharide effects on reactivity of guinea-pig airways. *J Pharmacol Exp Ther* 272: 1141–1150

13 Filep JG, Battistini B, Sirois P (1993) Induction by endothelin-1 of epithelium-dependent relaxation of guinea-pig trachea *in vitro*: role for nitric oxide. *Br J Pharmacol* 637–644

14 Fischer A, Mundel P, Mayer B, Preissler U, Philippin B, Kummer W (1993) Nitric oxide synthase in guinea-pig lower airway innervation. *Neuroscience Letters* 149: 157–160

15 Folkerts G, van der Linde HJ, Nijkamp FP (1995) Virus-induced airway hyperresponsiveness in guinea-pigs is related to a deficiency in nitric oxide. *J Clin Invest* 95: 26–30

16 Gao Y, Vanhoutte PM (1993) Attenuation of contractions to acetylcholine in canine bronchi by an endogenous nitric oxide-like substance. *Br J Pharmacol* 109: 887–891

17 Gaston B, Drazen JM, Jansen A, Sugarbaker DA, Loscalzo J, Richards W et al. (1994) Relaxation of human bronchial smooth muscle by S-nitrosothiols *in vitro*. *J Pharmacol Exp Ther* 268: 978–984

18 Gaston B, Reilly J, Drazen JM, Fackler J, Ramdev P, Arnelle D et al. (1993) Endogenous nitric oxides and bronchodilator S-nitrosothiols in human airways. *Proc Natl Acad Sci USA* 90: 10957–10961

19 Gruetter CA, Childres CE, Bosserman MK, Lemke SM, Ball JG, Valentovic MA (1989) Comparison of relaxation induced by glyceryl trinitrate, isosorbide dinitrate and sodium nitroprusside in bovine airways. *Am Rev Respir Dis* 139: 1192–1197

20 Gwyn DR, Lindeman KS, Hirshman CA (1996) Inhaled nitric oxide attenuated bronchoconstriction in canine peripheral airways. *Am J Respir Crit Care Med* 153: 604–609

21 Henry Y, Ducrocq C, Drapier JC, Servent D, Pellat C, Guissani A (1991) Nitric oxide, a biological effector: Electron paramagnetic resonance detection of nitrosyl-iron-protein complexes in whole cells. *Eur Biophys J* 20: 1–15

22 Hibbs JBJ, Taintor RR, Vavrin Z, Rachlin EM (1988) Nitric Oxide: a cytotoxic activated macrophage effector molecule. *Biochem Biophys Res Commun* 157: 87–94

23 Hogman M, Frostell C, Arnberg H, Hedenstierna G (1993) Inhalation of nitric oxide modulates methacholine-induced bronchoconstriction in the rabbit. *Eur Respir J* 6: 177–180

23 b Hogman M, Frostell CG, Hedenstrom H, Hedenstierna G (1993) Inhalation of nitric oxide modulates adult human bronchial tone. *Am Rev Respir Dis* 148: 1474–1478

24 Ignarro LJ (1989) Endothelium-derived nitric oxide: actions and properties. *FASEB J* 3: 31–36

25 Jamieson DD, Taylor KM (1979) Comparison of the bronchodilator and vasodilator activity of sodium azide and sodium nitroprusside in the guinea-pig. *Clin Exp Pharmacol Physiol* 6: 515–525

26 Jansen A, Drazen JM, Osborne JA, Brown R, Loscalzo J, Stamler JS (1992) The relaxant properties in guinea-pig airways of S-nitrosothiols. *J Pharmacol Exp Ther* 216: 154–160

27 Jorens PG, Van Overveld FJ, Bult H, Vermeire PA, Herman AG (1992) Synergism between interleukin-1 beta and interferon gamma, an inducer of nitric oxide synthase, in rat lung fibroblasts. *Eur J Pharmacol* 224: 7–12

28 Kacmarek RM, Ripple R, Cockrill BA, Bloch KJ, Zapol WM, Johnson DC (1996) Inhaled nitric oxide: A bronchodilator in mild asthmatics with methacholine-induced bronchospasm. *Am J Respir Crit Care Med* 153: 128–135

29 Katsuki S, Arnold WA, Murad F (1977) Effect of sodium nitroprusside, nitroglycerine, and sodium azide on levels of cyclic nucleotides and mechanical activity of various tissues. *J Cyclic Nucleotide Res* 3: 239–247

30 Katsuki S, Murad F (1976) Regulation of adenosine cyclic 3',5'-monophosphate and guanosine cyclic 3',5'-monophosphate levels and contractility in bovine tracheal smooth muscle. *Mol Pharmacol* 13: 330–341

31 Kishen R (1985) Some actions of sodium nitroprusside and glyceryl trinitrate on guinea-pig isolated trachealis muscle. *J Pharmacol* 37: 502–504

32 Kobzik L, Bredt DS, Lowenstein CJ, Drazen JM, Gaston B, Sugarbaker D et al (1993) Nitric oxide synthase in human and rat lung: immunocytochemical and histochemical localization. *Am J Respir Cell Mol Biol* 9: 371–377

33 Kuo HP, Liu S, Barnes PJ (1992) The effect of endogenous nitric oxide on neurogenic plasma exudation in guinea-pig airways. *Eur J Pharmacol* 221: 385–388

34 Li CG, Rand MJ (1991) Evidence that part of the NANC relaxant response of guinea-pig trachea to electrical field stimulation is mediated by nitric oxide. *Br J Pharmacol* 102: 91–94

35 Lilly CM, Stamler JS, Gaston B, Meckel C, Loscalzo J, Drazen JM (1993) Modulation of vasoactive intestinal peptide pulmonary relaxation by NO in tracheally superfused guinea-pig lungs. *Am J Physiol* 265: L410–L415

36 Lindeman KS, Aryana A, Hirshman CA (1995) Direct effects of inhaled nitric oxide on canine peripheral airways. *J Appl Physiol* 78: 1898–1903
37 Macquin-Mavier I, Levame M, Istin N, Harf A (1989) Mechanisms of endothelin-mediated bronchoconstriction in the guinea-pig. *J Pharmacol Exp Ther* 250: 740–745
38 Mehta S, Drazen JM, Lilly CM (1997) Endogenous nitric oxide and allergic bronchial hyperresponsiveness in guinea-pigs. *Am J Physiol* 273: L656–L662
39 Mehta S, Boudreau J, Lilly CM, Drazen JM (1998) The role of endogenous nitric oxide in the regulation of airway microvascular leak. *Am J Physiol* 275: L961–968
40 Mehta S, Lilly CM, Rollenhagen JE, Haley KJ, Asano K, Drazen JM (1997) The acute and chronic effects of allergic airway inflammation on pulmonary nitric oxide production. *Am J Physiol* 272: L124–131
41 Nijkamp FP, van der Linde HJ, Folkerts G (1993) Nitric oxide synthesis inhibitors induce airway hyperresponsiveness in the guinea-pig *in vivo* and *in vitro* – Role of the epithelium. *Am Rev Respir Dis* 148: 727–734
42 Persson MG, Gustafsson LE (1993) Allergen-induced airway obstruction in guinea-pigs is associated with changes in nitric oxide levels in exhaled air. *Acta Physiol Scand* 149: 461–466
43 Pfeffer KD, Ellison G, Robertson D, Day RW (1996) The effect of inhaled nitric oxide in pediatric asthma. *Am J Respir Crit Care Med* 153: 747–751
44 Putensen C, Rasanen J, Lopez FA (1995) Improvement in V/Q distributions during inhalation of nitric oxide in pigs with methacholine-induced bronchoconstriction. *Am J Respir Crit Care Med* 151: 116–122
45 Rimele TJ, Sturn RJ, Adams LM, Henry DE, Heaslip RJ, Weichman BM et al (1987) Interaction of neutrophils with vascular smooth muscle: Identification of a neutrophil-derived relaxing factor. *J Pharmacol Exp Ther* 345: 102–111
46 Robbins RA, Hamel FG, Floreani AA, Gossman GL, Nelson KJ, Belenky S et al (1993) Bovine bronchial epithelial cells metabolize L-arginine to L-citrulline: possible role of nitric oxide synthase. *Life Sci* 52: 709–716
47 Robbins RA, Springall DR, Warren JB, Kwon OJ, Buttery LKD, Wilson AJ et al (1994) Inducible nitric oxide synthase is increased in murine lung epithelial cells by cytokine stimulation. *Biochem Biophys Res Commun* 198: 835–843
48 Sanna A, Kurtansky A, Veriter C, Stanescu B (1994) Bronchodilator effect of inhaled nitric oxide in healthy men. *Am J Respir Crit Care Med* 150: 1702–1704
49 Schlemper V, Calixto JB (1994) Nitric oxide pathway-mediated relaxant effect of bradykinin in the guinea-pig isolated trachea. *Br J Pharmacol* 111: 83–88
50 Schmidt HHHW, Gagne GD, Nakane M, Pollock JS, Miller MF, Murad F (1992) Mapping of neural nitric oxide synthase in the rat suggests frequent co-localization with NADPH diaphorase but not with soluble guanylyl cyclase, and novel paraneural functions for nitrinergic signal transduction. *J Histochem Cytochem* 40: 1439–1456
51 Stamler JS, Simon DI, J Osborne A, Mullins ME, Jaraki O, Michel T et al (1992) S-nitrosylation of proteins with nitric oxide; Synthesis and characterization of biologically active compounds. *Proc Natl Acad Sci* 89: 444–448
52 Stuart-Smith K, Bynoe TC, Lindeman KS, Hirshman CA (1994) Differential effects of nitrovasodilators and nitric oxide on procine tracheal and bronchial muscle *in vitro*. *J Appl Physiol* 77: 1142–1147
53 Suzuki K, Kenzo T, Satake T, Sugiyama S, Ozawa T (1986) The relationship between tissue levels of cyclic GMP and tracheal smooth muscle relaxation in the guinea-pig. *Clin Exp Pharmacol Physiol* 13: 39–46
54 Tucker JF, Brave SR, Charalambous L, Hobbs AJ, Gibson A (1990) L-N^G-nitro-arginine inhibits NANC relaxations of guinea-pig isolated tracheal smooth muscle. *Br J Pharmacol* 100: 663–664
55 Ward JK, Belvisi MG, Fox AJ, Miura M, Yacoub MH, Barnes PJ (1993) Modulation of cholinergic neural bronchoconstriction by endogenous nitric oxide and vasoactive intestinal peptide in human airways *in vitro*. *J Clin Invest* 92: 736–742
56 Wright P, Ishihara Y, Bernard GR (1988) Effects of nitroprusside on lung mechanics and hemodynamics after endotoxemia in awake sheep. *J Appl Physiol* 64: 2026–2032

Nitric Oxide in Pulmonary Processes:
Role in Physiology and Pathophysiology of Lung Disease
ed. by M. G. Belvisi and J. A. Mitchell
© 2000 Birkhäuser Verlag Basel/Switzerland

CHAPTER 8
Role of Nitric Oxide in Airway Inflammation

El-Bdaoui Haddad

Department of Pharmacology, Rhône-Poulenc Rorer, Dagenham, Essex RM10 7XS, UK

1 Introduction
2 Role of Nitric Oxide (NO) in Airway Inflammation
3 Role of NO in Eosinophil Migration
4 Effect of NO on Eosinophil Apoptosis
5 Effect of NO on T Lymphocytes
6 Effect of NO on Mast Cells
7 Effect of NO on Macrophage Function
8 Conclusion
9 References

1. Introduction

Nitric oxide (NO) is generated from L-arginine by the enzyme NO synthase (NOS) [1]. NO production requires many cofactors, including nicotinamide dinucleotide phosphate (NADPH), flavin mononucleotide (FMN), flavin adenine dinucleotide (FAD) and tetrahydrobiopterin [1, 2]. Three genes encoding NO synthases are expressed as enzymes in mammals [3, 4]. These enzymes are denoted either by their historical order of cloning or by the cell type from which their cDNA was first cloned. Thus, the human genes encoding neuronal NOS (nNOS), inducible NOS (iNOS), and endothelial NOS (eNOS) are termed NOS1, NOS2, and NOS3, respectively. Of the three major NOS isoforms, eNOS and nNOS are calcium-dependent enzymes, and are generally but not invariably expressed constitutively and denoted therefore cNOS. NOS2 was named "iNOS" to connote its independence of elevated intracellular Ca^{2+}, the distingushing biochemical feature primarily responsible for conferring the capacity of this isoform for more sustained catalysis than typically exercised either by nNOS or eNOS. Because iNOS is expressed in most cells only after induction by immunologic and inflammatory stimuly, the "i" doubles for "inducible". cNOS has been localised in vascular endothelium (eNOS), platelets, and neurons (nNOS) of the central nervous system [1].

With regard to the airways, NO is an important mediator of biological functions in the lung and regulates airway smooth muscle contractility, pulmonary vascular tone, mucus glands secretion, mucociliary clearance through effects on ciliary beat frequency, and immune responses [5–9]. In the respiratory tract, NO is produced by autonomic neurons, fibroblasts, endothelial cells, vascular and airway smooth muscle cells, skeletal muscle cells, inflammatory cells and in airway epithelial cells [6]. NO is also an important mediator of inflammatory responses in the lungs and produces this effect by the formation of reactive nitrogen products that are released from a variety of inflammatory cells [10]. NOS is a key enzyme in the formation of NO and both the cNOS and iNOS isoforms have been described in human alveolar and bronchial epithelia cells [11]. The generation of NO by cNOS is rapid, occurring within seconds [12, 13]. cNOS produces small quantities of NO and is involved in a variety of normal physiological functions such as vasorelaxation, neurotransmission, platelet and leukocyte adhesion [14, 15]. On the other hand, the activity of iNOS can be increased several-fold by activation with cytokines or endotoxin [16–18]. Although maximal induction of iNOS requires several hours, cells will produce NO over a period of several days [17, 18]. NO produced by iNOS plays an important role in host defence mechanisms against bacteria and viruses [19, 20].

2. Role of NO in Airway Inflammation

There is increasing evidence that endogenously produced NO may have both beneficial and detrimental effects in asthma [21]. These differential properties have been attributed to a dual physiologic and pathologic role of NO, depending on the enzyme responsible for its generation. The constitutive isoforms (cNOS) are expressed in neurons and endothelial cells of the airway [22] and are involved in the physiologic regulation of the airway. iNOS is expressed in epithelial cells and inflammatory cells of the airway [16, 23], and may be responsible for the pathologic effects of NO in asthma. Biopsy samples from patients with bronchial asthma show increased iNOS expression in epithelial cells [24], and raised levels of NO are found in exhaled air of patients with bronchial asthma and allergic rhinitis [25–27]. NO has been reported to be increased in the exhaled air of asthmatics during late responses [28, 29]. These data suggest that increased NO production may represent a general feature of airway inflammation. Furthermore, exhaled NO levels rise further during asthma exacerbations [30] and are lowered after treatment with corticosteroids [26]. Recently, it has been demonstrated that eosinophils themselves are a source of NO production in eosinophilic inflammation [31]. In contrast to many other organs where iNOS is not expressed unless induced by cytokines [32], NO is continuously produced by iNOS in normal noninflamed upper and lower airway epithelium [33]. Placed in culture, the cells lose iNOS [33]. Thus, it is difficult to tell whether iNOS in airway epithelium is expressed "constitutively" or is continually "induced".

The pathophysiological consequences, however, of increased NO production in allergic diseases are not yet knwon. The mechanisms by which

NO may be deleterious in asthma are poorly understood, but there is evidence to suggest that excess NO generation may enhance the inflammatory processes underlying asthma [34] as well as producing epithelial cell shedding [35], a characteristic feature of asthma. In laboratory animals, several lines of evidence suggest that iNOS-derived NO is capable of potentiating neurogenic plasma leakage in airways [36, 37]. Furthermore, it has been demonstrated in rat airways, that under "physiological" conditions endogenous NO suppresses plasma leakage but when iNOS is expressed, after lipopolysaccharide (LPS) stimulation, the increased production of NO enhances plasma leakage [38]. We have shown that ozone inhalation induces iNOS expression *in vivo*, suggesting the possible involvement of NO generation in ozone-induced pulmonary inflammation or lung damage [39]. NO can have both direct effects on cell signalling as well as indirect actions mediated by the reaction products formed when NO interacts with other molecules such as oxygen or superoxide [5]. NO rapidly reacts with proteins or with superoxide anions to form peroxynitrite ($ONOO^-$). Most cytotoxic effects of high levels of NO are mediated by peroxynitrite [40–42]. Increased production of NO and superoxide, components of peroxynitrite, have been implicated in the pathogenesis of asthma [43–45]. Peroxynitrite formation has been shown to increase airway hyperresponsiveness, and to cause epithelial cell damage, and eosinophil activation in guinea-pigs [46]. In asthma, there is increased peroxynitrite formation in the airways, as evidenced by a strong immunoreactivity for nitrotyrosine in the airway epithelium and inflammatory cells [47]. The potent oxidant peroxynitrite may therefore contribute to airway obstruction and hyperresponsiveness and epithelial damage in asthma.

In contrast, there is also considerable evidence that NO may be bronchoprotective in asthma [21] and have mast cell-stabilizing properties [48, 49]. NO generated from nNOS is a neurotransmitter released by inhibitory nonadrenergic, noncholinergic (iNANC) nerves [7], counteracts cholinergic bronchoconstriction [50] and inhibits both basal and neurogenic mucus secretion in ferret trachea *in vitro* [51]. Low levels (5–300 ppm) of inhaled NO, or an aerosolised NO-releasing compound are potent bronchodilators in guinea-pigs. The onset of bronchodilation was rapid, beginning within 30 sec after commencing inhalation [52]. Furthermore, inhalation of high concentrations of NO has a small bronchodilating effect in patients with asthma [53, 54], and inhibition of its production with NOS inhibitors increased airway responsiveness in experimental animals and in patients with asthma [55–59].

3. Role of NO in Eosinophil Migration

There is considerable evidence to suggest that NO generated from iNOS is able to enhance the inflammatory processes underlying asthma. In experimental animals, inhaled allergen challenge produces a rapid increase in exhaled NO associated with acute bronchoconstriction, and this rise returns to baseline within 20 min despite continuing bronchoconstriction [60, 61]. This acute increase in NO in experimental animals is also observed after challenge with other spasmogens, such as histamine and leukotriene C_4 [58]. Furthermore, iNOS activity is increased in the lung tissue of sensitised and challenged guinea-pigs [62], suggesting that NO is important in the pathogenesis of allergic lung disorders. Furthermore, it has been shown that exposure of rats to antigen leads to the expression of inducible NO synthase in the epithelium of the airways of sensitised animals 8 hours after antigen challenge [63]. In the same study, little or no expression of mRNA and practically no protein expression for NO synthase was found in inflammatory cells in the airways or in lung lavage after antigen challenge despite the fact that NO synthase can be expressed on inflammatory cells [64, 65]. These data suggest that epithelial cells are the main source of increased expression of iNOS.

We have shown in Brown-Norway rats that there is enhanced iNOS gene expression in lung tissue following ovalbumin sensitisation alone, followed by a further increase in gene expression at 4 hours, with return towards baseline values by 24 hours after exposure to ovalbumin aerosol [66]. Immunohistochemical examination of the lungs revealed that the expression was predominantly in macrophages but not in airway epithelium. In addition, the increase in iNOS mRNA expression was preceded by an increase in NF-κB DNA-binding in the lung. Our data concerning the expression of iNOS following allergen challenge are complementary of those of Yeadon and Price [67] who demonstrated that allergen challenge in the same strain of rats induced increased levels of calcium-independent NOS activity in lung tissue at 6 and 24 hours after allergen exposure. Therefore, enhanced production of NO following allergen challenge is likely to be the result of an increase in iNOS mRNA and protein expression, together with increased NOS activity, particularly in macrophages. This increase in iNOS mRNA expression may be dependent on increased NF-κB binding. The increase in iNOS expression may underlie the increase in exhaled NO found after allergen challenge and may contribute to the development of allergen-induced airway hyperresponsiveness.

In our model, lung macrophages appear to be an important source of iNOS following allergen challenge. Lung macrophages are known to express iNOS and release NO following stimulation with endotoxin or various cytokines including interferon-γ (IFN-γ) interleukin (IL)1β and tumor necrosis factor-α (TNF-α) [17, 32, 68]. However, there is no direct evidence that macrophages release NO on direct activation with allergen. Exposure of sensitised Brown-Norway rats to inhaled allergen increases the number of low affinity immunoglobulin-(Ig)E receptor FCεRII (CD23) on alveolar macrophages [69], an effect probably mediated by the release of IL-4 [70]. Exposure of macrophages with upregulated CD23 expression on exposure to IgE/IgE complexes induces nitrite production [71, 72], supporting a direct effect of allergen in inducing iNOS expression in these cells. Although airway epithelial cells can be induced to express iNOS mRNA and to release nitrite on exposure to cytokines [16, 23], we found no increase in expression of iNOS following either allergen or endotoxin exposure in these cells. It is of interest that the pattern of expression of immunoreactive iNOS in the rats after endotoxin exposure [73] is different from that of allergen exposure.

More direct evidence for a role of NO in airway eosinophilia arises from experiments examining the role of NOS inhibitors on airway inflammation. It has been shown in allergic Balb/C mice that iNOS inhibitors abolish murine airway neutrophilia and eosinophilia following allergen challenge [74]. The inhibitory effect of the selective iNOS inhibitor AMT (2-amino-5,6-dihydro-6-methyl-4H-1,3-thiazine) on broncho-alveolar lavage (BAL) leukocyte accumulation was accompanied by a reduction of the lung mRNA levels of the chemokines lymphotactin, eotaxin, macrophage inflammatory protein (MIP) 1α, MIP-1β, MIP-2, Interferon inducible protein-10 (IP-10), monocyte chemotactic protein (MCP)1 and TCA 3 [75]. These data would suggest the effect of AMT may be mediated partly through inhibition of chemokine expression. It should be noted that the protein levels for IL-4 and IL-5 production from activated lung T cells were increased and IFN-γ production decreased in mice treated with AMT when compared to the control group [75]. Feder et al. [76] have also been able to show an inhibitory effect of non-selective NOS inhibitors on pulmonary eosinophilia in allergic B6D2F1/J mice. Thise response is not due to an effect on bone marrow precursors because NOS inhibitors do not block eosinophil release from the bone marrow. Furthermore, these authors have shown that the NO contributing to the eosinophilia is not generated through the activity of iNOS because the selective iNOS inhibitor, L-NG-(1-Iminoethyl) lysine (L-NIL), had no effect on eosinophil influx into the lungs. Contrary to the findings in allergic rats [66, 67], there was no increase in the level of iNOS protein or mRNA in the lungs or on the levels of nitrite in the (BAL) fluid [76]. However, serum nitrite levels were increased after ovalbumin (OVA) challenge. Similar findings have been reported in OVA-sensitised and challenged guinea-pigs where no detectable increase in NOS activity or mNRA was found in the lungs after antigen challenge even though increased NO was detected in the exhaled air [77]. The authors speculated that the localised production of NO, possibly from pulmonary vascular endothelial cells or mast cells, is involved in the extravasation of eosinophils from the circulation into the lung tissue. Indeed, mast cells have the capacity to synthesise NO [19, 78], and mast cells contribute to the development of pulmonary eosinophilia in allergic mice [79, 80]. NO derived from endothelial cells of lung capillaries and/or bronchial epithelial cells is under control of constitutive endothelial NOS [11, 81, 82] and may be a source of NO. Furthermore, there are several mechanisms by which NO may recruit eosinophils into the lungs following in allergic reaction. As well as having local effects such as increasing vascular permeability and oedema formation which may augment the migration of eosinophils from the blood into the lungs [83, 84], NO, under certain conditions, has also been demonstrated to increase the production of prostaglandings through an action on cyclooxygenase enzyme [85], which may further contribute to the inflammatory process. Additionally, NO is chemotactic for a variety of cell types including eosinophils [86] and may, thereby, play a role in the recruitment of these cells into the lungs of allergic mice. Indeed, in experimental animals chronic treatment with L-N^G-L-arginine methylester (L-NAME) inhibits eosinophil migration *in vivo* and *ex vivo* [87, 88], and this property appears to represent a direct effect of NO on the eosinophil itself.

4. Effect of NO on Eosinophil Apoptosis

Programmed cell death, or apoptosis, is an active process of cellular self destruction with unique morphologic and molecular characteristics including cell shrinkage, membrane blebbing, chromatin condensation, and DNA fragmentation [89]. Apoptotic cell death can result either from developmentally controlled activation of endogenous execution programs or from transduction of death signals triggered by a wide variety of external stimuli or by withdrawal of survival factors such as growth factors or cytokines [90]. A key part of the pathway leading to apoptosis involves the activation of a series of proteolytic enzymes known as the caspases [91].

Inhibition of eosinophil apoptosis has been proposed as a key mechanism for the development of blood and tissue eosinophilia in diseases such as bronchial asthma and other allergic disorders [92, 93]. The delay of eosinophil death might be due, at least in part, to overproduction of T cell-derived cytokines [93]. Besides cytokines, eosinophil apoptosis also seems to be regulated by members of the TNF/nerve growth factor (NGF) receptor superfamily, including the Fas receptor (CD95/APO-1) [94–97]. In allergic mice, the administration of an anti-Fas monoclonal antibody to the lungs produced a marked reduction in the number of eosinophils in the airways [98]. Furthermore, it was demonstrated that NO prevents Fas receptor-mediated apoptosis in freshly isolated human eosinophils through disruption of the Fas receptor-mediated death signalling pathways [99, 100]. These data suggest that NO concentrations within allergic inflammatory sites may be important in determining whether an eosinophil survives or undergoes apoptosis upon Fas ligand stimulation. Similar data also suggest that the Fas activity is under the control of the NO signalling pathway in human leukocytes [101, 102].

5. Effect of NO on T Lymphocytes

Beside a direct effect on eosinophil migration and survival, there is evidence to suggest that endogenously released NO increases eosinophil recruitment into the lungs by modulating the proliferation and the cytokine activity of T lymphocytes [34, 103]. NO inhibits the proliferation of cloned T-helper type 1 (Th$_1$) cells and their production of IL-2 and IFN-γ [104, 105]. By contrast, Th$_2$ cells neither produce nor are affected by NO [104]. The reduction in IL-2 production by NO was shown to be mediated through selective inactivation of the transcription factors NF-κB and NF-AT in the IL-2 promoter [106]. The reduction in IL-2 and IFN-γ production would result in increased antigen-driven proliferation of Th$_2$ cells as IFN-γ from Th$_1$ T cells can inhibit Th$_2$ cells [107]. In a human T cell line (Jurkat cells), the NO generating agent sodium nitroprusside induced a dramatic decrease of IFN-γ, while IL-10 was enhanced; and conversely the inhibition of iNOS activity using L-N^G-monomethyl argine (L-NMMA) induced a clear inhibition of IL-10 and IL-4, while IFN-γ was enhanced [108]. Thus, NO seems to be able to assume the polarisation of activated T cells to the type 2 profile. Furthermore, sodium nitroprusside and S-nitroso-N-acetylpenicillamine (SNAP) increased the secretion of IL-4 in Th$_2$ clones [106]. On the other hand, Th$_2$ cytokines such as IL-4, IL-10 and IL-13 can inhibit the induction of iNOS and in this way may allow some activity of Th$_1$ cells [23, 109, 110]. We have previously found that the sensitised and challenged Brown-Norway rat lung expresses the Th$_2$ cytokines, IL-4 and IL-5 with a reduction in the expression of the Th$_1$ cytokine, IFN-γ [111]. Thus, it is conceivable that the inhibition of IFN-γ expression in sensitised and exposed rats may be due to enhanced iNOS activity, in addition to the enhanced IL-4 expression in rat lung [66, 111]. Thus, iNOS may be involved in the complex balance between Th$_1$ and Th$_2$ cells in immune and inflammatory states, which ultimately favours a Th$_2$ cell outcome. It should be noted that in human T cells and human T cell clones, NO-donors, 3-morpholinosydnonimine (SIN-1) and SNAP, markedly inhibited the release of IFN-γ, IL-2, IL-5, IL-10 and IL-4 by anti-CD3 activated T cells [112]. Unlike in mice, preferential inhibition of Th$_2$-associated cytokines in activated human T cells *in vitro* was not observed [112, 113].

6. Effect of NO on Mast Cells

There is considerable evidence that endogenous NO regulates the reactivity of mast cells in experimental animals [48, 114]. NO is constitutively produced by mast cells [115]. IgE-mediated mast cell degranulation results in the release of a wide variety of spasmogenic mediators in addition to a number of proinflammatory cytokines [116]. IgE-stimulated mucosal mast cells expressed iNOS mRNA and protein and synthesised nitrites suggesting that NO derivatives generated by mast cells could participate in inflammatory reactions during allergic stimulation [117]. NOS inhibitors have been demonstrated not only to increase histamine release from activated rat mast cells *in vitro* [118] but also to produce all the features of mast cell-induced inflammation *in vivo* [119], suggesting that endogenous NO may protect against the effects of inhaled allergen. In inflamed venules, the mast cell-induced histamine-dependent rolling, platelet activating factor (PAF)-dependent adhesion, and albumin leakage were completely inhibited by the addition of the NO donor spermine NO [48]. Furthermore, anti-IgE-induced or ionophore A23187-induced histamine release from human basophils and rat peritoneal mast cells is inhibited by exogenous NO [120]. These data would suggest that NO donors may be a reasonable therapeutic approach to reducing mast cell-dependent inflammation. It should be noted that the mast cell-regulating properties of NO may not be functionally important *in vivo* since endogenous NO neither protects against nor contributes to the processes underlying airway responses to inhaled allergen [121].

7. Effect of NO on Macrophage Function

Alveolar macrophages are the predominant leukocytes found in the air space under homeostatic conditions, and most importantly, the alveolar macrophage has numerous regulatory characteristics [122]. Macrophages have the ability to make cytokines in response to both non-specific stimuli, such as endotoxin, and specific antigen stimulation via IgE-mediated pathways [122, 123].

NO, generated from DETA NONOate (2,2-(hydroxynitrosohydrazono)-bis-ethanamine) inhibited LPS-stimulated inflammatory cytokine production (TNF-α, IL-1β, MIP-1α) by human alveolar macrophages [124]. NO did not affect basal cytokine levels. These findings indicate that NO functions as antiinflammatory through downregulation of proinflammatory-cytokine secretion by stimulated normal human alveolar macrophages [124]. The release of macrophage proinflammatory cytokines is generally secondary to increased gene transcription, which is controlled by activation of transcription factors such as NF-κB [125, 126]. Interestingly, endogenous NO has been shown in human endothelial cells to inhibit the activation of NF-κB. This effect is mediated through increased mRNA expression, stabilisation and increased transcription of the NF-κB inhibitor, IκBα, by preventing its degradation from NF-κB [127, 128]. Similarly, the NO donors, decreased TNF-α-induced vascular cell adhesion molecule (VCAM)-1, intercellular cell adhesion molecule (ICAM)-1, and E-selectin expression through increased expression of IκBα [129]. For a full review of the effect of NO on macrophage function, the readers are invited to consult recent reviews [130, 131].

8. Conclusion

Whilst this simple inorganic gas plays an important role in the physiology and pathophysiology of airway diseases such as asthma, the true extent of this role has yet to be determined. iNOS expression is induced by signals associated with inflammation such as in asthma and rheumatoid arthritis. Therefore iNOS inhibitors might constitute a therapeutic target. However, NO possesses both pro- and antiinflammatory properties. The antiinflammatory role of iNOS emphasises the possibility of adverse consequences attendant on its inhibition. These dichotomies in NO function warrant caution but do not preclude therapeutic intervention with either iNOS inhibitors, iNOS, cDNAs, NO, or NO donors. The development of more specific iNOS inhibitors will undoubtedly allow a more precise definition of the pro- and antiinflammatory roles of this molecule in airway diseases.

9. References

1　Sessa WC (1994) The nitric oxide synthase family of proteins. *J Vasc Res* 31: 131–143
2　Nathan C, Xie Q-W (1994) Minireview: regulation of biosynthesis of nitric oxide. *J Biol Chem* 269: 13725–13728
3　Michel T, Xie Q-W, Nathan C (1996) Molecular biological analysis of nitric oxide synthases. In: Feelisch M, Stamler JS (eds) Methods in Nitric Oxide Research. Chichester: Wiley & Sons, 161–175
4　Förstermann U, Closs EI, Pollock JS, Nakane M, Scharz P, Gath I et al (1994) Nitric oxide synthase isoforms: characterization, purification, molecular cloning, and functions. *Hypertension* 23: 1121–1127
5　Schmidt HHHW, Walter U (1994) NO at work. *Cell* 78: 919–925
6　Barnes PJ, Belvisi MG (1993) Nitric oxide and lung disease. *Thorax* 48: 1034–1043
7　Belvisi MG, Stretton CD, Yacoub M, Barnes PJ (1992) Nitric oxide is the endogenous neurotransmitter of bronchodilator nerves in humans. *Eur J Pharmacol* 210: 221–222
8　Nijkamp FP, Folkerts G (1994) Nitric oxide and bronchial reactivity. *Clin Exp Allergy* 24: 905–914
9　Adler KB, Fischer BM, Li H, Choe NH, Wright DT (1995) Hypersecretion of mucin in response to inflammatory mediators by guinea-pig tracheal epithelial cells *in vitro* is blocked by inhibition of nitric oxide synthase. *Am J Respir Cell Mol Biol* 13: 526–530
10　Jorens PG, VanOverveld FJ, Butt H, Vermeire PA, Herman AG (1991) L-arginine-dependent production of nitric oxides by rat pulmonary macrophages. *Eur J Pharmacol* 200: 205–209
11　Asano K, Chee CBE, Gaston B, Lilly CM, Gerard C, Drazen JM et al (1994) Constitutive and inducible nitric oxide synthase gene expression, regulation and activity in human lung epithelial cells. *Proc Natl Acad Sci* 91: 10089–10093
12　Furchgott RF (1983) Role of endothelium in responses of vascular smooth muscle. *Circulation Res* 53: 557–573
13　Werner-Felmayer G, Werner ER, Fuchs D, Hausen A, Reibnegger G, Wachter H (1991) On multiple forms of NO synthase and their occurences in human cells. *Res Immunol* 142: 555–600
14　Moncada S, Higgs A (1993) The L-arginine-nitric oxide pathway. *N Eng J Med* 329: 2002–2012
15　Szabo C, Thiemermann C (1995) Regulation of the expression of the inducible isoform of nitric oxide synthase. *Adv Pharmacol* 34: 113–153
16　Robbins RA, Barnes PJ, Springall DR, Warren JB, Kwon OJ, Buttery LDK et al (1994) Expression of inducible nitric oxide synthase in human bronchial epithelial cells. *Biochem Biophys Res Commun* 203: 209–218

17 Stuehr DJ, Marletta MA (1987) Synthesis of nitrite and nitrate in murine macrophage cell lines. *Cancer Res* 47: 5590–5594

18 Marletta MA, Yoon PS, Iyengar R, Leaf CP, Wishnot JS (1988) Macrophage oxidation of L-arginine to nitrite and nitrate: nitric oxide is an intermedite. *Biochem* 27: 8706–8711

19 Nathan C (1992) Nitric oxide as a secretory product of mammalian cells. *FASEB J* 6: 3051

20 Hibbs J Jr (1991) Synthesis of nitric oxide from L-arginine: a recently discoverd pathway induced by cytokines with antitumor and antimicrobial activity. *Res Immunol* 142: 565–569

21 Barnes PJ (1996) NO or no NO in asthma? *Thorax* 51: 218–220

22 Kobzik L, Bredt DS, Lowenstein CJ, Drazen J, Gaston B, Sugarbaker D et al (1993) Nitric oxide synthase in human and rat lung: immunocytochemical and histochemical localization. *Am J Respir Cell Mol Biol* 9: 371–377

23 Berkman N, Robichaud A, Robbins RA, Roesems G, Haddad EB, Barnes PJ et al (1996) Inhibition of inducible nitric oxide synthase expression by interleukin-4 and interleukin-13 in human lung epithelial cells. *Immunology* 89: 363–367

24 Hamid Q, Springall DR, Riveros-Moreno V, Chanez P, Howarth P, Redington A et al (1993) Induction of nitric oxide synthase in asthma. *Lancet* 342: 1510–1513

25 Alving KE, Weitzberg E, Lundberg JM (1993) Increased amount of nitric oxide in exhaled air of asthmatics. *Eur Respir J* 6: 1268–1370

26 Kharitonov SA, Yates D, Robbins RA, Logan-Sinclair R, Shinebourne E, Barnes PJ (1994) Increased nitric oxide in exhaled air of asthmatic patients. *Lancet* 343: 133–135

27 Kharitonov SA, Rajakulasingam K, O'Connor BJ, Durham SR, Barnes PJ (1997) Nasal nitric oxide is increased in patients with asthma and allergic rhinitis and may be modulated by nasal glucocorticoids. *J Allergy Clin Immunol* 99: 58–64

28 Kharitonov SA, O'Connor BJ, Evans DJ, Barnes PJ (1995) Allergen-induced late asthmatic reactions are associated with elevation of exhaled nitric oxide. *Am J Respir Crit Care Med* 151: 1894–1899

29 Deykin A, Massaro AF, McGarry WP, McFadden CA, Drazen JM, Israel E (1995) Exhaled nitric oxide following allergen challenge in atopic patients with asthma. *Am J Respir Crit Care Med* 151: A699

30 Massaro AF, Gaston B, Kita D, Fanta C, Stamler J, Drazen JM (1995) Expired nitric oxide levels during treatment for acute asthma. *Am J Respir Crit Care Med* 152: 800–803

31 del Pozo V, de Arruda-Chaves E, de Andrés B, Cardaba B, Lopez-Farré A, Gallardo S et al (1997) Eosinophils transcribe and translate messenger RNA for inducible nitric oxide synthase. *J Immunol* 158: 859–864

32 Nathan CF, Xie QW (1994) Nitric oxide synthases: Roles, tools, and controls. *Cell* 78: 915

33 Guo FH, De Raeve HR, Rice TW, Stuehr DJ, Tunnissen FBJM, Erzurum SC (1995) Continuous nitric oxide synthesis by inducible nitric oxide synthase in normal human airway epithelium *in vivo*. *Proc Natl Acad Sci* 92: 7809–7813

34 Barnes PJ, Liew FW (1995) Nitric oxide and asthmatic inflammation. *Immunol Today* 16: 128–130

35 Heiss LN, Lancaster JR, Corbett JA, Goldman WE (1994) Epithelial autotoxicity of nitric oxide: role in the respiratory cytopathology of pertussis. *Proc Natl Acad Sci* 91: 267–270

36 Kageyama N, Miura M, Ichinose M, Tomaki M, Ishikawa J, Ohuchi Y et al (1997) Role of endogenous nitric oxide in airway microvascular leakage induced by inflammatory mediators. *Eur Respir J* 70: 13–19

37 Ohuchi Y, Ichinose M, Miura M, Kageyama N, Tomaki M, Endoh N et al (1998) Induction of nitric oxide synthase by lipopolysaccharide inhalation enhances substance P-induced microvascular leakage in guinea-pigs. *Eur Respir J* 12: 831–836

38 Bernareggi M, Mitchell JA, Barnes PJ, Belvisi MG (1997) Dual action of nitric oxide on airway plasma leakage. *Am J Respir Crit Care Med* 155: 869–874

39 Haddad E-B, Liu S, Salmon M, Koto H, Barnes PJ, Chung KF (1995) Expression of inducible nitric oxide synthase mRNA in Brown-Norway rats exposed to ozone: effect of dexamethasone. *Eur J Pharmacol* 293: 287–290

40 Ischiropoulos H, Zhu L, Beckman JS (1992) Peroxynitrite formation from macrophage-derived nitric oxide. *Arch Biochem Biophys* 298: 446–451

41 Lipton SA, Choi YB, Pan ZH, Lei SZ, Chen HS, Sucher NJ et al (1993) A redox-based mechanism for the neuroprotective and neurodestructive effects of nitric oxide and related nitroso-compounds. *Nature* 364: 626–632

42 Radi R, Beckman JS, Bush KM, Freeman BA (1991) Peroxynitrite oxidation of sulf-hydryls. The cytotoxic potential of superoxide and nitric oxide. *J Biol Chem* 4244–4250

43 Calhoun WJ, Reed HE, Moest DR, Stevens CA (1992) Enhanced superoxide production by alveolar macrophages and airspace cells, airway inflammation and alveolar macro-phage density changes after segmental antigen bronchoprovocation in allergic subjects. *Am Rev Respir Dis* 145: 317–325

44 Barnes PJ (1996) Pathophysiology of asthma. *Br J Clin Pharmacol* 42: 3–10

45 Teramoto S, Shu CY, Ouchi Y, Fukuchi Y (1996) Increased spontaneous production and generation of superoxide anion by blood neutrophils in patients with asthma. *J Asthma* 33: 149–155

46 Sadeghi-Hashjin G, Folkerts G, Henricks PAJ, Verheyen AKCP, Linde HJ, Ark I et al (1996) Peroxynitrite induces airway hyperresponsiveness in guinea-pigs *in vitro* and *in vivo*. *Am J Respir Crit Care Med* 153: 1697–1701

47 Saleh D, Ernst P, Lim S, Barnes PJ, Giaid A (1998) Increased formation of the potent oxidant peroxynitrite in the airways of asthmatic patients is associated with induction of nitric oxide synthase: effect of inhaled glucocorticoid. *FASEB J* 12: 929–937

48 Gaboury JP, Niu XF, Kubes P (1996) Nitric oxide inhibits numerous features of mast cell induced inflammation. *Circulation* 93: 318–326

49 Valentovic MA, Ball JG, Morenas M, Szarek JL, Gruetter CA (1992) Influence of nitrovasodilators on bovine pulmonary histamine release. *Pulmonol Pharmacol* 5: 97–102

50 Ward JK, Belvisi MG, Fox AJ, Miura M, Tadjkarimi S, Yacoub MH et al (1993) Modulation of cholinergic neural bronchoconstriction by endogenous nitric oxide and vasoactive intestinal peptide in human airways *in vitro*. *J Clin Invest* 92: 736–743

51 Ramnarine SI, Khawaja AM, Barnes PJ, Rogers DF (1996) Nitric oxide inhibition of basal and neurogenic mucus secretion in ferret trachea *in vitro*. *Br J Pharmacol* 118: 998–1002

52 Dupuy PM, Shore SA, Drazen JM, Frostell C, Hill WA, Zapol WM (1992) Bronchodilator action of inhaled nitric oxide in guinea-pigs. *J Clin Invest* 90: 421–428

53 Hogman M, Frostell C, Arnberg H, Hedenstierna G (1993) Inhalation of nitric oxide modulates methacholine-induced bronchoconstriciton in the rabbit. *Eur Respir J* 6: 177–180

54 Hogman M, Frostell CG, Hedenstrom H, Hadenstierna G (1993) Inhalation of nitric oxide modulates adult human bronchial tone. *Am Rev Respir Dis* 148: 1474–1478

55 Nijkamp FP, Van der Linde HJ, Folkerts G (1993) Nitric oxide synthesis inhibitors induce airway hyperresponsiveness in the guinea-pig *in vivo* and *in vitro*. *Am Rev Respir Dis* 148: 727–734

56 Ricciardolo FLM, Geppetti P, Mistretta A, Nadel JA, Sapienza MA, Bellofiore S et al (1996) Randomized double-blind placebo-controlled study of the effect of inhibition of nitric oxide synthesis in bradykinin-induced asthma. *Lancet* 348: 374–377

57 Ricciardolo FLM, Nadel JA, Yoshihara S, Geppetti P (1994) Evidence for reduction of bradykinin-induced bronchoconstriction in guinea-pigs by release of nitric oxide. *Br J Pharmacol* 113: 1147–1152

58 Persson MG, Friberg SG, Gustafsson LE, Hedqvist P (1995) The promotion of patent airways and inhibition of antigen-induced bronchial obstruction by endogenous nitric oxide. *Br J Pharmacol* 116: 2957–2962

59 Mehta S, Lilly CG, Rollenhagen JE, Haley KJ, Asano K, Drazen JM (1997) Acute and chronic effects of allergic airway inflammation in pulmonary nitric oxide production. *Am J Physiol* 272: L124–L31

60 Persson MG, Gustafson LE (1993) Allergen-induced airway obstruction in guinea-pigs is associated with changes in nitric oxide levels in exhaled air. *Acta Physiol Scand* 149: 461–466

61 Persson MG, Wiklund NP, Gustafsson LE (1993) Endogenous nitric oxide in single exhalations and the change during exercise. *Am Rev Respir Dis* 148: 1210–1214

62 Yan Z-Q, Hansson GK, Skoogh B-E, Lötvall JO (1995) Induction of nitric oxide synthase in a model of allergic occupational asthma. *Allergy* 50: 760–764

63 Renzi PM, Sebastiao N, Al Assaad AS, Giaid A, Hamid Q (1997) Inducible nitric oxide synthase mRNA and immunoreactivity in the lungs of rats eight hours after antigen challenge. *Am J Respir Cell Mol Ciol* 17: 36–40

64 Bissonnette EY, Hogaboam CM, Wallace JL, Befus AD (1991) Potentiation of tumor necrosis factor-α-mediated cytoxicity of mast cells by their production of nitric oxide. *J Immunol* 147: 3060–3065

65 Holt PG, Olivier J, Bilyk N, McMenamin C, McMenamin PG, Kraal G et al (1993) Down-regulation of the antigen presenting cell function(s) of pulmonary dendritic cells *in vivo* by resident alveolar macrophages. *J Exp Med* 177: 397–407

66 Liu SF, Haddad E-B, Adcock IM, Salmon M, Koto H, Gilbey T et al (1997) Inducible nitric oxide synthase after sensitization and allergen challenge of Brown Norway rat lung. *Br J Pharmacol* 121: 1241–1246

67 Yeadon M, Price R (1995) Induction of calcium-independent nitric oxide synthase by allergen challenge in sensitized rat lung *in vivo. Br J Pharmacol* 116: 2545–2546

68 Modolell M, Corraliza IM, Link F, Soler G, Eichmann K (1995) Reciprocal regulation of the nitric oxide synthase/arginase balance in mouse bone marrow-derived macrophages by TH1 and TH2 cytokines. *Eur J Immunol* 25: 1101–1104

69 Mencia Huerta JM, Dugas B, Boichot E, Petit Frere C, Paul Eugene N, Lagente V et al (1991) Pharmacological modulation of the antigen-induced expression of the low-affinity IgE receptor (Fc epsilon RII/CD23) on rat alveolar macrophages. *Int Arch Allergy Appl Immunol* 94: 295–298

70 Paul-Eugene N, Kolb JP, Calenda A, Gordon J, Kikutani H, Kishimoto T et al. (1993) Functional interaction between β_2-adrenoceptor agonists and interleukin-4 in the regulation of CD23 expression and release and IgE production in human. *Mol Immunol* 30: 157–164

71 Paul-Eugene N, Kolb JP, Damais C, Dugas B (1994) Heterogenous nitrite production by IL-4-stimulated human monocytes and peripheral blood mononuclear cells. *Immunology Letters* 42: 31–34

72 Becherel PA, Mossalayi MD, Ouaaz F, Le Goff L, Dugas B, Paul-Eugene N et al (1994) Involvement of cyclic AMP and nitric oxide in immunoglobulin E-dependent activation of FcεRII/CD23$^+$ normal human keratinocytes. *J Clin Invest* 93: 2275–2279

73 Liu S, Adcock IM, Old RW, Barnes PJ, Evans TW (1993) Lipopolysaccharide treatment *in vivo* induces widespread tissue expression of inducible nitric oxide synthase mRNA. *Biochem Biophys Res Commun* 196: 1208–1213

74 Trifilieff A, Fujitani Y, Fuentes M, Bertrand C (1996) Inducible nitric oxide synthase (iNOS) inhibitors inhibit airway eosinophilia following allergen challenge in mice. *Eur Resp J* 9: 35F

75 Trifilieff A, Fujitani Y, Fuentes M, Bertrand C (1998) Inducible nitric oxide synthase (iNOS) inhibitors inhibit airway leukocyte infiltration in a murine model of lung inflammation: down-regulation of chemokine mRNA levels. *Am J Resp Crit Care Med* 157: A713

76 Feder LS, Stelts D, Chapman RW, Manfra D, Crawley Y, Jones H et al (1997) Role of nitric oxide on eosinophilic lung inflammation in allergic mice. *Am J Respir Cell Mol Biol* 17: 436–442

77 Mehta S, Lilly CM, Haley KH, Asano K, Massaro AF, Drazen JM (1996) Increased nitric oxide production during actue allergic bronchoconstriction. *Am J Respir Crit Care Med* 153: A796

78 Moncada S, Palmer RMJ, Higgs EA (1991) Nitric oxide physiology, pathophysiology and pharmacology. *Pharmacol Rev* 43: 109

79 Kung TT, Stelts D, Zurcher J, Jones H, Umland SP, Kreutner W et al (1995) Mast cells modulate allergic pulmonary eosinophilia in mice. *Am J Respir Cell Mol Biol* 12: 404–409

80 Wardlaw AJ, Dunnette S, Gleich GJ, Collins JV, Kay AB (1988) Eosinophils and mast cells in bronchoalveolar lavage in subjects with mild asthma. *Am Rev Respir Dis* 173: 62 69

81 Shaul RW, North AJ, Wu LC, Wells LB, Brannon TS, Lau KS et al (1994) Endothelial nitric oxide synthase is expressed in cultured human bronchial epithelium. *J Clin Invest* 94: 2231–2236

82 Ignarro LJ, Byrns RE, Buga GM, Wood KS (1987) Endothelium-derived relaxing factor from pulmonary artery and vein possesses pharmacologic and chemical properties identical to those of nitric oxide radical. *Circ Res* 61: 866–879

83 Kuo H-P, Liu S, Barnes PJ (1992) The effect of endogenous nitric oxide on neurogenic plasma exudation in guinea-pig airways. *Eur J Pharmacol* 221: 385–388

84 Li X-Y, Donaldson K, MacNee W (1998) Lipopolysaccharide-induced alveolar epithelial permeability: The role of nitric oxide. *Am J Respir Crit Care Med* 157: 1027–1033

85 Salvemini D, Misko TP, Masferrer JL, Currie MG, Needleman P (1993) Nitric oxide activates cyclooxygenase enzymes. *Proc Natl Acad Sci* 90: 7240–7244

86 Belenky SN, Robbins RA, Rennard SI, Gossman GL, Nelson KJ, Rubinstein I (1993) Inhibitors of nitric oxide synthase attenuate human neutrophil chemotaxis *in vitro. J Lab Clin Med* 122: 388–394

87 Ferreira HHA, Madeiros MV, Lima CSP, Flores CA, Sannomiya P, Antunes E et al (1996) Inhibition of eosinophil chemotaxis by chronic blockade of nitric oxide biosynthesis. *Eur J Pharmacol* 310: 201–207

88 Zanardo RC, Costa E, Ferreira HH, Antunes E, Martins AR, Murad F et al (1997) Pharmacological and immunohistochemical evidence for a functional nitric oxide synthase system in rat peritoneal eosinophils. *Proc Natl Acad Sci* 94: 14111–14114

89 Cohen JJ (1993) Apoptosis. *Immunol Today* 14: 126–130

90 Steller H (1995) Mechanisms and genes of cellular suicide. *Science* 267: 1445–1449

91 Henkart PA (1996) ICE family proteases: Mediators of all apoptotic cell death? *Immunity* 4: 195

92 Simon HU, Blaser K (1995) Inhibition of programmed eosinophil death: a key pathogenic event for eosinophilia? *Immunol Today* 16: 53–55

93 Simon H-U, Yousefi S, Schranz C, Schapowall A, Bachert C, Blaser K (1997) Direct demonstration of delayed eosinophil apoptosis as a mechanism causing tissue eosinophilia. *J Immunol* 158: 3902–3908

94 Matsumoto K, Schleimer RP, Saito H, Iikura Y, Bochner BS (1995) Induction of apoptosis in human eosinophils by anti-Fas antibody treatment *in vitro*. *Blood* 86: 1437–1443

95 Druilhe A, Cai Z, Hailé S, Chonaib S, Petrolani M (1996) Fas-mediated apoptosis in cultured human eosinophils. *Blood* 87: 2822–2830

96 Baker SJ, Reddy EP (1996) Transducers of life and death: TNF receptor superfamily and associated proteins. *Oncogene* 12: 1

97 Nagata S (1997) Apoptosis by death factor. *Cell* 88: 355

98 Tsuyuki S, Bertrand C, Erard F, Trifilieff A, Tsuyuki J, Wesp M et al (1995) Activation of the Fas receptor on lung eosinophils leads to apoptosis and the resolution of eosinophilic inflammation of the airways. *J Clin Invest* 96: 2924–2931

99 Hebestreit H, Dibbert B, Balatti I, Braun D, Schapowal A, Blaser K et al (1998) Disruption of Fas receptor signaling by nitric oxide in eosinophils. *J Exp Med* 187: 415–425

100 Hebestreit H, Yousefi S, Balatti I, Weber M, Crameri R, Simon D et al (1996) Expression and function of the Fas receptor on human blood and tissue eosinophils. *Eur J Immunol* 26: 1775–1780

101 Beauvais F, Michel L, Dubertret L (1995) The nitric oxide donors, azide and hydroxylamine, inhibit the programmed cell death of cytokine-deprived human eosinophils. *FEBS Lett* 361: 229–232

102 Mannick JB, Miao XQ, Stamler JS (1997) Nitric oxide inhibits Fas-induced apoptosis. *J Biol Chem* 272: 24125–24128

103 Liew FY (1995) Nitric oxide in infectious and autoimmune diseases. *Ciba Found Symp* 195: 234–239

104 Taylor-Robinson AW, Liew FY, Severn A, Xu D, McSorley SJ, Garside P et al (1994) Regulation of the immune response by nitric oxide differentially produced by T helper type 1 and T helper type 2 cells. *Eur J Immunol* 24: 980–984

105 Taylor-Robinson AW (1997) Counter-regulation of T helper 1 cell proliferation by nitric oxide and interleukin-2. *Biochem Biophys Res Commun* 233: 14–19

106 Chang RH, Feng MH, Liu WH, Lai MZ (1997) Nitric oxide increased interleukin-4 expression in T lymphocytes. *Immunology* 90: 364–369

107 Gajewski TF, Fitch FW (1988) Anti-proliferative effect of IFN-gamma in immune regulation. I. IFN-γ inhibits the proliferation of Th2 but not Th1 murine helper T lymphocyte clones. *J Immunol* 140: 4245–4248

108 Benbernou N, Esnault S, Shin HCK, Fekkar H, Guenounou M (1997) Differential regulation of INF-gamma IL-10 and inducible nitric oxide synthase in human T cells by cyclic AMP-dependent signal transduction pathway. *Immunology* 91: 361–368

109 Liew FY, Li Y, Severn A, Millott S, Schmidt J, Salter M et al (1991) A possible novel pathway of regulation by murine T helper type-2 (Th2) cells of a Th1 cell activity via the modulation of the induction of nitric oxide synthase on macrophages. *Eur J Immunol* 21: 2489–2494

110 Cunha FQ, Moncada S, Liew FY (1992) Interleukin-10 (IL-10) inhibits the induction of nitric oxide synthase by interferon-gamma in murine macrophages. *Biochem Biophys Res Commun* 182: 1155–1159

111 Haczku A, MayAry P, Haddad E-B, Huang TJ, Kemeny M, Moqbel R et al (1996) Expression of Th-2 cytokines IL-4 and IL-5 and of Th-1 cytokine IFN-γ in ovalbumin-exposed sensitised Brown-Norway rats. *Immunology* 88: 247–251

112 Bauer H, Jung T, Tsikas D, Stichtenoth DO, Frolich JC, Neumann C (1997) Nitric oxide inhibits the secretion of T-helper 1- and T-helper 2-associated cytokines in activated human T cells. *Immunology* 90: 205–211

113 Shoker AS, Yang H, Murabit MA, Jamil H, Al Ghoul A, Okasha K (1997) Analysis of the *in vitro* effect of exogenous nitric oxide on human lymphocytes. *Mol Cell Biochem* 171: 75–83

114 Salvemini D, Masini E, Pistelli A, Mannaioni PF, Vane JR (1991) Nitric oxide: a regulatory mediator of mast cell reactivity. *J Cardiovasc Pharmacol* 17: S258

115 Hogaboam CM, Befus AD, Wallace JL (1993) Modulation of rat mast cell reactivity by IL-1β: divergent effects on nitric oxide and platelet-activating factor release. *J Immunol* 151: 3767–3774

116 Galli SJ (1993) New concepts about the mast cell. *N Engl J Med* 328: 257–265

117 Bidri M, Ktorza S, Vouldoukis L, Le-Goff L, Debre P, Guillosson JJ et al (1997) Nitric oxide pathway is induced by FcεRI and up-regulated by stem cell factor in mouse mast cells. *Eur J Immunol* 27: 2907–2913

118 Masini E, Salvemini D, Pistelli A, Mannaioni PF, Vane JR (1991) Rat mast cells synthesize a nitric oxide like-factor which modulates the release of histamine. *Agents Actions* 33: 61–63

119 Kanwar S, Wallace JL, Befus AD, Kubes P (1994) Nitric oxide synthesis inhibition increases epithelial permeability via mast cells. *Am J Physiol* 266: 222–229

120 Iikura M, Takaishi T, Hirai K, Yamada H, Iida M, Koshino T et al (1998) Exogenous nitric oxide regulates the degranulation of human basophils and rat peritoneal mast cells. *Int Arch Allergy Immunol* 115: 129–136

121 Taylor DA, Mcgrath JL, O'Connor BJ, Barnes PJ (1998) Allergen-induced early and late asthmatic responses are not affected by inhibition of endogenous nitric oxide. *J Am J Respir Crit Care Med* 158: 99–106

122 Lukacs NW, Strieter RM, Kunkel SL (1995) Leukocyte infiltration in allergic airway inflammation. *Am J Respir Cell Mol Biol* 13: 1–6

123 Kelly J (1990) Cytokines of the lung. *Am Rev Respir Dis* 141: 765–788

124 Thomassen MJ, Buhrow LT, Connors MJ, Kaneko FT, Erzurum SC, Kavuru MS (1997) Nitric oxide inhibits inflammatory cytokine production by human alveolar macrophages. *Am J Respir Cell Mol Biol* 17: 279–283

125 Baeuerle PA, Henkel T (1994) Function and activation of NF-κB in the immune system. *Annu Rev Immunol* 12: 141–179

126 Barnes PJ, Karin M (1997) Nuclear factor-κB: a pivotal transcription factor in chronic inflammatory diseases. *N Engl J Med* 336: 1066–1071

127 Zeiher AM, Fisslthaler B, Schray-Utz B, Busse R (1995) Nitric oxide modulates the expression of monocyte chemoattractant protein 1 in cultured human endothelial cells. *Circ Res* 76: 980–986

128 Peng HB, Libby P, Liao JK (1995) Induction and stabilization of IκBα by nitric oxide mediates inhibition of NF-κB. *J Biol Chem* 270: 14214–14219

129 Spiecker M, Peng HB, Liao JK (1997) Inhibition of endothelial vascular cell adhesion molecule-1 expression by nitric oxide involves the induction and nuclear translocation of IκBα. *J Biol Chem* 272: 30969–30974

130 MacMicking J, Yie QW, Nathan C (1997) Nitric oxide and macrophage function. *Ann Rev Immunol* 15: 323–350

131 Nathan C (1997) Inducible nitric oxide synthase: What difference does it make? *J Clin Invest* 100: 2417–2423

Therapeutic Potential of Inhaled Nitric Oxide and Nitric Oxide Synthase Inhibitors in Lung Disease

Nitric Oxide in Pulmonary Processes:
Role in Physiology and Pathophysiology of Lung Disease
ed. by M. G. Belvisi and J. A. Mitchell
© 2000 Birkhäuser Verlag Basel/Switzerland

CHAPTER 9
Nitric Oxide in Exhaled Air: Relevance in Inflammatory Lung Disease

Peter J. Barnes and Sergei A. Kharitonov

Department of Thoracic Medicine, National Heart and Lung Institute, Imperial College School of Medicine, Dovehouse Street, London SW3 6LY, UK

1   Introduction
2   How is Nitric Oxide (NO) in Exhaled Air Measured?
3   Factors Affecting Exhaled NO in Normal Individuals
4   Source of NO in Exhaled Air
5   Functional Relevance of Exhaled NO
6   Effect of Disease on Exhaled NO
6.1 Asthma
6.2 Bronchiectasis
6.3 Chronic Airways Disease
6.4 Vascular Disease
6.5 Infections
6.6 Nasal Disease
7   Effects of Therapy
8   Future Directions
9   References

1. Introduction

Nitric oxide (NO) is produced by many cells within the respiratory tract and endogenous NO may play an important signalling role in the physiological control of airway function and in the pathophysiology of airway diseases [1–3]. All three isoforms of NO synthase (NOS) exist within the respiratory tract [4–6]. The endothelial constitutive isoform (eNOS) is localised to bronchial endothelial cells and to epithelial cells [7] and the neuronal isoform (nNOS) to parasympathetic nerves and to epithelial cells [8, 9]. Inducible NOS (iNOS) may be localised to several cell types, including epithelial cells and macrophages [10–12] and may be expressed even in the normal human respiratory tract (Fig. 1).

Gustafsson and colleagues first demonstrated that NO can be deteced in the exhaled air of animals and normal human subjects [13] and this has subsequently been confirmed in many studies [14–20]. Furthermore, the concentration of exhaled NO is increased in patients with inflammatory diseases of the airways, such as asthma [15, 16, 21] and bronchiectasis [22] and is reduced by glucocorticoid therapy [23, 24]. This suggests that ex-

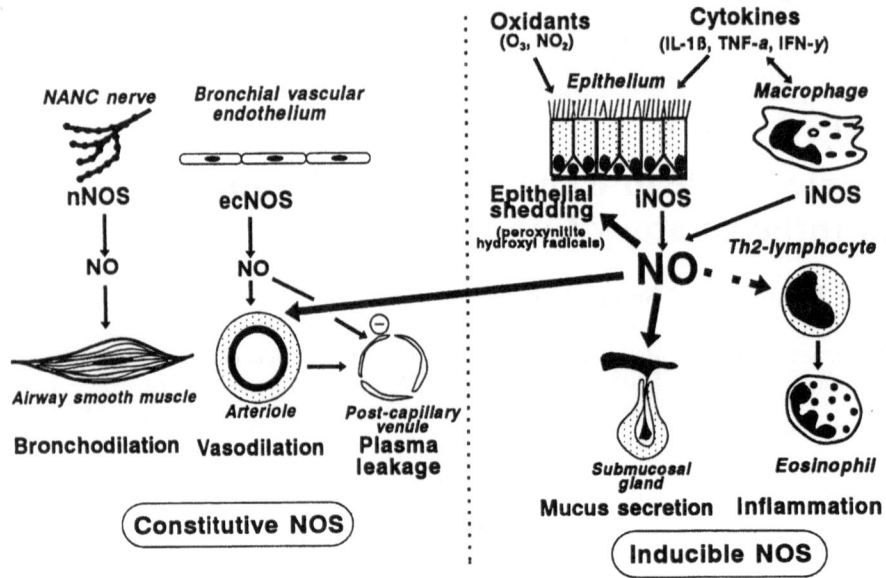

Figure 1. Sources of nitric oxide (NO) in the airways. NO is derived from constitutive (eNOS, nNOS) and inducible isoforms (iNOS) of NO synthase.

haled NO may provide a non-invasive means of monitoring inflammation in the respiratory tract and the measurement of exhalend NO has attracted increasing interest [25].

2. How is NO in Exhaled Air Measured?

Most studies have measured NO in exhaled air by chemiluminescence and detection depends on the photochemical reaction between NO and ozone generated in the analyser [26]. The specificity of exhaled NO measurements by chemiluminescence has recently been confirmed using gas chromatography-mass spectrometry [19]. Several NO analysers are now commercially available, but may need to be converted for on-line measurement of NO in exhaled air. Most analysers are sensitive to < 1 part per billion (ppb) of NO and this is adequate for studies of exhaled air. NO may be detected by direct expiration into the analyser (Fig. 2) or by collection into an impermeable reservoir or balloon for later analysis.

Several technical factors may affect the measurement of exhaled NO and it is important that the technique should be specified, so that comparisons between studies is possible. Breath-holding results in an increase in exhaled NO, which may reflect accumulation of NO in the upper or lower respiratory tracts [17, 27]. High concentrations of NO have been detected in the upper respiratory tract and nasopharynx, with particularly high con-

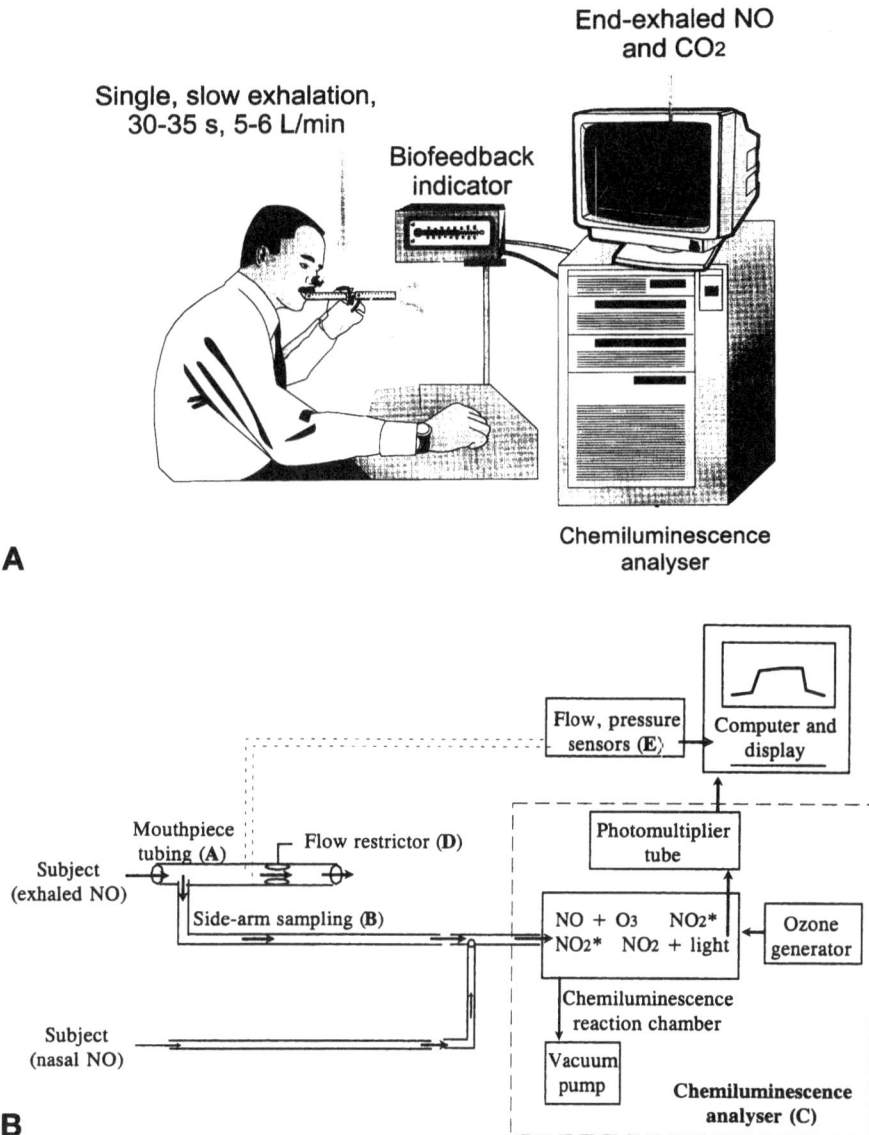

Figure 2. Measurement of exhaled nitric oxide (NO) by chemiluminescence analyser using a single slow expiration. *A:* Seated subject expires slowly into the mouthpiece keeping flow and pressure constant. *B:* Schematic diagram of the chemiluminescence analyser.

centrations in the paranasal sinuses [12, 28, 29]. This has suggested that exhaled NO may largely reflect NO derived from the upper airways, rather than the lower airways. The manoeuvres that block the upper respiratory tract markedly reduce exhaled NO concentrations [30] and much lower levels of NO are recorded from the lower respiratory tract of patients with

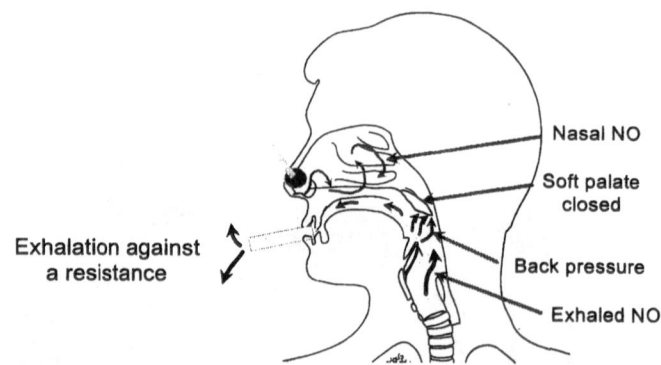

Figure 3. Expiration against resistance causes a closure of the soft palate and thus prevents conta-mination of exhaled air with the high concentration of nitric oxide (NO) within the nose.

tracheostomies that exclude the upper respiratory tract [28, 29]. Expiration against a resistance prevents any nasal contamination, as this leads to iso-lation of the nasopharynx from the oropharynx by elevation of the soft palate (Fig. 3). Thus slow expiration against resistance produces levels of exhaled NO in the expired air that are identical to those measured by direct sampling via a bronchoscope from the lower respiratory tract in both nor-mal and asthmatic patients [31]. During quiet tidal breathing, however, there may be nasal contamination of the exhaled NO as there is a commu-nication between the nasopharynx and oropharynx. This means that collec-tion of expired air in a reservoir during tidal breathing may overestimate exhaled NO levels from the lower respiratory tract due to nasal contamina-tion.

3. Factors Affecting Exhaled NO in Normal Individuals

Breath-holding causes a marked rise in exhaled NO [17, 31] and values recorded with a nose-clip may be higher due to increased diffusion of NO from the upper respiratory tract into the nasopharynx. Flow, but not pres-sure, have an effect on exhaled NO, and increasing flow results in lower values of exhaled NO [27, 32]. In normal individuals there is marked ele-vation of NO in exhaled air with upper respiratory tract infections [33]. This may be a reflection of iNOS induction by virus infection in the upper airways. In normal subjects orally administered L-arginine results in an increase in exhaled NO, presumably reflecting increased synthesis due to provision of more substrate for NOS [34].

The effect of exercise is complex, with a progressive fall in exhaled NO with increasing exercise but correction for increased ventilation shows an increased production of NO [17, 35]. Hyperventilation at rest also in-creases exhaled NO, albeit to a lesser extent than exercise [17]. The mechanism for increased exhaled NO during exercise and hyperventilation is not yet certain, but may involve increased entrainment of NO from the upper respiratory tract.

Chronic cigarette smokers have lower levels of exhaled NO than non-smokers [21, 36, 37] and there is a close correlation between the reduction in exhaled NO and the number of cigarettes smoked [37]. Active smoking causes a further, but transient, fall in exhaled NO, indicating that exhaled NO is reduced by acute and chronic effects of cigarette smoking. Since cigarettes generate a very high concentrations of NO, it is possible that this is due to downregulation of NOS by NO, as has been demonstrated for both the constitutive and inducible enzymes [38–40]. The inhibition of endogenous NO production in the respiratory tract may contribute to reduced mucociliary clearance in smokers, as endogenous NO appears to be important in ciliary beating [41] and possibly to an increased susceptibility to lower respiratory tract infections.

Ethanol also has an effect on exhaled NO. Although there is no effect on exhaled NO in normal individuals, a significant decrease has been reported in asthmatic patients, suggesting that ethanol may inhibit iNOS expression [42]. This is consistent with the demonstration that ethanol decreases iNOS expression in alveolar macrophages [43]. This is associated with decreased killing of microorganisms and might contribute to the increases susceptibility to infection with chronic alcoholism.

4. Source of NO in Exhaled Air

The cellular source of NO in the lower respiratory tract is not yet certain. Studies with perfused porcine lungs suggest that exhaled NO originates at the alveolar surface, rather than from the pulmonary circulation [44], and may be derived from eNOS expressed in the alveolar walls of normal lungs [4]. Studies in ventilated perfused lungs of guinea-pigs show that exhaled NO is reduced during perfusion with calcium-free solutions, suggesting that NO is derived from a constitutive NOS, which is calcium-dependent [18]. Airway epithelial cells may also express both eNOS and nNOS and therefore contribute to NO in the lower respiratory tract [7, 9]. In inflammatory diseases, it is likely that the increase in exhaled NO is due to induction of iNOS. Indeed increased NOS activity has been demonstrated in lung tissue of patients with asthma, cystic fibrosis and obliterative bronchiolitis [45]. In asthmatic patients there is evidence for increased expression of iNOS in airway epithelial cells [10], although even epithelial cells from normal individuals appear to express iNOS [11]. Proinflammatory cytokines induce the expression of iNOS in murine epithelial cells and cultured human airway epithelial cells [9, 46, 47] and it is likely that these same cytokines are released in asthmatic inflammation. iNOS may be expressed in other cell types, such as alveolar macrophages and other inflammatory cells. Furthermore, glucocorticoids inhibit the induction of iNOS in epithelial cells *in vitro* [46, 47] and *in vivo* [48] and reduce exhaled NO levels in asthmatic patients to normal [24]. In bronchiectasis there is some evidence for iNOS expression in macrophages of affected lung [6].

The levels of NO in the nose and nasopharynx are much higher than those recorded in expiration at the mouth, suggesting that upper airway may be the major contributor to exhaled NO, at least in normal individuals [28–31, 49]. However, the lower respiratory tract is likely to contribute some of the exhaled NO, even in normal individuals. NO has been detected in the exhaled air of tracheotomised rabbits, rats, guinea-pigs and humans [13, 28] and via bronchoscopy in normal individuals [31, 50]. The products of NO metabolism, nitrite and nitrothiols are also present in bronchoalveolar lavage (BAL) of normal subjects [51]. Simultaneous measurement of expired CO_2 and NO demonstrate that the peak in exhaled NO precedes the peak value of CO_2 (end-tidal), suggesting that NO is derived from airways rather than alveoli [17]. Although it is likely that nasal NO contributes to the levels of exhaled NO in normal individuals, it is unlikely to contribute to the elevated levels found in inflammatory airway disease. Direct sampling via fibreoptic bronchoscopy in asthmatic patients shows a similar elevation of NO in trachea and main bronchi to that recorded at the mouth, thus indicating that the elevated levels in asthma are derived from the lower airways [31, 50].

5. Functional Relevance of Exhaled NO

NO gas may be a useful marker of airway and pulmonary disease, but it may also play a physiological and pathophysiological role. Endogenous NO may have both beneficial and deleterious effects on the airways [52] (Fig. 1). The high concentrations of NO generated in the paranasal sinuses may have a sterilising effect in the sinuses and upper respiratory tract, since NO is toxic to bacteria, parasites and viruses [53]. NO derived from the lower respiratory tract may also contribute to host defence and the fact that iNOS can be rapidly expressed in airway epithelial cells provides a rapid non-specific defence mechanisms in the respiratory tract. Targeted disruption ("knock-out") of the iNOS gene in mice results in marked increase in susceptibility to infections [54, 55].

NO in the respiratory tract may also have an effect on the bronchial and pulmonary circulations [56–59]. NO is a potent vasodilator and the increased production of NO in asthmatic airways may underlie the hyperaemia seen in asthmatic airways. Inhalation of high concentrations of NO from the upper respiratory tract and that derived from the lower respiratory tract may have effects on ventilation-perfusion (V/Q) matching within the lungs. Thus in inflammatory conditions, such as asthma, there may be increased V/Q matching due to pulmonary vasodilatation in response to autoinhalation of endogenously generated NO, resulting in increased hypoxaemia due to shunting. The role of endoenous NO in V/Q matching remains to be determined.

Although endogenous NO appears to be the major bronchodilator neurotransmitter in humans [60, 61], high concentrations of inspired NO have only weak bronchodilator and bronchoprotective effects [62–64], so it is unlikely that endogenous NO is an important determinant of airway calibre. Indeed marked inhibition of endogenous NO production by nebulised NOS inhibitors has no detectable effect on airway function, even in patients with asthma [23, 65].

6. Effect of Disease on Exhaled NO

The level of NO in exhaled air is altered in several diseases (Tab. 1).

Table 1. Factors affecting exhaled nitric oxide (NO)

Increased NO	Decreased NO
Breath-holding	Cigarette smoking
Exercise/hyperventilation	Pulmonary hypertension
L-arginine (oral)	Kartagener's syndrome
Upper respiratory tract infections	Cystic fibrosis
Asthma	Glucocorticoids
Allergen challenge (late response)	NOS Inhibitors
Bronchiectasis	
Lower respiratory tract infection	
Endotoxin	

6.1. Asthma

Several studies have reported an elevation of exhaled NO in patients with asthma [15, 16, 21, 66] (Fig. 4). The increase in exhaled NO does not appear to be related to asthma severity or to airway responsiveness (measured by methacholine challenge) and exhaled NO is not elevated in asthmatic patients controlled with inhaled steroids [16]. Changes in bronchial calibre have no effect on exhaled NO as neither bronchoconstriction with histamine or methacholine, nor bronchodilatation with salbutamol have any effect on the measurement in asthmatic patients [67–69]. Immunocytochemical staining of bronchial biopsies has demonstrated increased expression of iNOS in epithelial cells in asthmatic compared to non-asthmatic subjects [10], suggesting that proinflammatory cytokines present in asthmatic airways have induced its expression, resulting in increased NO production in the lower airways. After inhaled allergen challenge in asthmatic patients there is no change of exhaled NO during the early

EXHALED NITRIC OXIDE

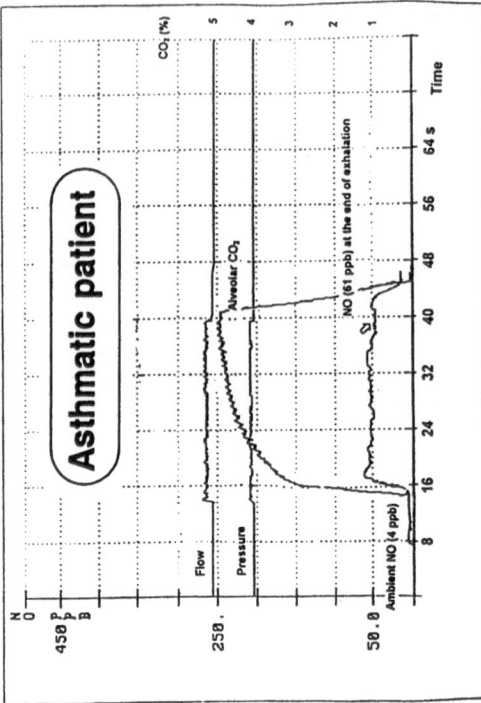

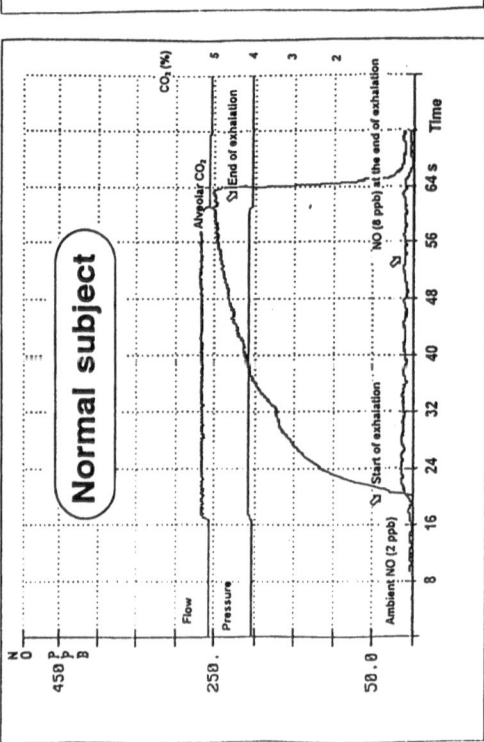

Figure 4. Increased exhaled nitric oxide (NO) in patients with asthma. *Left panel* shows a tracing from a normal subject (exhaled NO 8 ppb); *Right panel* from a patient with asthma (exhaled NO 61 ppb)

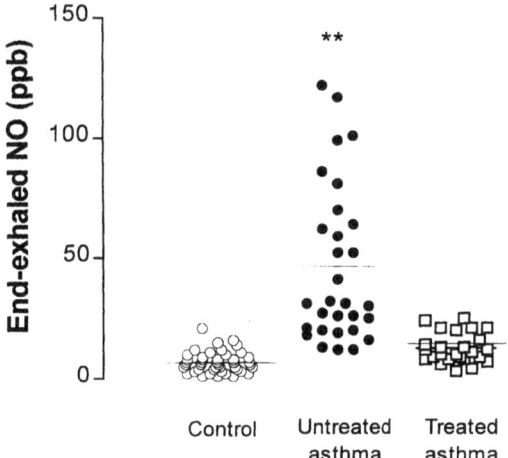

Figure 4 (continued). This panel shows data from a group of normal control subjects (○), untreated asthmatic patients (●) and asthmatic patients treated with inhaled steroids (□).

bronchoconstrictor response, but a progressive elevation during the late response [67]. In patients who have no late response to allergen (single responders), there is no change in exhaled NO throughout the study period. The suggests that increased NO is associated with the inflammatory late response and may be a reflection of iNOS expression in response to inflammatory cytokines. In sensitised guinea-pigs allergen challenge is associated with increased NO production during the late response and this is preceded by iNOS mRNA expression [70]. Whether increased NO production is merely a marker of the cytokine-mediated inflammation, or contributes to the airway narrowing (secondary to vasodilatation and increased plasma exudation) during the late response is not yet certain and studies with NOS inhibitors are needed. There is also an increse in exhaled NO during exacerbations of asthma [71, 72] and when the dose of inhaled glucocorticoids is reduced [73]. By contrast, there is no increase in exhaled NO after bronchoconstriction induced by histamine (direct effect on airway smooth muscle) or by adenosine (via activation of airway mast cells [67, 74]. These findings suggest that exhaled NO may reflect airway inflammation in asthma and may be used as a means of monitoring inflammatory events in the lower airways.

6.2. Bronchiectasis

Elevated levels of exhaled NO has also been detected in patients with bronchiectasis and the level of NO is related to the extent of disease, as measured by a computerised tomography score [22]. As in asthma, the elevation of exhaled NO is not seen in patients treated with inhaled steroids

[22]. This suggests that exhaled NO in bronchiectasis may reflect active inflammation in the lower airways and may be used to monitor disease activity.

6.3. Chronic Airways Disease

Although the airways are inflamed in cystic fibrosis, surprisingly there is no elevation of exhaled NO [75, 76]. Indeed there appears to be a decrease in nasal NO in children with cystic fibrosis [76] and in exhaled NO in adults [77]. It is possible that exhaled NO levels become elevated during infective exacerbations and there are also anecdotal reports of elevated exhaled NO in association with lower respiratory tract infections [15].

In patients with chronic bronchitis and chronic obstructive pulmonary disease (COPD) there is an active inflammatory process, with a predominantly neutrophilic inflammation [78]. Surprisingly exhaled NO has been reported to be normal in these patients [66, 79]. This may be because neutrophilic inflammation is not associated with increased iNOS expression or that cigarette smoking may block any tendency for iNOS expression. However, it does suggest that exhaled NO might be used to discriminate asthma from COPD.

6.4. Vascular Disease

In patients with pulmonary hypertension, secondary to systemic sclerosis, there is a reduction in exhaled NO compared to normal subjects and to patients with interstitial lung disease without pulmonary hypertension [80]. This may be a reflection of the reduced eNOS expression described in patients with pulmonary hypertension [81]. The reduced endogenous production in the vessels of patients with pulmonary hypertension may contribute to the vasoconstriction of pulmonary vessels and to the increased proliferation of vascular smooth muscle cells in this condition [82].

A reduction in exhaled NO has also been reported in systemic hypertension [36]; this is more difficult to explain, but may reflect a generalised defect in endothelial NOS function.

6.5 Infections

Endotoxin induces iNOS in animal lungs [83] and preliminary studies show that lipopolysaccharide inhalation in normal individuals results in an increase in exhaled NO [84]. Exhaled NO is also increased in an animal model of sepsis, suggesting that it may be useful in the early management of adult respiratory distress syndrome.

6.6. Nasal Disease

High concentrations of NO have been detected in the nose of normal individuals [28–30, 49] and very high concentrations in the paranasal sinuses [12]. This may be inhaled into the lower respiratory tract and exhaled and may contribute to the exhaled NO measured at the mouth. It was suggested that the high concentrations of NO may be derived from bacteria which colonise the nose, as higher values were found in patients with penicillinase-resistant *Staphylococcus aureus* [28]. Bacteria may stimulate the local production of NO by induction of NO synthase [85] and bacteria themselves may synthesise NO [86, 87]. However, treatment of normal subjects with a course of antibiotics fails to reduce nasal NO concentrations [29].

Elevated nasal NO has been described in patients with allergic and perennial rhinitis [88, 89] and may be due to allergic inflammation in the nose. This may reflect the increased expression of iNOS in epithelial cells of patients with allergic rhinitis [5]. Very low levels of NO have been detected in the nose of patients with Kartagner's syndrome, in which there is a congenital defect in ciliary activity [29]. Endogenous NO appears to be important in ciliary beating [41] and in the absence of NO there may be ciliary stasis.

7. Effects of Therapy

Exhaled NO levels are significantly lower in patients with asthma and bronchiectasis who are treated with inhaled glucocorticoids, suggesting that inhaled steroids reduce exhaled NO [16, 22]. An oral glucocorticoid prednisolone (30 mg for 3 days) has no effect on exhaled NO in normal individuals, but decreases the elevated levels of exhaled NO in asthmatic patients [23]. This suggests that the exhaled NO in normal subjects is derived from constitutive NOS (unaffected by steroids), whereas the elevated levels in asthma are derived from iNOS, which is inhibited by glucocorticoids. In asthmatic patients a double-blind study of inhaled budesonide shows a progressive reduction in exhaled NO down to normal values after three weeks of therapy [24]. The reduction in exhaled NO is progressive and may reflect direct inhibitory effects of glucocorticoids on induction of iNOS, via an direct blockade of the transcription factor nuclear factor-kappa B (NF-κB) and an indirect effect due to reduced synthesis of the pro-inflammatory cytokines that lead to iNOS expression in airway epithelia cells. Biopsy studies have confirmed that iNOS expression in asthmatic airway epithelial cells in reduced in patients treated with inhaled steroids [48]. NO production in rhinitic patients, measured by the concentration of nitrite and nitrate in nasal lavage fluid, is apparently unaffected by topical glucocorticoids, suggesting that nasal NO may not be derived from iNOS or originates from cells that cannot be reached by topically applied steroids [90]. However, measurement of nasal NO shows a reduction after topical steroids, although the reduction is relatively small in magnitude, suggesting that only a fraction of nasal NO is derived from the steroid-repressible iNOS expressed in the nasal mucosa [89]. NO is produced in high concentrations by an enzyme expressed in paranasal sinuses that has similarities to iNOS, but does not appear to be repressed by glucocorticoids [12].

Neither short-acting nor long-acting inhaled β_2-agonists reduce exhaled NO in asthmatic patients [69]. This is in keeping with other studies show-ing no antiinflammatory effect of inhaled β_2-agonists in asthma [91, 92] and add further support to the view that exhaled NO may be useful in asses-sing antiinflammatory effect of inhaled asthma treatments.

Several analogues of L-arginine, such as N^G-monomethyl-L-arginine (L-NMMA) and N^G-nitro-L-arginine methylester (L-NAME) act as false substrates and block NOS activity. These NOS inhibitors have been in-valuable in investigating the role of endogenous NO in animal models and may have some therapeutic potential. Single inhalations of L-NMMA and L-NAME (via a nebuliser) result in reduced exhaled NO in normal and asthmatic patients [16, 23, 93]. Interestingly, there is no fall in forced ex-pired volume in one second (FEV_1), even in asthmatic patients with highly reactive airways, suggesting that basal production of NO is not important in basal airway tone. Although infusion of L-NMMA in normal subjects causes an increase in blood pressure [94, 95], neither nebulised L-NAME nor L-NMMA have any effect on heart rate or blood pressure, suggesting that inhibition of NOS is confined to the respiratory tract. While L-NMMA and L-NAME are non-selective inhibitors of constitutive NOS and iNOS, aminoguanidine has some selectivity for iNOS [96, 97]. Inhalation of aminoguanidine has no effect on exhaled NO in normal subjects, but sig-nificantly reduces exhaled NO in patients with asthma [65], adding further support to the view that the elevated exhaled NO in asthma is derived form iNOS.

8. Future Directions

The measurement of exhaled NO has excited considerable interest as it may provide a simple noninvasive means of measuring airway inflammation. There is now persuasive evidence that levels of NO are increased in asso-ciation with airway inflammation and are decreased with antiinflammatory treatments. Correlation of exhaled NO with more direct measurements of inflammation in the airways, such as induced sputum, BAL and bronchial biopsies, is now needed. There is a correlation between exhaled NO and the number of eosinophil in induced sputum of asthmatic patients, but this is only a weak correlation and it is unlikely that expression of iNOS will reflect all of the inflammatory changes present in asthmatic airways [98].

The great advantage of exhaled NO is that the measurement is completely non-invasive and can therefore by performed repeatedly and also in children [75, 76] and patients with severe airflow obstruction [71], where more invasive techniques are not possible. The measurement, however, is not specific and exhaled NO is increased in inflammation due to asthma, bronchiectasis and respiratory tract infections. This means that absolute values are less important than serial measurements in individual patients. The value of this approach has been demonstrated in asthmatic patients where the dose of inhaled steroid is changed, resulting in increased levels when the dose is reduced and lower levels when the dose is increased [73]. Because exhaled NO is reduced by antiinflammatory treatments, it may be useful for monitoring whether therapy is adequate. The technique may also have application in the monitoring of antiinflammatory effects of new antiasthma drugs, such as selective phosphodiesterase inhibitors, leukotriene antagonists and synthesis inhibitors and immunomodulators. Because the measurement is precise and reasonably reproducible, it may facilitate the measurement of dose-response effects with antiinflammatory treatments, that is difficult at present. Thus, it is possible to discriminate effects of budesonide 100 µg daily from 400 µg daily on exhaled NO which would be difficult using other clinical parameters unless very large numbers of patients were selected [99].

The currently available analysers for exhaled NO are expensive, but in the future it is likely that technological advances will make it possible to miniaturise these analysers, so that they are portable and may even be used at home in conjunction with peak flow meters. This may lead to their application in epidemiological studies and this may be a useful screening measurement for community studies.

9. References

1 Barnes PJ, Belvisi MG (1993) Nitric oxide and lung disease. *Thorax* 48: 1034–1043
2 Gaston B, Drazen JM, Loscalzo J, Stamler JS (1994) The biology of nitrogen oxides in the airways. *Am J Respir Crit Care Med* 149: 538–551
3 Barnes PJ, Liew FY (1995) Nitric oxide and asthmatic inflammation. *Immunol Today* 16: 128–130
4 Kobzik L, Bredt DS, Lowenstein CJ, Drazen J, Gaston D, Sugarbaker D et al (1993) Nitric oxide synthase in human and rat lung: immunocytochemical and histochemical localization. *Am J Resp Cell Mol Biol* 9: 371–377
5 Furukawa K, Harrison DG, Saleh D, Shennib H, Chagnon FP, Giaid A (1996) Expression of nitric oxide synthase in human nasal mucosa. *Am J Respir Crit Care Med* 153: 847–850
6 Tracey WR, Xue C, Klinghoffer V, Barlow J, Pollock JS, Förstermann U et al (1994) Immunocytochemical detection of inducible NO synthase in human lung. *Am J Physiol* 266: L722–727
7 Shaul PW, North AJ, Wu LC, Wells LB, Brannon TS, Lau KS et al (1994) Endothelial nitric oxide synthase is expressed in cultured bronchiolar epithelium. *J Clin Invest* 94: 2231–2236
8 Ward JK, barnes PJ, Springall DR, Abelli L, Tadjkarimi S, Yacoub MH et al (1995) Human iNANC bronchodilatation and nitric oxide-immunoreactive nerves are reduced in distal airways. *Am J Resp Cell Mol Biol* 13: 175–184

9 Asano K, Chee CBE, Gaston B, Lilly CM, Gerard C, Drazen JM et al (1994) Constitutive and inducible nitric oxide synthase gene expression, regulation and activity in human lung epithelial cells. *Proc Natl Acad Sci USA* 91: 10089–10093

10 Hamid Q, Springall DR, Riveros-Moreno V, Chanez P, Howarth P, Redington A et al (1993) Induction of nitric oxide synthase in asthma. *Lancet* 342: 1510–1513

11 Guo FH, de Raeve HR, Rice TW, Stuehr DJ, Thunnissen FBJM, Erzurum SC (1995) Continuous nitric oxide synthesis by inducible nitric oxide synthase in normal human airway epithelium *in vivo. Proc Natl Acad Sci USA* 92: 7809–7813

12 Lundberg JON, Farkas-Szallasi T, Weitzberg E, Rinder J, Lidholm J, Anggard A et al (1995) High nitric oxide production in human paranasal sinuses. *Nature Med* 1: 370–373

13 Gustaffsson LE, Leone AM, Persson M, Wiklund NP, Moncada S (1991) Endogenous nitric oxide is present in the exhaled air of rabbits, guinea-pigs and humans. *Biochem Biophys Res Commun* 181: 852–857

14 Borland C, Cox Y, Higenbottam T (1993) Measurement of exhaled nitric oxide in man. *Thorax* 48: 1160–1162

15 Alving K, Weitzberg E, Lundberg JM (1993) Increased amount of nitric oxide in exhaled air of asthmatics. *Eur Respir J* 6: 1268–1270

16 Kharitonov SA, Yates D, Robbins RA, Logan-Sinclair R, Shinebourne E, Barnes PJ (1994) Increased nitric oxide in exhaled air of asthmatic patients. *Lancet* 343: 133–135

17 Persson MG, Wiklund NP, Gustafsson LE (1993) Endogenous nitric oxide in single exhalation, and the change during exercise. *Am Rev Respir Dis* 148: 1210–1214

18 Persson MG, Midtvedt T, Leone AM, Gustafsson LE (1994) Ca^{2+}-dependent and Ca^{2+}-independent exhaled nitric oxide, presence in germ-free animals and inhibition by arginine analogues. *Eur J Pharmacol* 264: 13–20

19 Leone AM, Gustafsson LE, Francis PL, Persson MG, Wiklund NP, Moncada S (1994) Nitric oxide in exhaled breath in humans: direct GC-MS confirmation. *Biochem Biophys Res Commun* 201: 883–887

20 Robbins RA, Floreani AA, Von Essen SG, Sisson JH, Hill GE, Rubinstein I et al (1996) Measurement of nitric oxide by three different techniques. *Am J Respir Crit Care Med* 153: 1631–1635

21 Persson MG, Zetterstrom O, Argenius V, Ihre E, Gustafsson LE (1994) Single-breath oxide measurements in asthmatic patients and smokers. *Lancet* 343: 146–147

22 Kharitonov SA, Wells AU, O'Connor BJ, Cole PJ, Hansell DM, Logan-Sinclair RB, Barnes PJ (1995) Elevated levels of exhaled nitric oxide in bronchiectasis. *Am J Resp Crit Care Med* 151: 1889–1893

23 Yates DH, Kharitonov SA, Robbins RA, Thomas PS, Barnes PJ (1995) Effect of a nitric oxide synthase inhibitor and a glucocorticosteroid on exhaled nitric oxide. *Am J Resp Crit Care Med* 152: 892–896

24 Kharitonov SA, Yates DH, Barnes PJ (1996) Regular inhaled budesonide decreases nitric oxide concentration in the exhaled air of asthmatic patients. *Am J Resp Crit Care Med* 153: 454–457

25 Barnes PJ, Kharitonov SA (1996) Exhaled nitric oxide: a new lung function test. *Thorax* 51: 218–220

26 Archer S (1993) Measurement of nitric oxide in biological models. *FASEB J* 7: 349–360

27 Kharitonov SA, Barnes PJ (1997) There is no nasal contribution to exhaled NO during exhalation against resistance or during breath-holding. *Am J Respir Crit Care Med* 155: A824

28 Gerlach H, Rossaint R, Pappert D, Knorr M, Falke KJ (1994) Autoinhalation of nitric oxide after endogenous synthesis in nasopharynx. *Lancet* 343: 518–519

29 Lundberg JON, Weitzberg E, Nordvall SL, Kuylenstierna R, Lundberg JM, Alving K (1994) Primarily nasal origin of exhaled nitric oxide and absence in Kartagener's syndrome. *Eur Resp J* 8: 1501–1504

30 Kimberley B, Nejadnik B, Giraud GD, Holden WE (1996) Nasal contribution to exhaled nitric oxide at rest and during breathholding in humans. *Am J Respir Crit Care Med* 153: 829–836

31 Kharitonov S, Chung KF, Evans DJ, O'Connor BJ, Barnes PJ (1996) Increased exhaled nitric oxide in asthma is derived from the lower respiratory tract. *Am J Respir Crit Care Med* 153: 1773–1780

32 Sato K, Sakamaki T, Sumino H, Sakamoto H, Hoshino J, Masuda H et al (1996) Rate of nitric oxide release in the lung and factors influencing the concentration of exhaled nitric oxide. *Am J Physiol* 14: L914–L920

33 Kharitonov SA, Yates D, Barnes PJ (1995) Increased nitric oxide in exhaled air of normal human subjects with upper respiratory tract infections. *Eur Resp J* 8: 295–297

34 Kharitonov SA, Lubec G, Lubec B, Hjelm M, Barnes PJ (1995) L-Arginine increase exhaled nitric oxide in normal human subjects. *Clin Sci* 88: 135–139

35 Massaro AF, Drazen JM (1996) Exhaled nitric oxide during exercise: site of release and modulation by ventilation and blood flow. *J Appl Physiol* 80: 1863–1864

36 Schilling J, Holzer P, Guggenbach M, Gyurech D, Marathia K, Geroulanos S (1994) Reduced endogenous nitric oxide in the exhaled air of smokers and hypertensioners. *Eur Resp J* 7: 467–471

37 Kharitonov SA, Robbins RA, Yates D, Keatings V, Barnes PJ (1995) Acute and chronic effects of cigarette smoking on exhaled nitric oxide. *Am J Resp Crit Care Med* 152: 609–612

38 Buga GM, Griscavage JM, Rogers NE, Ignarro LJ (1993) Negative feedback regulations of endothelial cell function by nitric oxide. *Circ Res* 73: 808–812

39 Assrevy J, Cunha FQ, Liew FY, Moncada S (1993) Feedback inhibition of nitric oxide synthase by nitric oxide. *Br J Pharmacol* 108: 833–837

40 Rengasamy A, Johns RA (1993) Regulation of nitric oxide synthase by nitric oxide. *Mol Pharmacol* 44: 124–128

41 Jain B, Lubinstein I, Robbins RA, Leise KL, Sisson JH (1993) Modulation of airway epithelial cell ciliary beat frequency by nitric oxide. *Biochem Biophys Res Commun* 191: 83–88

42 Yates DH, Kharitonov SA, Barnes PJ (1996) The effect of alcohol ingestion on exhaled nitric oxide. *Eur Respir J* 9: 1130–1133

43 Xie J, Kolls J, Bagby G, Greenberg SS (1995) Independent suppression of nitric oxide and TNF-α in the lung of conscious rata by ethanol. *FASEB J* 9: 253–261

44 Cremona G, Higenbottam J, Takao M, Hall L, Bower EA (1995) Exhaled nitric oxide in isolated pig lungs. *J Appl Physiol* 78: 59–63

45 Belvisi MG, Barnes PJ, Larkin S, Yacoub MH, Tadjkarimi S, Williams T et al (1995) Nitric oxide synthase activity is elevated in inflammatory lung diseases in humans. *Eur J Pharmacol* 283: 252–258

46 Robbins RA, Springall DR, Warren JB, Kwon OJ, Buttery LKD, Wilson AJ et al (1994) Inducible nitric oxide synthase is increased in murine lung epithelial cells by cytokine stimulation. *Biochem Biophys Res Commun* 198: 1027–1033

47 Robbins RA, Barnes PJ, Springall DR, Warren JB, Kwon OJ, Buttery LKD et al (1994) Expression of inducible nitric oxide synthase in human bronchial epithelial cells. *Biochem Biophys Res Commun* 203: 209–218

48 Springall DR, Meng Q, Redington A, Howarth PH, Evans TJ, Polak JM (1995) Inducible nitric oxide synthase in asthmatic airway epithelium is reduced by corticosteroid therapy. *Am J Respir Crit Care Med* 151: A833

49 Du Bois AB, Douglas JS, Leaderer BP, Mohsenin V (1994) The presence of nitric oxide in the nasal cavity of normal humans. *Am J Respir Crit Care Med* 149: A197

50 Massaro AF, Mehta S, Lilly CM, Kobzik L, Reilly JJ, Drazen JM (1996) Elevated nitric oxide concentrations in isolated lower airway gas of asthmatic subjects. *Am J Respir Crit Care Med* 153: 1510–1514

51 Gaston B, Reilly J, Drazen JM, Fackler J, Ramdev P, Arnelle D et al (1993) Endogenous nitric oxides and bronchodilator S-nitrosolthiols in human airways. *Proc Natl Acad Sci USA* 90: 10957–10961

52 Barnes PJ, Liew FY (1995) Nitric oxide and asthmatic inflammation. *Immunology Today* 16: 128–130

53 Liew FY, Cox FF (1991) Nonspecific resistance mechanisms: the role of nitric oxide. *Immunology Today* 12: A17–A21

54 Wei X, Charles IG, Smith A, Ure J, Feng GJ, Huang FP et al (1995) Altered immune responses in mice lacking inducible nitric oxide synthase. *Nature* 375: 408–411

55 Laubach VE, Shesely EG, Smithies O, Sherman PA (1995) Mice lacking inducible nitric oxide synthase are not resistant to lipopolysaccharide induced death. *Proc Natl Acad Sci USA* 92: 10688–10692

56 Higenbottam TW (1995) Lung disease and pulmonary endothelial nitric oxide. *Exp Physiol* 134: 855–864
57 Crawley DF, Liu SF, Evans TW, Barnes PJ (1990) Inhibitory role of endothelium-derived nitric oxide in rat and human pulmonary arteries. *Br J Pharmacol* 101: 166–170
58 Liu SF, Crawley DE, Barnes PJ, Evans TW (1991) Endothelium derived nitric oxide inhibits pulmonary vasoconstriction in isolated blood perfused rat lungs. *Am Rev Respir Dis* 143: 32–37
59 Martinez C, Cases E, Vila JM, Aldasoro M, Medina P, Marco V et al (1995) Influence of endothelial nitric oxide on neurogenic contraction of human pulmonary arteries. *Eur Respir J* 8: 1328–1332
60 Belvisi MG, Stretton CD, Yacoub MH, Barnes PJ (1992) Nitric oxide is the endogenous neurotransmitter of bronchodilator nerves in human airways. *Eur J Pharmacol* 210: 221–222
61 Ward JK, Belvisi MG, Fox AJ, Miura M, Tadjkarimi S, Yacoub MH et al (1993) Modulation of cholinergic neural bronchoconstriction by endogenous nitric oxide and vasoactive intestinal peptide in human airways *in vitro. J Clin Invest* 92: 736–743
62 Högman M, Frostell CG, Hedenström H, Hedenstierna G (1993) Inhalation of nitric oxide modulates adult human bronchial tone. *Am Rev Respir Dis* 148: 1474–1478
63 Sanna A, Kurtansky A, Veriter C, Stanescu D (1994) Bronchodilator effect of inhaled nitric oxide in healthy men. *Am J Respir Crit Care Med* 150: 1702–1709
64 Kacmarek RM, Ripple R, Cockrill BA, Bloch KJ, Zapol WM, Johnson DC (1996) Inhaled nitric oxide: a bronchodilator in mild asthmatics with methacholine-induced bronchospasm. *Am J Respir Crit Care Med* 153: 128–135
65 Yates DH, Kharitonov SA, Thomas PS, Barnes PJ (1996) Endogenous nitric oxide is decreased after inhalation of a specific inhibitor of inducible nitric oxide synthase in asthmatic but not in normal subjects. *Am J Respir Crit Care Med* 151: A699
66 Robbins RA, Floreani AA, Von Essen SG, Sisson JH, Hill GE, Rubinstein I et al (1996) Measurement of exhaled nitric oxide by three different techniques. *Am J Respir Crit Care Med* 153: 1631–1635
67 Kharitonov SA, O'Connor BJ, Evans DJ, Barnes PJ (1995) Allergen-induced late asthmatic reactions are associated with elevation of exhaled nitric oxide. *Am J Resp Crit Care Med* 151: 1894–1899
68 Garnier P, Fajac I, Dessanges JF, Dall'Ava-Santucci J, Lockhart A, Dinh-Xuan AT (1996) Exhaled nitric oxide during acute changes in airways calibre in asthma. *Eur Respir J* 9: 1134–1138
69 Yates DH, Kharitonov SA, Scott DM, Worsdell M, Barnes PJ (1995) Short and long acting b2-agonists do no alter exhaled nitric oxide in asthma. *Am J Respir Crit Care Med* 151: A129
70 Endo T, Uchida Y, Nomura A, Ninomiya H, Sakamoto T, Hasegawa S (1995) Increased production of nitric oxide in the immediate and late response models of guinea-pig experimental asthma. *Am J Respir Crit Care Med* 151: A177
71 Massaro AF, Gaston B, Kita D, Fanta C, Stamler J, Drazen JM (1995) Expired nitric oxide levels during treatment of acute asthma. *Am J Respir Crit Care Med* 152: 800–803
72 Kharitonov SA, Yates D, Robbins RA, Logan-Sinclair R, Shinebourne EA, Barnes PJ (1994) Endogenous nitric oxide is increased in the exhaled air of asthmatic patients. *Am J Respir Crit Care Med* 149: A198
73 Kharitonov SA, Yates DH, Chung KF, Barnes PJ (1996) Changes in the dose of inhaled steroid affect exhaled nitric oxide levels in asthmatic patients. *Eur J Respir Dis* 9: 196–201
74 Kharitonov SA, Evans DJ, Barnes PJ, O'Connor BJ (1995) Bronchial provocation challenge with histamine or adenosine 5' monophosphate does not alter exhaled nitric oxide in asthma. *Am J Respir Crit Care Med* 151: A125
75 Lundberg JON, Nordvall SL, Weitzberg E, Kollberg H, Alving K (1996) Exhaled nitric oxide in paediatric asthma and cystic fibrosis. *Arch Dis Child* 75: 323–326
76 Balfour-Lynn IM, Laverty A, Dinwiddic R (1996) Reduced upper airway nitric oxide in cytic fibrosis. *Arch Dis Child* 75: 319–322
77 Thomas SR, Kharitonov SA, Hodson ME, Barnes PJ (1997) Exhaled and nasal nitric oxide levels are reduced in patients with cystic fibrosis. *Am J Respir Crit Care Med* 155: A198
78 Keatings VM, Collins PD, Scott DM, Barnes PJ (1996) Differences in interleukin-8 and tumor necrosis factor-a in induced sputum from patients with chronic obstructive pulmonary disease or asthma. *Am J Respir Crit Care Med* 153: 530–534

79 Rutgers SR, Postma DS, Van der Mark TW, Koeter GH (1996) Nitric oxide in exhaled air in COPD. *Eur Respir J* 9 (Suppl 23): 13S

80 Cailes JB, Kharitonov S, Yates D, Barnes P, DuBois RM (1995) Decreased endogenous nitric oxide in the exhaled air of systemic sclerosis patients. *Thorax* 50: 452P

81 Giaid A, Saleh D (1995) Reduced expression of endothelial nitric oxide synthase in the lungs of patients with pulmonary hypertension. *New Engl J Med* 333: 214–221

82 Barnes PJ, Liu S (1995) Regulation of pulmonary vascular tone. *Physiol Rev* 47: 87–118

83 Liu S, Adcock IM, Old RW, Barnes PJ, Evans TW (1993) Lipopolysacharide treatment *in vivo* induces widespread expression of inducible nitric oxide synthase mRNA. *Biochem Biophys Res Commun* 196: 1208–1213

84 Kharitonov SA, Nightingale JA, Chung KF, Barnes PJ (1997) Inhaled bacterial lipopoly-saccharide increases exhaled nitric oxide in normal and asthmatic subjects. *Am J Respir Crit Care Med* 155: A946

85 Heiss LN, Lancaster JR, Corbett JA, Goldman WE (1994) Epithelial autotoxicity of nitric oxide: role in the respiratory cytopathology of pertussis. *Proc Natl Acad Sci USA* 91: 267–270

86 Vosswinkel R, Neidt I, Bothe H (1991) The production and utilization of nitric oxide by a new denitrifying strain of Pseudomonas aeuruginosa. *Arch Microbiol* 156: 62–69

87 Cannons AC, Barber MJ, Solomonson LP (1993) Expression and characterization of the home-binding domain of Chlorella nitrate reductase. *J Biol Chem* 268: 3268–3271

88 Martin U, Bryden K, Devoy M, Howarth PH (1996) Increased levels of exhaled nitric oxide during nasal or oral breathing in subjects with seasonal rhinitis. *J Allergy Clin Immunol* 97: 768–772

89 Kharitonov SA, Rajakulasingam K, O'Connor BJ, Durham SR, Barnes PJ (1997) Nasal nitric oxide is increased in patients with asthma and allergic rhinitis and may be modulated by nasal glucocorticoids. *J Allergy Clin Immunol* 99: 58–64

90 Garrelds IM, van Amsterdam JGC, de Graaf-In't Veld C, van Wijk G, Zijlstra MN (1995) Nitric oxide metabolites in nasal lavage fluid of patients with house dust mite allergy. *Thorax* 50: 275–279

91 Laitinen LA, Laitinen A, Haahtela T (1992) A comparative study of the effects of an inhaled corticosteroid, budesonide, and of a β_2 agonist, terbutaline, on airway inflammation in new-ly diagnosed asthma. *J Allergy Clin Immunol* 90: 32–42

92 Gardiner PV, Ward C, Booth H, Allison A, Hendrick DJ, Walters EH (1994) Effect of eight weeks of treatment with salmeterol on bronchoalveolar lavage inflammatory indices in asth-matics. *Am J Resp Crit Care Med* 150: 1006–1011

93 Yates DH, Kharitonov SA, Worsdell M, Thomas PS, Barnes PJ (1995) Exhaled nitric oxide is decreased after inhalation of a specific inhibitor of inducible nitric oxide synthase, in asthmatic but not in normal subjects. *Am J Resp Crit Care Med* 152: 892–896

94 Haynes WG, Noon JP, Walker BR, Webb DJ (1993) Inhibition of nitric oxide synthesis increases blood pressure in healthy humans. *J Hypertension* 11: 1375–1380

95 Stammler JS, Loh E, Roddy M, Currie XE, Creager MA (1994) Nitric oxide regulates broad systemic and pulmonary vascular resistance in normal humans. *Circulation* 89: 2035–2040

96 Misko TP, Moore WM, Kasten TP, Nickols GA, Corbett JA, Tilton RG et al (1993) Selec-tive inhibition of inducible nitric oxide synthase by aminoguanidine. *Eur J Pharmacol* 233: 119–125

97 Hasan K, Heesen BJ, Corbett JA, McDaniel ML, Chang K, Allison W et al (1993) Inhibi-tion of nitric oxide formation by guanidines. *Eur J Pharmacol* 249: 101–106

98 Jatakanon A, Lim S, Chung KF, Barnes PJ (1997) Correlation between exhaled nitric oxide, sputum eosinophils and methacholine responsiveness. *Am J Respir Crit Care Med* 155: 819

99 Kharitonov SA, Jatakanon A, Lim S, O'Connor BJ, Barnes PJ (1997) Dose-dependent reduction in exhaled nitric oxide in patients with asthma regularly treated with 100 mg, 400 mg budesonide in double-blind placebo-controlled parallel group study. *Am J Respir Crit Care Med* 155: A290

Nitric Oxide in Pulmonary Processes:
Role in Physiology and Pathophysiology of Lung Disease
ed. by M. G. Belvisi and J. A. Mitchell
© 2000 Birkhäuser Verlag Basel/Switzerland

CHAPTER 10
Luminal Nitric Oxide in the Upper Airways: Implications for Local and Distal Sites of Action

Kjell Alving[1], Jon O. N. Lundberg[1], Johan Rinder[2] and Eddie Weitzberg[2]

[1] *Department of Physiology and Pharmacology, Karolinska Institute, S-171 77 Stockholm, Sweden*
[2] *Department of Surgical Sciences, Karolinska Hospital, S-171 76 Stockholm, Sweden*

1   Introduction
2   Measurements of Nasal Nitric Oxide (NO)
3   Anatomical Origin of NO in Normal Airways
4   Nature of NO Formation in the Airways
5   Regulation of NO Production in the Airways
6   Physiological Role of Upper Airway NO Production
6.1 Host Defence
6.2 Inflammation
6.3 Aerocrine Messenger
7   Conclusions and Future Research
8   References

1. Introduction

The nose has probably developed primarily to serve as a protection barrier for the lower airways and lungs. The sense of smell is also located in the nose, but may not be vital for the human species. The well-known protective functions of the nose are heating, humidification and filtration of inhaled air. Recently, other protective and regulating functions pertaining to the nasal airways and the paranasal sinuses have been proposed, which involve high nitric oxide (NO) production in the paranasal sinus mucosa. Because this NO can travel with the airstream during inhalation it may play a physiological role not only in the sinuses themselves but also in other parts of the respiratory tract, including the lungs.

2. Measurements of Nasal NO

Airborne NO in the nasal airways can easily be measured with the use of chemiluminescence analysers [1, 2]. A simple approach has been to aspirate air from one nostril directly into the NO analyser by introducing a nasal olive connected to non-absorbing tubings [3]. This can be done during breathhold or during normal tidal breathing, but the measured NO levels will be higher during breathhold, probably due to less admixture of air from the oral cavity, which contains much lower concentrations of NO [2]. To ensure that no contamination of air from the lower respiratory tract occurs, simultaneous measurement of carbon dioxide in air sampled from the nose may be performed [4]. Sampling at a fixed flow rate is advantageous, as the rate of NO release in the nasal airways can be calculated: the NO concentration in air aspirated from the nasal cavity will be inversely proportional to sampling flow rate [5]. Continuous sampling during breathhold from one nostril at a rather high flow rate (0.7–0.8 L/min) will give NO concentrations that are representative of NO release per time unit in the nasal airways [6]. Measurements using this method indicate that NO concentration ranges between 200–400 parts per billion (ppb) in the nasal cavity of healthy subjects. All concentrations of NO given in this chapter are from studies using this method unless otherwise stated.

As a measure of the actual NO concentration in the nasal cavity at a given time, a small volume not exceeding total nasal cavity volume can be aspirated in a syringe during breathhold and then injected into the NO analyser [6, 7]. The NO concentration obtained using this technique correlates negatively with nasal cavity volume, indicating that NO concentration in the nose depends not only on release rate but also on nasal cavity volume [6]. However, the NO release rate, as measured by continuous sampling at a relatively high sampling flow rate, will be much less influenced by changes in nasal cavity volume [6].

The principle of sampling a small volume of air from a body cavity where air exchange is low, and to measure the actual concentration of NO in this sample, can also be applied elsewhere, e.g. in the maxillary sinus [8], the intestines [9], and in the urinary bladder [10].

3. Anatomical Origin of NO in Normal Airways

The presence of NO in exhaled air was discovered in 1991 [11], and some of the early follow-up studies suggested that the peripheral airways and the lungs might be the main origin of exhaled NO [12, 13]. However, it soon became clear that the major source of airborne NO in the respiratory tract of healthy subjects was to be found in the upper airways [2, 3, 14]. Thus, in intubated or tracheostomized patients only very low concentrations of NO were found in exhaled air [2, 3, 15, 16], and the search for the source of exhaled NO was concentrated to the nose. The exact site of origin of NO in the nose was at first difficult to establish, however, and the early finding that nasal administration of N^G-nitro-L-arginine methylester (L-NAME), an NO-synthase (NOS) inhibitor, did not reduce nasal NO levels, was unexpected [8]. It had previously been shown that a topically administered nasal decongestant is unable to reach the paranasal sinuses [17]. Thus, one plausible explanation for the finding that intranasal administration of an

NOS inhibitor did not reduce nasal NO levels might be that the inhibitor did not reach the paranasal sinuses, and that these were the major site of NO production [8, 18]. This hypothesis was then tested. One of the maxillary sinuses in healthy volunteers was punctured and air was aspirated via a catheter: this air showed very high concentration of NO, levels that sometimes approached the highest permissible atmospheric pollution levels (25 ppm). Furthermore, an ongoing production was shown. Repeated aspiration of the total sinus air volume gave the same high concentrations of NO without any sign of decline [8]. The release of NO in one maxillary sinus (approximately 20 nmol/min) greatly exceeds the total release in the lower respiratory tract (5 nmol/min) [19].

The possible contribution of sinus NO to the levels found in the nasal airways was then examined. When air was aspirated from the maxillary sinus via the catheter the concentration of NO in the ipsilateral nasal cavity fell, whereas if air was instead injected into the sinus, there was a marked peak in nasal cavity NO concentration [18]. This clearly showed that the maxillary sinus is an important source of NO in the nasal airways. Since a high NO concentration has also been found in the sphenoid sinus [8], the paranasal sinuses are indicated as the major site of NO production in the upper airways. NO also seems to be produced in the nasal mucosa, albeit in much smaller quantities [8]. Interestingly, NO production in the upper airways can be detected directly after birth in humans [8, 20], in spite of the fact that the paranasal sinuses are poorly developed at this age.

4. Nature of NO Formation in the Airways

The human inducible NOS (iNOS) has been cloned and characterized in e.g. hepatocytes [21] and chondrocytes [22]. Human iNOS was first believed to be expressed only in the presence of proinflammatory cytokines such as interleukin-1β and tumour necrosis factor-α as had been described previously for rodent macrophage iNOS [23]. However, iNOS seems to be constitutively expressed in the epithelium of the human airways [8, 24, 25], although it can also be upregulated in inflammatory conditions [26, 27]. Despite this constitutive enzyme expression, healthy individuals show only minor release of NO in the lower airways, whereas high concentrations of NO are found in the upper airway lumen. This could be explained by the reported differences in the localization and density of iNOS in the epithelial cell layer in the upper and lower airways. Thus, this enzyme seems to be primarily basally located in the lower airways [25], whereas it is densely expressed in the apical part of the epithelium in the upper airways, especially in the paranasal sinuses [8].

Even though this airway NOS is constitutively expressed, it closely resembles iNOS with regard to antigenicity and mRNA sequence [8], and, like iNOS, its activity is Ca^{2+}-independent [28]. The existence of several closely related iNOS gene products has been suggested by studies at the molecular level. First, multiple iNOS-like sequences were found in the human genome, even mapped to different chromosomes [29]. Interestingly, this iNOS gene duplication seems to have occurred very recently in primate evolution, with an almost identical pattern in the chimpanzee and in human. This also fits well with the findings of large NO production in the upper airways of certain higher primates [30, 31], but not in other mammals [31, 32]. Second, several sites of alternative splicing have been found in human iNOS mRNA from airway epithelial cells, with an increase in alternative splicing of iNOS mRNA after stimulation with cytokines [33]. Thus, different forms of iNOS may be present in the same cell. Third, structural diversity of iNOS at the protein level has also been suggested [34]. In the latter study, antigenic differences at the amino terminus were found between a soluble and a membrane-associated iNOS in mouse macrophages. This heterogeneity could be due to differences in the amino acid sequence or to post-translational modification. However, no antigenic diversity was found among the soluble and particulate forms of iNOS when antibodies directed against the carboxyl terminus were used. In the human sinus epithelium, in studies that also used antibodies directed against the carboxyl terminus of iNOS, strong apical staining closely related to the cell membrane was found as well as weaker staining in the cytosol [8]. Future studies will hopefully show precisely which forms of iNOS are expressed in the human upper airways epithelium, but functional data indicate that at least one form in the paranasal sinus mucosa is different from the classical iNOS. The picture has now become even more complicated, since some groups have also reported the expression of endothelial NOS in the nasal epithelium [35, 36]. However, since iNOS produces NO at a much higher rate than endothelial NOS, iNOS may still be the most important source of NO in the upper airways.

An alternative explanation for the difference in upper and lower airway NO release could be that NO reacts rapidly with glutathione [37], which is present at much higher concentrations in the epithelial lining fluid in the lower respiratory tract [38] than in the upper airways [39]. A simple reabsorption of NO into the lower airways mucosa does not seem to be an adequate explanation for low levels of exhaled NO, as it has been shown that NO is not absorbed to any great extent in the dead space area [40].

It has also been suggested that the NO in the upper airways could be of bacterial origin [14], as some bacteria can produce NO by reducing nitrite [41]. However, several studies have shown no effect of antibiotics on nasal NO levels in normal subjects [3, 42], indicating that bacterial NO production is probably only of minor importance.

Another source of NO in the upper airways is the oropharynx, where non-enzymatic NO formation from nitrite in the saliva has been shown [43]. It is also clear, that air from the stomach contributes with high amounts of NO in the case of regurgitation, since nitrite in swallowed saliva is effectively reduced to NO in the acidic environment of the stomach [44].

5. Regulation of NO Production in the Airways

In certain inflammatory diseases, such as allergic asthma and rhinitis, iNOS expression is induced in both upper [26] and lower [27] airways epithelium. This expression has been shown to be sensitive to glucocorticoid treatment [45], which thus leads to reduced NO release in the airways [46–49]. Local glucocorticoid treatment also reduces iNOS expression [24] and NO production [42] in normal lower airways, indicating a minor cytokine-induced iNOS expression even in healthy subjects. However, the major part of normal NO production in the upper airways of healthy subjects is glucocorticoid-resistant and remains more or less intact after both short term [50] and long term [28] systemic steroid treatment. This, again, indicates the unique features of the iNOS-like enzyme primarily found in the paranasal sinus epithelium.

NO production by the iNOS isoenzyme is generally considered to be regulated by changing the expression of the enzyme, whereas the activity of the classical constitutive NO synthases – endothelial and neuronal NOS – is regulated by intracellular Ca^{2+} levels. The NOS described in the paranasal sinus mucosa is constitutively expressed and Ca^{2+}-independent, suggesting that this enzyme has been adapted for continuous production of large amounts of NO. Normally, the substrates for NO synthesis (L-arginine, nicotinamide dinucleotide phosphate (NAL-argininePH) and O_2) are present in excess, but for iNOS, which is a high-rate NO-producing enzyme, substrate concentration may be a rate-limiting factor. This seems to be the case for sinus NO production, since intravenous L-arginine infusion results in increased nasal NO concentration [28]. There are at least two common situations in which blood flow and hence substrate supply to the paranasal sinus epithelium may be greatly reduced. First, during and directly after heavy physical exercise, both nasal [51] and sinus [52] mucosal blood flow are significantly reduced, most probably due to increased sympathetic tone. Second, the use of α-adrenergic nasal decongestants also reduces nasal mucosal blood flow [53]. Because the arterial supply to the sinus mucosa first passes through the nasal mucosa and the ostia [54], it is not surprising that intranasal administration of a nasal decongestant also reduces blood flow in the sinus mucosa, even though the aerosol does not reach the paranasal simuses [53]. Thus, in these two situations substrate supply to the sinus epithelial iNOS may be insufficient and, indeed, heavy physical exercise acutely reduces nasal [5, 7, 55, 56] and sinus [7] NO concentration, an effect that seems to be only partly due to increased nasal cavity volume [7]. We have recently also shown that nasally administered α-adrenergic agonists acutely reduce nasal NO release, again probably due to reduced blood flow into the sinus mucosa [6].

It has previously been suggested that physical exercise increases NO output in the lower respiratory tract [13, 57]. These studies, which measured NO content in orally exhaled air, actually showed reduced concentrations of NO. However, when exhaled volume was taken into account and total NO output was calculated, an increase was found. Such an increase can also be seen during voluntary hyperventilation at rest but not during dobutamine infusion which increases cardiac output but not ventilation, suggesting that increased exhaled NO output during physical exercise is more closely related to increased ventilation than to increased pulmonary blood flow [56]. Furthermore, increased exhalation flow rate during a controlled single-breath exhalation manoeuvre also results in an increase in the calculated release rate of NO [58]. This indicates that the process of adapting the pulmonary circulation to higher blood flow during physical exercise does not involve increased NO production in the lungs, at least not as measured in exhaled air. Instead, due to increased exhalation flow rate, increased amounts of NO are released from the airways mucosa per time unit. The increased release rate could be due to a more marked gradient for NO concentration between the airways mucosa and luminal air, or possibly to more turbulent airflow at higher exhalation flow rates.

6. Physiological Role of Upper Airway NO Production

Over the last few years it has been shown convincingly that there is a substantial NO production in the normal human upper airways, primarily in the paranasal sinuses, but what is the possible role of these high luminal NO concentrations? Already, several functions for NO in the respiratory tract have been suggested, and although epithelially-derived luminal NO may not play a vital role in every instance, some of these proposed functions are presented below (see also Figure 1).

6.1. Host Defense

One of the first functions of NO to be described was in primary host defence. It was discovered that activated mouse macrophages produce large amounts of NO, and that much of the antimicrobial activity of these cells against fungal, helminthic protozoal and bacterial pathogens depends on NO production [59]. Later, NO was also demonstrated to have antiviral activity [60]. The human nasal cavity normally carries a rich bacterial flora whereas the paranasal sinuses are considered to be sterile. This correlates well with the fact that the NO concentrations in the paranasal sinuses are higher than in the nasal cavity, where the exchange of air is more rapid. Furthermore, gaseous NO in concentrations relevant for the paranasal sinuses has been reported to have a bacteriostatic effect on *Staphylococcus aureus* [61], a common bacterial strain found in the nasal mucosa. This points towards a bacteriostatic role for NO in the human respiratory tract, at least within the paranasal sinuses.

Children with Kartagener's syndrome, a triad consisting of *situs inversus*, sinusitis and bronchiectasis, have been found to have very low levels of nasal NO (<20 ppb) [3]. Also, intermediate nasal NO concentrations (50–100 ppb) were found in patients with cystic fibrosis [48, 62], a disease characterised by e.g. chronic sinusitis. The intermediate nasal NO levels found in cystic fibrosis, which approximate those found in patients with acute or chronic sinusitis described below, may be the result of impaired NO diffusion from the paranasal sinuses. On the other hand, the very low NO levels found in patients with Kartagener's syndrome may represent a primary NO deficiency in the paranasal sinuses rather than a diffusion block, since low nasal NO concentrations are also found in patients whose sinuses have been shown to be open by radiographic examinations [84]. As patients with both Kartagener's syndrome and cystic fibrosis suffer from recurrent airways infections, a host defence role for NO is again indicated.

Patients with Kartagener's syndrome also suffer from ciliary dysfunction, and in patients with chronic sinusitis, a correlation was found between nasal NO levels and mucociliary function [63]. In pharmacological studies, NO has been shown to be involved in the regulation of ciliary motility, first in bovine epithelium *in vitro* [64] and recently also in human nasal mucosa *in vivo* [65]. Thus, NO may be involved in airways host defence in several ways.

The bacteriostatic and mucociliary activity stimulating properties of NO in the airways may together constitute a significant contribution to the primary host defence, at least in the upper airways. In humans, and possibly also in other higher primates in the upright body posture, the maxillary sinus ostia are in an unfavourable position: mucociliary clearance is more difficult due to gravital forces. Thus, sinus NO production may have developed to help resist infections in the more vulnerable sinuses in these species. However, paranasal sinus NO may also exert protective effects in the lower respiratory tract, since this NO will be present in air inhaled through the nose. Indeed, a relation between very low nasal NO levels and the presence of atelectasis or bronchiectasis has been observed [63]. Furthermore, a high incidence of aspirates and radiographic abnormalities in the paranasal sinuses, which may lead to reduced nasal NO concentrations, has been found in patients with acute asthma [66], again suggesting a protective effect of sinus NO in the lower airways.

NO in normal human respiratory tract.

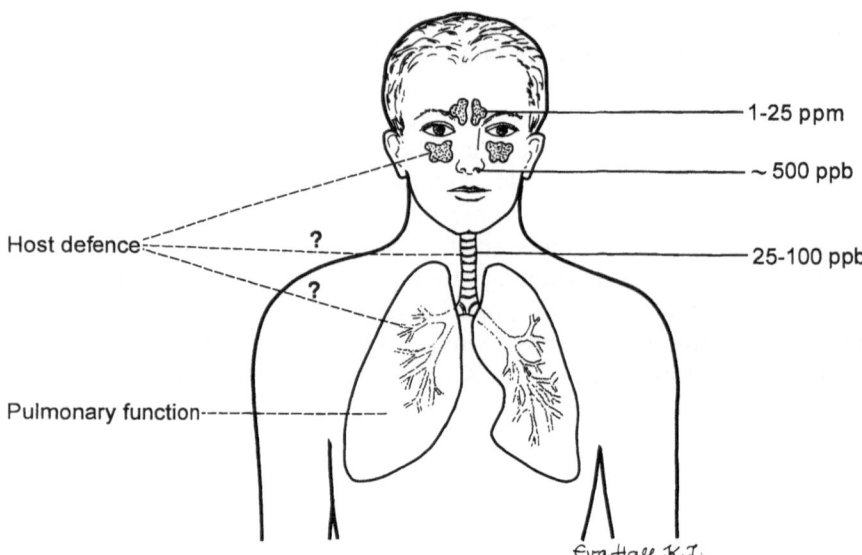

Figure 1. Principal drawing showing concentrations and proposed functions of endogenous air-borne NO in the normal human respiratory tract. High NO production in the paranasal sinuses has been demonstrated and this NO travels during nasal breathing with inhaled air to the lower respiratory tract. Approximate maximal concentrations of NO in the paranasal sinuses, nasal cavity and trachea during normal tidal breathing are given. Maximal alveolar concentrations are probably low due to rapid binding to haemoglobin in this compartment. The most apparent candidate roles for luminal NO in the airways are to take part in the host defence in the parana-sal sinuses, and to improve pulmonary function. However, a host defence function in other part of the airways cannot be excluded. Mechanisms for the host defence function may include direct bacteriostasis and stimulation of ciliary beat. In the lungs, inhaled nasal NO may help to opti-mise the matching of ventilation and perfusion.

6.2. Inflammation

In some individuals, certain pathogens are able to invade the paranasal sinuses and cause acute sinusitis. During acute sinusitis in children [67], markedly reduced nasal NO concentrations have been found. It is not known whether these reduced NO levels preceded the development of acute sinusitis or if they are a result of the sinusitis. Since the NO con-centration within the sinuses under these conditions has not yet been re-ported, we cannot tell if the lower nasal NO concentration during sinusitis is due to impaired NO production in the sinus mucosa, or is just a sign of blocked communication between the sinuses and the nasal cavity, although the rapid restoration of nasal NO concentration with 15 days of antibiotic treatment suggests that the reduction in NO was caused by sinus blockage [67]. However, in patients with chronic sinusitis, where reduced nasal NO levels have also been reported [68], a primary NO deficiency could possibly be the cause of these chronic symptoms. It is at least theoretically possible that an initial infection or inflammation has caused permanent damage to sinus NOS activity. Although the reason for reduced nasal NO levels in sinusitis is presently unknown, it can be concluded that infection/inflammation in the upper airways can sometimes lead to reduced nasal NO levels, which would not be expected in these situations. Furthermore, in upper respiratory tract infections of viral origin, without any symptoms of sinusitis, nasal NO concentrations were not increased, but unchanged in both adults [68, 69] and children [67]. In contrast, both upper [70] and lower [2] respiratory tract infections increase NO release from the lower airways as measured in orally exhaled air, probably indicating an induction of iNOS expression in the tracheobronchial epithelium. This again, illustrates the different nature of the upper airway NOS compared to the iNOS in the lower airways.

In allergic rhinitis, another inflammatory condition of the upper airways, conflicting data have been reported. In children with allergic rhinitis and asthma, there was no difference in nasal NO concentrations compared to those in nonallergic controls, in spite of clearly increased NO levels in orally exhaled air [48]. However, other studies in adults with allergic rhinitis have shown increased nasal NO concentrations [49, 71]. The results remain to be explained, but the difference may be due to a functional difference between children and adults, or possibly, to the different methods used. Interestingly, in patients with acute rhinitis with clear-cut symptoms, nasal NO concentration is lower than in nonsymptomatic rhinitis patients [49, 71]. This may be due to reduced communication between the paranasal sinuses and the nasal cavity in symptomatic rhinitis; this contention is further supported by the finding that treatment with a nasal decongestant increased nasal NO concentrations in patients with symptoms, probably by improving communication from the sinus, whereas in non-symptomatic patients a reduction was found [71]. The latter effect is similar to what is seen in healthy subjects [6].

It must be stressed that the nasal NO concentration depends on many processes: nasal cavity NO release; paranasal sinus NO release; transport of NO from the sinuses to the nasal cavity; and nasal cavity volume. This makes interpretations of nasal NO measurements difficult and it may be impossible – based on the relatively simple methods used to date – to draw any conclusions from minor changes in nasal NO concentration.

If NO production is really increased in inflammation in the upper airways, what would be the role of epithelially-derived NO in the inflammatory process? An autotoxic effect of epithelial NO production has been suggested, primarily based on studies on *Bordetella pertussis* infections, but these mechanisms may also be relevant for the epithelial damage seen in asthma [72]. However, as discussed above, there is also a constitutive expression of iNOS in the airways epithelium generating large amounts of NO, at least in the paranasal sinuses, without any sign of epithelial damage. It may be that the sinus epithelial cells have developed resistance to high intracellular concentrations of NO, or that this NO is primarily being released extracellularly and thus, that the build-up of toxic intracellular NO levels is avoided. Another explanation could be that NO does not in fact have any toxic effects in the airways mucosa, but instead serves as a cytoprotective agent, mainly by reacting with and neutralizing reactive oxygen species [73].

An alternative proinflammatory role for NO could be to potentiate vascular leakage, since it has been shown that intranasal administration of an NOS inhibitor reduces plasma protein extravasation induced by allergen or histamine challenge in the nasal mucosa [74]. However, other studies suggest that NO may act to suppress protein extravasation in the airways mucosa [75], again suggesting that NO can act as a pro- or antiinflammatory agent, depending on the circumstances.

6.3. Aerocrine Messenger

A few years after the identification of NO as the endothelium-derived relaxing factor (EDRF), the vasodilatory property of NO was put to use. Inhaled exogenous NO gas was used to selectively relax the pulmonary circulation after experimental induction of pulmonary hypertension [76, 77]. In these early studies rather high concentrations of NO were used (40–80 ppm), but it was later shown that inhalation of as little as 100 ppb of NO causes near maximal pulmonary vascular relaxation and improvement of arterial oxygenation in patients with severe pulmonary disease [78].

In a parallel line of research, large amounts of NO were found in the nasal airways of normal subjects [2, 3], and it was soon suggested that inhalation of nasal NO, leading to NO concentrations of 25–100 ppb at the level of the trachea, may have pulmonary effects [3, 14]. Indeed, in intubated and mechanically-ventilated patients we were able to show clear-cut improvement of arterial oxygenation and, in some subjects, pulmonary vascular relaxation after reintroducing nasal air to the respiratory system [79, 80]. Although inhalation of low doses of NO causes vasodilation in the pulmonary and also in the bronchial circulation [81], NO gas even in high doses (90 ppm) does not seem to cause any vasodilation in the nasal vascular bed [6], which of course is an advantage, as vasodilation would lead to nasal congestion.

We have also shown that in normal volunteers, nasal breathing results in higher arterial oxygen levels compared to oral breathing, even though ventilation was kept constant as monitored by end-tidal CO_2 concentration [80]. This could explain the improved endurance experienced by e.g. football players who apply plasters onto the nose to facilitate nasal breathing, since this may lead to increased inhalation of nasal NO and hence possibly to improved arterial oxygenation. It may also give a background to the widely held belief that deep inhalation through the nose followed by exhalation through the mouth would enhance mental concentration, e.g. during the course of meditation: this breathing pattern will optimise the delivery of nasal NO to the lungs and thus improve arterial oxygenation [80]. This apparent use of NO as an aerocrine messenger to improve pulmonary function is a very recent development in mammals, and one can only speculate about the reasons for such an adaptation. However, since the mammalian lung developed for about 200 million years to function primarily in a horizontal position, and since high nasal NO concentrations are found above all in higher primates with an upright body posture, it may be speculated that the lung needed extra help to function properly in this new vertical position. Endogenous production and release of the airborne vasodilator NO at one site (the paranasal sinuses) and transportation with inhaled air to its site of action would be an ingenious way to achieve optimal matching of ventilation and perfusion in the lung.

The possible importance of nasal NO for pulmonary function in humans indicates that the reintroduction of nasal NO into the air inhaled by intubated patients may be of prophylactic value, not least with regard to the possible bacteriostatic effects of NO. In addition, the introduction of nasal NO in these situations may help to counteract the rebound pulmonary hypertension often seen after the withdrawal of higher concentrations of exogenous NO [82].

7. Conclusions and Future Research

Several studies point towards an important role for NO as a protective agent in the airways. This role may include direct bacteriostasis and improved clearance by stimulation of ciliary beat. Furthermore, NO may act as an aerocrine hormone to optimise pulmonary function. The primary site of NO production in normal airways is the paranasal sinuses, at least with regard to delivery into luminal air. However, the exact gene product responsible for the very rapid NO synthesis in the upper airways has not yet been identified, and future molecular studies should focus on the apparent diversity of iNOS-like enzymes in the airways of higher primates including humans.

Since upper airway NO seems to possess several protective properties, situations in which NO delivery from the sinuses is impaired should be considered to entail an increased risk of complications in the respiratory tract. For example, there are indications of a correlation between low nasal NO concentrations and the development of pulmonary disease in children. As yet, we cannot tell if these low nasal NO levels are the cause or the result of airways disease and further studies are needed. For these studies, the nasal air sampling method must be further developed and standardised:

indeed the first steps have already been taken [83]. With a standardised method, results from different studies can be compared, and the significance of reduced nasal NO for the development of airways disease, especially in children, may soon emerge. Already, measurements of nasal NO are used in the diagnosis of patients with suspected Kartagener's syndrome: in patients without *situs inversus* (50% of all patients with Kartagener's syndrome), the correct diagnosis is often delayed for several years.

In the situation of tracheal intubation, when the nasal source of NO is effectively by-passed, the reintroduction of nasal NO may be advantageous. We have already shown that reintroduction of nasal air improves pulmonary oxygen uptake, and future studies will show if nasal NO is also able to reduce the high incidence of lower respiratory tract infections in intubated patients.

Even though NO derived from the paranasal sinuses seems to have mainly favourable effects, increased NO production in other parts of the airways during the course of inflammation may promote the inflammatory response, for example by causing damage to the epithelial cell layer. Since gaseous NO is already used for treatment of respiratory complications and as a diagnostic marker of inflammation in the lower airways, the various factors that control the end results of endogenous NO synthesis and exogenous NO delivery in the airways must be thoroughly studied in the future.

8. References

1 Archer S (1992) Measurement of nitric oxide in biological models. *FASEB J* 7: 349–360
2 Alving K, Weitzberg E, Lundberg JM (1993) Increased amount of nitric oxide in exhaled air of asthmatics. *Eur Resp J* 6: 1368–1370
3 Lundberg JON, Weitzberg E, Nordvall SL, Kuylenstierna R, Lundberg JM, Alving K (1994) Primarily nasal origin of exhaled nitric oxide and absence in Kartagener's syndrome. *Eur Resp J* 7: 1501–1504
4 Kimberly B, Nejadnik B, Giraud GD, Holden WE (1996) Nasal contribution to exhaled nitric oxide at rest and during breathholding in humans. *Am J Respir Crit Care Med* 153: 829–836
5 Imada M, Iwamoto J, Nonaka S, Kobayashi Y, Unno T (1996) Measurement of nitric oxide in human nasal airway. *Eur Resp J* 9: 556–559
6 Rinder J, Lundberg JON, Änggård A, Alving K, Lundberg JM (1996) Effects of topical nasal decongestants, L-arginine and nitric oxide synthase inhibition, on nasal cavity nitric oxide levels and nasal cavity comume in man. *Am J Rhinol* 10: 399–408
7 Lundberg JON, Rinder J, Weitzberg E, Alving K, Lundberg JM (1997) Heavy physical exercise decreases nitric oxide levels in the nasal airways in humans. *Acta Physiol Scand* 159: 51–57
8 Lundberg JON, Farkas-Szallasi T, Weitzberg E, Rinder J, Lidholm J, Änggård A et al (1995) High nitric oxide production in paranasal sinuses. *Nature Med* 1: 370–373
9 Lundberg JON, Hellström P, Lundberg JM, Alving K (1994) Greatly increased luminal nitric oxide in ulcerative colitis. *Lancet* 344: 1673–1674
10 Lundberg JON, Ehrén I, Jansson O, Adolfson J, Lundberg JM, Weitzberg E et al (1996) Elevated nitric oxide in the urinary bladder in infectious and noninfectious cystitis. *Urology* 48: 700–702
11 Gustaffson LE, Leone AM, Persson MG, Wiklund NP, Moncada S (1991) Endogenous nitric oxide is present in exhaled air of rabbits, guinea-pigs and humans. *Biochem Biophys Res Comm* 181: 852–857

12 Borland C, Cox Y, Higenbottam T (1993) Measurement of exhaled nitric oxide in man. *Thorax* 48: 1160–1162

13 Persson MG, Wiklund NP, Gustafsson LE (1993) Endogenous nitric oxide in single exhalations and the change during exercise. *Am Rev Resp Dis* 148: 1210–1214

14 Gerlach H, Rossaint R, Pappert D, Knorr M, Falke KJ (1994) Autoinhalation of nitric oxide after endogenous synthesis in nasopharynx. *Lancet* 343: 518–519

15 Schedin U, Frostell C, Persson MG, Jakobsson J, Andersson G, Gustafsson LE (1995) Contribution from the upper and lower airways to exhaled endogenous nitric oxide in humans. *Acta Anaesthesiol Scand* 39: 327–332

16 Münch C, Monchi M, Fierobe L, Brunet F, Dhainaut JF, Tuan Dinh-Xuan A (1994) Absence of nitric oxide in airways of ventilated patients. *Lancet* 343: 1232–1233

17 Hardy JG, Lee SW, Wilson CG (1985) Intranasal drug delivery by spray and drops. *J Pharmaceut Pharmacol* 37: 294–297

18 Lundberg JON, Rinder J, Weitzberg E, Lundberg JM, Alving K (1994) Nasally exhaled nitric oxide in humans originates mainly in the paranasal sinuses. *Acta Physiol Scand* 152: 431–432

19 Trolin G, Andén T, Hedenstierna G (1994) Nitric oxide in expired air at rest and during exercise. *Acta Physiol Scand* 151: 159–163

20 Schedin U, Norman M, Gustafsson LE, Herin P, Frostell C (1996) Endogenous nitric oxide in the upper airways of healthy newborn infants. *Pediatr Res* 40: 148–151

21 Geller DA, Lowenstein CJ, Shapiro RA, Nussler AK, Di Silvio M, Wang SC et al (1993) Molecular cloning and expression of inducible nitric oxide synthase from hepatocytes. *Proc Natl Acad Sci USA* 90: 3491–3495

22 Charles IG, Palmer RM, Hickery MS, Bayliss MT, Chubb AP, Hall VS et al (1993) Cloning characterization, and expression of a cDNA encoding an inducible nitric oxide synthase from the human chondrocyte. *Proc Natl Acad Sci USA* 90: 11419–11423

23 Knowles RG, Moncada S (1994) Nitric oxide snytheses in mammals. *Biochem J* 298: 249–258

24 Guo FH, De Raeve HR, Rice TW, Stuehr DJ, Thunnissen FBJM, Erzurum SC (1995) Continuous nitric oxide synthesis by inducible nitric oxide synthase in normal human airway epithelium *in vivo*. *Proc Natl Acad Sci USA* 92: 7809–7813

25 Kobzik L, Bredt DS, Lowenstein CJ, Drazen J, Gaston B, Sugarbaker D et al (1993) Nitric oxide synthase in human and rat lung: immunocytochemical and histochemical localization. *Am J Respir Cell Mol Biol* 9: 371–377

26 Springall DR, Mason NA, Redington AE, Meng Q-H, Howarth PH, Polak JM (1996) Inducible nitric oxide synthase is upregulated in nasal epithelium in perennial allergic rhinitis. *Am J Respir Crit Care Med* 153: A800

27 Hamid Q, Springall DR, Riveros-Moreno V, Chanez P, Howarth P, Redington A et al (1993) Induction of nitric oxide synthase in asthma. *Lancet* 342: 1510–1513

28 Lundberg JON, Weitzberg E, Rinder J, Rudehill A, Jansson O, Wiklund NP et al (1996) Calcium-independent and steroid-resistant nitric oxide synthase activity in human paranasal sinus mucosa. *Eur Resp J* 9: 1344–1347

29 Xu W, Charles IG, Liu L, Koni PA, Moncada S, Emson P (1995) Molecular genetic analysis of the duplication of human inducible nitric oxide synthase (NOS-2) sequences. *Biochem Biophys Res Comm* 212: 466–472

30 Douglas JS, Stitt JT, DuBois AB (1995) Nasal and lung nitric oxide production in human and animals: Effect of endotoxin. *Am J Respir Crit Care Med* 151: A44

31 Schedin U, Frostell C, Gustafsson LE (1995) Nitric oxide occurs in high concentrations in monkey upper airways. *Acta Physiol Scand* 155: 473–474

32 Lewandowski K, Busch T, Lewandowski M, Keske U, Gerlach U, Falke KJ (1996) Evidence of nitric oxide in the exhaled gas of Asian elephants (*Elephas maximus*). *Respir Physiol* 106: 91–98

33 Eissa NT, Strauss AJ, Haggerty CM, Choo EK, Chu SC, Moss J (1996) Alternative splicing of human inducible nitric oxide synthase mRNA: tissue-specific regulation and induction by cytokines. *J Biol Chem* 271: 27184–27187

34 Ringheim GE, Pan J (1995) Particulate and soluble isoforms of the inducible nitric oxide synthase are distinguishable at the amino terminus in RAW 264.7 macrophage cells. *Biochem Biophys Res Comm* 210: 711–716

35 Sakai M, Sawada T, Nishimura T, Nagatsu I (1996) Expression of nitric oxide syntheses in the mouse and human nasal mucosa. *Acta Histochem Cytochem* 29: 177–179

36 Furukawa K, Harrison DG, Saleh D, Shennib H, Chagnon FP, Giaid A (1996) Expression of nitric oxide synthase in the human nasal mucosa. *Am J Respir Crit Care Med* 153: 847–850

37 Wink DA, Mims RW, Darbyshire JF, Christodoulou D, Hanbauer I, Cox GW et al (1994) Reaction kinetics for nitrosylation of cysteine and glutathione in aerobic nitric oxide solutions at neutral pH. Insights into the fate and physiological effects of intermediates in the NO/O_2 reaction. *Chem Res Toxicol* 7: 519–525

38 Cantin AM, North SL, Hubbard RC, Crystal RG (1987) Normal alveolar epithelial lining fluid contains high levels of glutathione. *J Appl Physiol* 63: 152–157

39 Testa B, Mesolella M, Testa D, Giuliano A, Costa G, Marione F et al (1995) Glutathione in the upper respiratory tract. *Anno Oto Rhinol Laryngol* 104: 117–119

40 Borland CDR, Higenbottam TW (1989) A simultaneous single breath measurement of pulmonary diffusing capacity with nitric oxide and carbon monoxide. *Eur Resp J* 2: 56–63

41 Ji X, Hollocher TC (1989) Nitrite reductase of *Escherichia coli* as a NO-producing nitrite reductase. *Biochem Arch* 5: 61–66

42 Dillon WC, Hampl V, Shultz PJ, Rubins JB, Archer SL (1996) Origins of breath nitric oxide in humans. *Chest* 110: 930–938

43 Zetterquist W, Pedroletti C, Lundberg JON, Alving K (1999) Salivary contribution to exhaled nitric oxide. *Eur Resp J* 13: 327–333

44 Lundberg JON, Weitzberg E, Lundberg JM, Alving K (1994) Intragastric nitric oxide production in humans: measurements in expelled air. *Gut* 35: 1543–1546

45 Springall DR, Meng Q-H, Redington A, Howarth PH, Evans TJ, Polak JM (1995) Inducible nitric oxide in asthmatic airway epithelium is reduced by corticosteroid therapy. *Am J Respir Crit Care Med* 151: A833

46 Kharitonov SA, Yates DH, Barnes PJ (1996) Inhaled glucocorticoids decrease nitric oxide in exhaled air of asthmatic patients. *Am J Respir Crit Care Med* 153: 454–457

47 Kharitonov SA, Yates D, Robbins RA, Logan-Sinclair R, Shinebourne EA, Barnes PJ (1994) Increased nitric oxide in exhaled air of asthmatic patients. *Lancet* 343: 133–135

48 Lundberg JON, Nordvall SL, Weitzberg E, Kollberg H, Alving K (1996) Exhaled nitric oxide in paediatric asthma and cystic fibrosis. *Arch Dis Child* 75: 323–326

49 Kharitonov SA, Rajakulasingam K, O'Connor B, Durham SR, Barnes PJ (1997) Nasal nitric oxide is increased in patients with asthma and allergic rhinitis and may be modulated by nasal glucocorticoids. *J Allergy Clin Immunol* 99: 58–64

50 Sato K, Sumino H, Sakamaki T, Sakamoto H, Nakamura T, Ono Z et al (1996) Lack of inhibitory effect of dexamethasone on exhalation of nitric oxide by healthy humans. *Internal Med* 35: 356–361

51 Ohki M, Hasegawa M, Kurita N, Watanabe I (1987) Effects of exercise on nasal resistance and nasal blood flow. *Acta Otolaryngol* 104: 328–333

52 Falck B, Aust R, Svanholm H, Bäcklund L (1989) The effect of physical work on the mucosal blood flow and gas exchange in the human maxillary sinus. *Rhinology* 27: 241–250

53 Åkerlund A, Bende M, Arfors K-E, Intaglietta M (1993) Effect of oxymetazolin on nasal and sinus mucosal blood flow in the rabbit as measured with laser-Doppler flowmetry. *Ann Otol Rhinol Laryngol* 102: 123–126

54 Kumlien J, Schiratzki H (1985) The vascular arrangement of the sinus mucosa – a study in rabbits. *Acta Otolaryngol* 99. 122–132

55 Rinder J, Lundberg JON, Weitzberg E, Lundberg JM, Alving K (1995) Nitric oxide in human nasal airways decreases during exercise. *Endothelium* 3: S82

56 Phillips CR, Giraud GD, Holden WE (1996) Exhaled nitric oxide during exercise: site of release and modulation by ventilation and blood flow. *J Appl Physiol* 80: 1865–1871

57 Iwamoto J, Pendergast DR, Suzuki H, Krasney JA (1994) Effect of graded exercise on nitric oxide in expired air in humans. *Respir Physiol* 97: 333–345

58 Silkoff PE, Mcclean PA, Slutsky AS, Furlott HG, Hoffstein E, Wakita S et al (1997) Marked flow-dependence of exhaled nitric oxide using a new technique to exclude nasal nitric oxide. *Am J Respir Crit Care Med* 155: 260–267

59 Nathan CF, Hibbs Jr J (1991) Role of nitric oxide synthesis in macrophage antimicrobial activity. *Curr Opin Immunol* 3: 65–70

60 Croen KD (1993) Evidence for an antiviral effect of nitric oxide. Inhibition of Herpes Simplex type I replication. *J Clin Invest* 91: 2446–2452

61 Mancinelli RL, McKay CP (1983) Effects of nitric oxide and nitrogen dioxide on bacterial growth. *Appl Environ Microbiol* 46: 198–202

62 Lundberg JON, Nordvall SL, Weitzberg E, Kollberg H, Alving K (1995) Exhaled nitric oxide in paediatric asthma and cystic fibrosis. *Endothelium* 3: S113

63 Lindberg S, Cervin A, Runer T (1997) Low levels of nasal nitric oxide (NO) correlate to impaired mucociliary function in the upper airways. *Acta Otolaryngol* 117: 728–734

64 Jain B, Rubinstein L, Robbins RA, Leise KL, Sisson JH (1993) Modulation of airway epithelial cell ciliary beat frequency by nitric oxide. *Biochem Biophys Res Comm* 191: 83–88

65 Runer T, Lindberg S (1998) Effects of nitric oxide on blood flow and mucociliary activity in the human nose. *Ann Otol Rhinol Laryngol* 107: 40–46

66 Rossi OVJ, Pirilä T, Laitinen J, Huhti E (1994) Sinus aspirates and radiographic abnormalities in severe attacks of asthma. *Int Arch Allergy Immunol* 103: 209–213

67 Baraldi E, Azzolin NM, Biban P, Zacchello F (1997) Effect of antibiotic therapy on nasal nitric oxide concentration in children with acute sinusitis. *Am J Respir Crit Care Med* 155: 1680–1683

68 Lindberg S, Cervin A, Runer T (1997) Nitric oxide (NO) production in the upper airways is decreased in chronic sinusitis. *Acta Otolaryngol* 117: 113–117

69 Ferguson EA, Eccles R (1996) Changes in nasal nitric oxide concentration associated with symptoms of common cold and treatment with a topical nasal decongestant. *Br J Clin Pharmacol* 42: 657P

70 Kharitonov SA, Yates DH, Barnes PJ (1995) Increased nitric oxide in exhaled air of normal subjects with upper respiratory tract infections. *Eur Resp J* 8: 295–297

71 Arnal J-F, Didier A, Rami J, M'Rini C, Charlet J-P, Serrano E et al (1997) Nasal nitric oxide is increased in allergic rhinitis. *Clin Exp Allergy* 27: 358–362

72 Flak TA, Goldman WE (1996) Autotoxicity of nitric oxide in airway disease. *Am J Respir Crit Care Med* 154: S202–S206

73 Wink DA, Hanbauer I, Laval F, Cook JA, Krishna MC, Mitchell JB (1994) Nitric oxide protects against the cytotoxic effects of reactive oxygen species. *Ann New York Acad Sci* 738: 265–278

74 Dear JW, Scadding GK, Foreman JC (1996) Reduction by N^G-nitro-L-arginine methyl ester (L-NAME) of antigen-induced nasal airway plasma extravasation in human subjects *in vivo*. *Br J Pharmacol* 116: 1720–1722

75 Erjefält JS, Erjefält I, Sundler F, Persson CG (1994) Mucosal nitric oxide may tonically suppress airways plasma exudation. *Am J Respir Crit Care Med* 150: 227–232

76 Frostell C, Fratacci M-D, Wain JC, Jones R, Zapol WM (1991) Inhaled nitric oxide. A selective pulmonary vasodilator reversing hypoxic pulmonary vasoconstriction. *Circulation* 83: 2038–2047

77 Frostell CG, Blomqvist H, Hedenstierna G, Lundberg JM, Zapol WM (1993) Inhaled nitric oxide selectively reverses human hypoxic pulmonary vasoconstriction without causing systemic vasodilatation. *Anesthesiology* 78: 427–435

78 Puybasset L, Rouby J, Mourgeon E, Stewart T, Cluzel P, Arthaud M et al (1994) Inhaled nitric oxide in acute respiratory failure: dose-response curves. *Intensive Care Med* 20: 319–327

79 Lundberg JON, Lundberg JM, Settergren G, Alving K, Weitzberg E (1995) Nitric oxide, produced in the upper airways, may act in an "aerocrine" fashion to enhance pulmonary oxygen uptake in humans. *Acta Physiol Scand* 155: 467–468

80 Lundberg JON, Settergren G, Gelinder S, Lundberg JM, Alving K, Weitzberg E (1996) Inhalation of nasally derived nitric oxide modulates pulmonary function in humans. *Acta Physiol Scand* 158: 343–347

81 Alving K, Fornhem C, Lundberg JM (1993) Pulmonary effects of endogenous and exogenous nitric oxide in the pig: relation to cigarette smoke inhalation. *Br J Pharmacol* 110: 739–746

82 Miller OI, Tang SF, Keech A, Celermajer DS (1995) Rebound pulmonary hypertension on withdrawal from inhaled nitric oxide. *Lancet* 346: 51–52

83 Kharitonov SA, Alving K, Barnes PJ (1997) Exhaled and nasal nitric oxide measurements: Recommendations. The European Respiratory Society Task Force. *Eur Resp J* 10: 1683–1693

84 Amal J-F, Flores P, Rami J, Murris-Espin M, Bremont F, Pasto I, Aguilla M, Serrano E, Didier A (1999). Nasal nitric oxide concentration in paranasal sinus inflammatory diseases. *Eur Resp J* 13: 307–312

Nitric Oxide in Pulmonary Processes:
Role in Physiology and Pathophysiology of Lung Disease
ed. by M. G. Belvisi and J. A. Mitchell
© 2000 Birkhäuser Verlag Basel/Switzerland

CHAPTER 11
Inhaled Nitric Oxide as a Therapy for Diseases of the Pulmonary Vasculature

Helen M. Marriott and Timothy W. Higenbottam

Section of Respiratory Medicine, Clinical Sciences Division (CSUHT), University of Sheffield, Sheffield S10 2PX, UK

1   Nitric Oxide (NO) and the Pulmonary Circulation
2   History of Inhaled NO
3   Therapeutic Use of Inhaled NO
3.1 Persistent Pulmonary Hyertension of the Neonate
3.2 Acute Respiratory Distress Syndrome (ARDS)
3.3 Airway Disease
3.4 Primary Pulmonary Hypertension (PPH)
4   Precautions with the Use of Inhaled NO
5   Future of Inhaled NO Therapy
6   References

1. Nitric Oxide (NO) and the Pulmonary Circulation

NO is a potent vasodilator found in the exhaled breath of humans and animals [1]. Its importance in the normal regulation of pulmonary vascular tone was realised when NO was identified as the endothelium-derived relaxing factor (EDRF) [2]. The endogenous synthesis of NO is achieved by the enzyme NO synthase (NOS) from the substrates L-arginine and molecular oxygen (O_2). This enzyme exists in three forms, neuronal NOS (nNOS), inducible NOS (iNOS) and endothelial (eNOS), which have been identified in different cell types [3]. eNOS and nNOS are constitutively expressed in endothelial cells and nerves, and are distinguished by a dependency on calcium/calmodulin. By comparison, iNOS is expressed in many cells including the airway epithelial cells. It is calcium independent and its expression is induced by endotoxin and cytokines [3].

It is possible to measure NO gas of the lower and upper airways of both healthy subjects and patients with respiratory disease. The maxillary sinuses of the nose have the highest concentration of NO production in the respiratory tract. The high concentration of NO in these sinuses is an example of the host defence role of NO as it is thought to maintain sterility through its bacteriocidal activity [5].

The overall view is that the endothelium of arterial segments of the pulmonary circulation produce NO in functionally active levels [1]. This endothelial production of NO is responsive to the alveolar oxygen tension [6] and contributes in certain species, including humans [1], to the basal pulmonary vascular tone. Therefore, the endothelial NO system in the lungs may offer a complementary system to hypoxic vasoconstriction in ensuring the matching of the distribution of ventilation and perfusion.

There is evidence to suggest that defective endothelial NO production causes hypertension [7]. Patients with pulmonary hypertension have reduced expression of eNOS [8]. However, in contrast Ca^{2+}-dependent NOS is increased in inflammatory lung disease [9].

2. History of Inhaled NO

In the isolated lung model, it has been shown that inhaled NO is not only taken up into the circulating red blood cells in the alveolar capillaries but also enters vascular smooth muscle cells of resistance arteries to reduce pulmonary vascular resistance (PVR) [10]. The first studies of the therapeutic effects of inhaled NO were undertaken in patients with cardiac disease or severe primary pulmonary hypertension (PPH) undergoing diagnostic right heart catheterisation. A comparison was made between the inhalation of a concentration of 80 parts per million (ppm) NO in air and an intravenous infusion of prostacyclin (PGI_2), a powerful short-acting vasodilator [11]. Pepke-Zaba et al. found that NO acted as a selective pulmonary vasodilator in these patients and, unlike prostacyclin, had no effect on the cardiac output or systemic artery pressure [12]. In the PPH patients there was a significant fall in the PVR equivalent in response to the maximum dose of PGI_2. The absence of any effect on the systemic circulation is because inhaled NO is principally taken up in the red blood cells circulating in the alveolar capillaries [13]. The inactivation is a result of the reaction of NO with oxyhaemoglobin to ultimately form nitrate anions and methaemoglobin (metHb). The metHb reductase in the red blood cells reduces metHb to haemoglobin, whilst the nitrate is excreted in the urine [14]. Some of the inhaled NO enters the urea cycle, up to 20% of the inhaled dose, but the pathways involved have not been fully elucidated [15]. Nitrate anions do not exert any vasorelaxation, thus confining the effects of inhaled NO to the pulmonary circulation.

NO reacts with the haem moiety of the soluble guanylate cyclase enzyme in vascular smooth muscle cells [16]. Soluble guanylate cyclase is activated by NO to increase the intracellular concentration of cyclic guanine monophosphate (cGMP). The second messenger cGMP causes relaxation and reduction in tone of the smooth muscle cell [17]. The anatomical location of the pre-capillary resistance arteries within the acini of the lungs is closely associated with the bronchioli and alveoli. This means that the diffusion distance for the inhaled NO between the alveoli and the vascular smooth muscle cells is short. Inhaled NO therefore gains access to the resistance pulmonary arteries [10]. In addition to activation of guanylate cyclase, NO has also been shown to initiate smooth muscle relaxation directly through activation of calcium-dependent potassium channels in smooth muscle [18].

3. Therapeutic Use of Inhaled NO

3.1. Persistent Pulmonary Hypertension of the Neonate

Persistent pulmonary hypertension of the neonate (PPHN) is a major cause of mortality in the newborn. These infants have a marked increase in pulmonary resistance which causes right to left shunting of blood across the patent ductus arteriosus and foramen ovale. Conventional treatment of PPHN has proved difficult as there are a number of separate causes and the natural history of the condition varies greatly. Intravenous vasodilators reduce pulmonary vascular resistance, however as they also reduce systemic vascular resistance, the right to left shunt is usually worsened. They can also lessen ventilation–perfusion (V/Q) matching which further contributes to the hypoxaemia. As a result of the "shunting" systemic oxygenation is not greatly improved with inhalation of 100% oxygen. The invasive approach to improve oxygenation with extra-corporeal membrane oxygenation (ECMO) is an effective treatment of these infants, but is associated with a significant morbidity and is expensive [19].

As inhaled NO is a selective pulmonary vasodilator it decreases PVR, whilst systemic vascular resistance remains unaltered, and should thus reduce right to left shunt. Inhaled NO causes a rapid increase in systemic oxygenation in many infants with PPHN, but although inhaled NO significantly reduces the incidence of ECMO use and the associated mortality in PPHN it has no effect on overall mortality [19]. There are, however, a large number of infants that fail to improve with inhaled NO therapy. There are several reasons why this may be the case; poor lung inflation could result in inadequate delivery of NO to the pulmonary vasculature; thickening of the pulmonary arteries could continue to restrict the flow of blood even when relaxed by NO; inhaled NO could worsen ventilation-perfusion matching [19, 20].

Other causes of pulmonary hypertension in neonates, such as respiratory distress syndrome or congenital diaphragmatic hernia, can also be treated with inhaled NO. Again, although inhaled NO reduces the need for ECMO, it has no effect on mortality [21]. There are also indications that inhaled NO may be used in the treatment of hypoxaemia and pulmonary hypertension in premature neonates. However, as inhaled NO has been shown to increase the bleeding time in animals and healthy adults [22] there is the danger that giving inhaled NO to premature neonates will increase their risk of intracranial haemorrhaging [23]. Also, studies in lambs have shown that inhaled NO of concentrations of 80 and 200 ppm causes damage to the pulmonary surfactant system [24].

The Federal Drugs Administration (FDA) is considering approval of inhaled NO for the treatment of PPHN and infantile respiratory distress syndrome.

3.2. Acute Respiratory Distress Syndrome (ARDS)

Acute respiratory distress syndrome (ARDS) is initially associated with acute pulmonary hypertension. The main pathophysiological change is the marked mismatch of the V/Q ratio and intra-pulmonary right to left shunting of venous blood. This is a result of the alveolar inundation with an inflammatory exudate and the reduced lung compliance as a result of inflammatory infiltration and oedema of the interstitium of the lungs.

Treatment with intravenous vasodilators, such as prostacyclin reduce the elevated pulmonary artery pressure, but can cause serious systemic hypotension, and disturb the matching between the distribution of ventilation and perfusion by dilating poorly ventilated regions of the lung. Normally hypoxic pulmonary vasoconstriction limits the disturbance of the matching between the ventilation and perfusion, but systemically delivered vasodilators override this effect with a fall in systemic oxygenation.

By contrast inhaled NO in ARDS, which is accessible only to ventilated regions of the lungs, increases perfusion of these regions. This effectively improves gas exchange and lessens the intra-pulmonary shunting. By using the multiple inert gas elimination technique (MIGET) it has been shown that the improvement in systemic oxygenation seen when inhaled NO is used to treat ARDS, is due to an increase in V/Q matching. Redistribution of blood flow from poorly ventilated regions of the lung to well ventilated regions is achieved by inhaled NO. The reduction in PVR increases flow through the pulmonary vasculature, thus reducing right to left shunt of venous blood [25]. The large variation in the response to inhaled NO in ARDS, is probably associated with cause and severity of the disease. The dose of inhaled NO required to improve gas exchange in ARDS is lower than the dose necessary to reduce pulmonary artery pressure in PPHN [26]. With lower doses of NO there is probably selective vasodilation of well-ventilated regions of the lung, improving V/Q matching. The effective treatment regime may, therefore, depend upon the underlying cause of the disease.

3.3. Airway Disease

Patients with inflammatory airways diseases, such as asthma, have increased levels of exhaled NO [27]. This is due to the increased production of NO in the lower airways. Selective inhibition of iNOS causes a decrease in exhaled NO in asthma, but not in normal control subjects, whereas non-selective NOS inhibition causes a decrease in NO production in both groups [28]. However the picture is not clear as in the severe inflammatory airways disease cystic fibrosis there is reduced expression of iNOS in the airway epithelium [29]. Besides acting on vascular smooth muscle cells, inhaled NO has also been shown to exert a weak bronchodilatory effect in bronchial asthma [30]. Inhalation of NO by patients with mild asthma during methacholine-induced bronchospasm resulted in a minor but significant reduction in airway tone [31].

Patients with chronic obstructive pulmonary disease (COPD) have irreversible symptomatic airflow obstruction, which can cause hypoxaemia in those patients where the forced expired volume in one second (FEV_1) is less than one litre. The disease is a major cause of mortality and morbidity. In those patients with persistent hypoxaemia where the arterial oxygen tension (PaO_2) is less than 7.3 kPa, long-term oxygen therapy (LTOT) improves survival and quality of life [32]. Patients with COPD and secondary pulmonary hypertension tend to respond poorly to vasodilators. Treatment with inhaled NO can reduce the secondary pulmonary hypertension in COPD patients [33]. However in most patients with COPD inhaled NO has been associated with a worsening of arterial oxygenation possibly resulting from an overall vasodilation of the pulmonary vasculature adversely affecting V/Q matching [33]. New delivery systems are needed to overcome widespread distribution of inhaled NO throughout the aerated lung. Delivery of NO at the beginning of the breath may limit the exposure of high ventilated regions of the lungs to the inhaled NO, which whilst achieving vasodilation will not adversely affect gas exchange [34].

3.4. Primary Pulmonary Hypertension (PPH)

The term primary pulmonary hypertension is used when pulmonary artery pressure is increased without a demonstrable cause. It is more common in females than in males (1.7 to 1), and the mean age of onset is 42 years [35]. There are several risk factors associated with PPH including anorectic use [36], and HIV infection [37]. The tendency to develop PPH can also be transmitted genetically as an autosomal dominant trait with incomplete penetrance [38]. Inhaled NO is effective in reducing pulmonary artery pressure in PPH whilst systemic pressure remains unaltered [12]. Although it is relatively simple to deliver precise concentrations of NO to patients on mechanical ventilation, this is not the case with spontaneously breathing patients. By giving NO as a bolus during inspiration with an oxygen delivery device it has been possible to give inhaled NO therapy to ambulatory patients with PPH [39].

4. Precautions with the Use of Inhaled NO

In air NO reacts with oxygen to form nitrogen dioxide (NO_2). This is a second order reaction with respect to NO and thus the time it takes to yield the recommended upper limit for NO_2 inhalation of 5 ppm depends upon the initial concentration of NO [40]. In an inhaled delivery system both the NO and NO_2 concentration need to be closely monitored. To reduce the formation of NO_2 the amount of time that NO is an contact with oxygen should be minimised, and the inspiratory O_2 should not be higher than clinically indicated.

Abrupt withdrawal of inhaled NO therapy can lead to a dramatic reduction in arterial oxygenation and increase in pulmonary artery pressure [41]. This may be due in part to a reduction of endogenous NO production to levels below that required to maintain normal vasculature tone. In cultured endothelial cells, NO release functions as a negative feedback mechanism by inhibiting NOS [42], and may be the mechanism by which exogenous NO inhibits endogenous NO production. Disruption of ventilation-perfusion matching could also cause the rapid fall in arterial saturation associated with the cessation of treatment. The rebound phenomenon has been shown to be alleviated by the gradual weaning of the patient from NO [41].

5. Future of Inhaled NO Therapy

Many of the problems associated with NO therapy can be overcome by giving NO as a short bolus during inspiration [34]. Giving a 6.7 ml bolus of 100 ppm NO has been shown to be as effective as continuous 40 ppm NO in reducing pulmonary artery pressure in the isolated blood free perfused pig lung whilst reducing the amount of NO given over 20-fold [34]. As NO is only in contact with oxygen for a short time within inspiration there is no problem with the formation of NO_2, and so the need for NO_2 monitoring is eliminated. Reducing the volume of NO used also overcomes the need for continual NO monitoring. This method of administration not only improves the safety of inhaled NO in ventilated patients, but also provides a delivery system for use by ambulatory patients. This strategy has been used successfully in the long term treatment a group of PPH patients [40].

6. References

1 Cremona G, Wood AM, Hall LW, Bower EA, Higenbottam TW (1994) Effect of inhibitors of nitric oxide release and action on vascular tone in isolated lungs of pig, sheep, dog and man. *J Physiol* 81: 185–195
2 Palmer RM, Ferrige AG, Moncada S (1987) Nitric oxide release accounts for the biological activity of endothelium derived relaxing factor. *Nature* 327: 524–526
3 Förstermann U, Kleinert H (1995) Nitric oxide synthase: expression and expressional control of the three isoforms. *Naunyn-Schmiedeberg's Arch Pharmacol* 352: 351–364

4 Schedin U, Frostell C, Persson MG, Jakobsson J, Andersson G, Gustafsson LE (1995) Contribution from upper and lower airways to exhaled endogenous nitric oxide in humans. *Acta Anaesthesiol* 39: 327–332

5 Lundberg JON, Farkas-Szallasi T, Weitzberg E, Rinder J, Lindholm J, Änggård A et al (1995) High nitric oxide production in human paranasal sinuses. *Nature Medicine* 1: 370–373

6 Cremona G, Higenbottam T, Takao M, Hall L, Bower EA (1995) Exhaled nitric oxide in isolated pig lungs. *J Appl Physiol* 78: 59–63

7 Ferro CJ, Webb DJ (1997) Endothelial dysfunction and hypertension. *Drugs* 53: 30–41

8 Giaid A, Saleh D (1995) Reduced expression of endothelial nitric oxide synthase in the lungs of patients with pulmonary hypertension. *N Engl J Med* 333: 214–221

9 Belvisi MG, Barnes PJ, Larkin S, Yacoub M, Tadjkarimi S, Williams TJ et al (1995) Nitric oxide synthase activity is elevated in inflammatory lung disease in humans. *Eur J Pharmacol* 283: 255–258

10 Cremona G, Higenbottam T, Takao M, Bower EA, Hall L (1997) Nature and site of action of endogenous nitric oxide in vasculature of isolated pig lungs. *J Appl Physiol* 82: 23–31

11 Higenbottam TW, Spiegelhalter D, Scott JP, Fuster V, Dinh-Xuan AT, Caine N et al (1993) Prostacyclin (epoprostenol) and heart lung transplantation as a treatment for severe pulmonary hypertension. *Br Heart J* 70: 366–370

12 Pepke-Zaba J, Higenbottam TW, Dinh-Xaun AT, Stone D, Wallwork J (1991) Inhaled nitric oxide as a cause of selective pulmonary vasodilation in pulmonary hypertension. *Lancet* 338: 1173–1174

13 Borland CDR, Higenbottam TW (1989) Simultaneous single breath measurement of pulmonary diffusing capacity with nitric oxide and carbon monoxide. *Eur Resp J* 2: 56–63

14 Wennmalm A, Benthin G, Edlund A, Jungersten L, Keiler-Jensen N, Lundin S et al (1993) Metabolism and Excretion of nitric oxide in humans. *Cir Res* 73: 1121–1127

15 Yoshida K, Kasama K, Kitabatake M, Imai M (1983) Biotransformation of nitric oxide, nitrate, and nitrite. *Int Arch Occup Envir Health* 52: 103–115

16 Ignarro LJ, Harbison RG, Wood KS, Kadowitzt PJ (1986) Activation of purified soluble guanylate cyclase by endothelium derived relaxing factor from intrapulmonary artery and vein: stimulation by acetylcholine, bradykinin and arachidonic acid. *J Pharmacol Exp Ther* 237: 893–900

17 Ignarro LJ (1990) Haem-dependant activation of guanylate cyclase and cyclic GMP formation by endogenous nitric oxide: a unique transduction mechanism for transcellular signalling. *Pharmacol Toxicol* 67: 1–7

18 Bolotina VM, Najibi S, Palacino JJ, Pagano PJ, Cohen RA (1994) Nitric oxide directly activates calcium-dependent potassium channels in vascular smooth muscle. *Nature* 368: 850–853

19 Roberts JD, Fineman JR, Morin FC, Shaul PW, Rimar SR, Schreiber MD et al (1997) Inhaled nitric oxide and persistent pulmonary hypertension of the newborn. *N Eng J Med* 336: 605–610

20 Kinsella JP, Abman SH (1996) Clinical pathophysiology of persistent pulmonary hypertension of the newborn and the role of inhaled nitric oxide. *J Perinat* 16: S24–S27

21 The inhaled nitric oxide study group (1997) Inhaled nitric oxide in full term and nearly full term infants with hypoxic respiratory failure. *N Eng J Med* 336: 597–604

22 Hogman M, Fostell C, Amberg H, Hedenstierna G (1993) Bleeding time prolongation and NO inhalation. *Lancet* 341: 1664–1665

23 Peliowski A, Finer NN, Etches PC, Tierny AJ, Ryan CA (1995) Inhaled nitric oxide for premature infants after prolonged rupture of the membranes. *J Pediat* 126: 450–453

24 Matalon S, DeMarco V, Haddad J, Myles C, Skimming JW, Schürch S et al (1996) Inhaled nitric oxide injures the pulmonary surfactant system of lambs *in vivo*. *Am J Physiol* 270 (*Lung Cell Mol Physiol* 14): L273–L280

25 Rossiant R, Falke KJ, Lopez F, Slama K, Pison U, Zapol WM (1993) Inhaled nitric oxide for the adult respiratory distress syndrome. *N Engl J Med* 328: 399–405

26 Puybasset L, Rouby JJ, Mourgeon E, Stewart TE, Cluzel P, Arthaud M et al (1994) Inhaled nitric oxide in acute respiratory failure: dose-response curves. *Int Care Med* 20: 319–327

27 Alving K, Weittzberg E, Lundberg JM (1993) Increased amount of nitric oxide in exhaled air of asthmatics. *Eur Respir J* 6: 1368–1370

28 Yates-DH, Kharitonov SA, Thomas PS, Barnes PJ (1996) Endogenous nitric oxide is decreased in asthmatic patients by an inhibitor of inducible nitric oxide synthase. *Am J Respir Crit Care Med* 154: 247–250

29 Springall DR, Meng QH, Yacoub MH, Polak JM (1997) Attenuated inducible nitric oxide synthase expression in airway epithelium accompanies CFTR gene mutation. *Am J Respir Crit Care Med* 155: A198

30 Hogman M, Fostell C, Hendenstrom H, Hedenstierna G (1993) Inhalation of nitric oxide modulates adult human bronchial tone. *Am Rev Respir Dis* 148: 1474–1478

31 Kacmarek RM, Ripple R, Cockrill BA, Bloch KJ, Zapol WM, Johnson DC (1996) Inhaled nitric oxide. A bronchodilator in mild asthmatics with methacholine induced bronchospasm. *Am J Resp Crit Care Med* 153: 128–135

32 Medical Research Council (1981) Long term domiciliary oxygen therapy in chronic hypoxic cor pulmonale complicating chronic bronchitis and emphysema. *Lancet* 1: 681–686

33 Barbera JA, Roger N, Roca J, Rovira I, Higenbottam TW, Rodrifuez-Roisin R (1996) Worsening of pulmonary gas exchange with nitric oxide inhalation in chronic obstructive pulmonary disease. *Lancet* 347: 436–440

34 Marriott H, Akamine S, Heller B, McCormack K, Brown B, Higenbottam T (1997) Minimising the dose of inhaled nitric oxide. *Am J Respir Crit Care Med* 155: A629

35 D'Alonzo GE, Barst RJ, Ayres SM, Bergofski EH, Brundage BH, Detre KM et al (1991) Survival in patients with primary pulmonary hypertension. Results from a national prospective registry. *Ann Intern Med* 115: 343–349

36 Brenot F, Herve P, Pretitpretz P, Parent F, Duroux P, Simmoneau G (1993) Primary pulmonary hypertension and fenfluramine use. *Br Heart J* 70: 537–541

37 Morse JH, Barst RJ, Itescu S, Flaster ER, Sinha G, Zhang Y et al (1996) Primary pulmonary hypertension in HIV infection. *Am J Crit Care Med* 153: 1299–1301

38 Lloyd JE, Primm RK, Newman JH (1984) Familial primary pulmonary hypertension: Clinical patterns. *Am Rev Respir Dis* 129: 194–197

39 Channick RN, Newhart JW, Johnson FW, Williams PJ, Auger WR, Fedullo PF et al (1996) Pulsed delivery of inhaled nitric oxide to patients with pulmonary hypertension. *Chest* 109: 1545–1549

40 Foubert L, Fleming B, Latimer R, Jonas M, Oduro A, Borland C et al (1992) Safety guidelines for use of nitric oxide. *Lancet* 339: 1615–1616

41 Lavoie A, Hall JB, Olson DM, Wylam ME (1996) Life-threatening effects of discontinuing inhaled nitric oxide in severe respiratory failure. *Am J Respir Crit Care Med* 153: 1985–1987

42 Assreuy J, Cunha FQ, Liew FY, Moncada S (1993) Feedback inhibition of nitric oxide synthase activity by nitric oxide. *Br J Pharmacol* 108: 833–837

Nitric Oxide in Pulmonary Processes:
Role in Physiology and Pathophysiology of Lung Disease
ed. by M. G. Belvisi and J. A. Mitchell
© 2000 Birkhäuser Verlag Basel/Switzerland

CHAPTER 12
Combined Use of Nitric Oxide and Nitric Oxide Synthase Inhibitors as a Possible Therapeutic Approach

Christoph Thiemermann

The William Harvey Research Institute, St. Bartholomew's Medical College, Charterhouse Square, London EC1M 6BQ, UK

1   Introduction
1.1 Biosynthesis of Nitric Oxide (NO)
1.2 Physiological Role of NO (cardiovascular system)
2   NO and the Pathophysiology of Septic Shock
2.1 NO and Circulatory Failure
2.2 NO and Multiple Organ Failure
3   Modulation of NO Formation in Shock
3.1 Prevention of Inducible Nitric Oxide Synthase (iNOS) Expression
3.2 Non-Selective, Competitive Inhibitors of NOS Activity
3.3 Relatively Selective Inhibitors of iNOS Activity
3.4 Combination of Inhibitors of NOS Activity of NO Donors
3.5 Combination of Inhibitors of NOS Activity with NO Gas Inhalation
4   Concluding Remarks
5   References

1. Introduction

Since the discovery in 1987 that endothelium-derived relaxant factor (EDRF) is identical to the gaseous mediator nitric oxide (NO), we have learned that NO serves as a ubiquitous signalling molecule in the cardiovascular, central nervous and immune systems. NO regulates vascular tone and prevents the adhesion of blood-borne cells to the endothelium. In the lung, the formation of NO by the NO synthase (NOS) located in the endothelium (eNOS) helps to maintain a low vascular resistance and acts to oppose hypoxic pulmonary vasoconstriction. An enhanced formation of NO following the induction of the inducible isoform of NOS (iNOS), however, contributes to the pathophysiology of several diseases including circulatory shock. Although the inhibition of NO formation with agents which non-selectively inhibit all isoforms of NOS exerts some beneficial effects (due to the inhibition of iNOS activity), they also exert side effects, which are secondary to the inhibition of eNOS activity. Using circulatory shock as one example of a disease associated with a significant overproduction of NO, this article reviews the effects and side effects of pharmacological approaches aimed at enhancing (e.g. NO gas, NO donors) or reducing (NOS inhibitors) the formation and/or availability of NO. In addition, results of therapeutic approaches designed to limit the side effects of non-selective inhibitors of NOS activity by combining these agents with either the administration of NO donors or NO inhalation will be discussed.

1.1. Biosynthesis of NO

NO is generated from L-arginine by a family of enzymes collectively called NOS. The oxidation of one of the guanidino nitrogen atoms of this semi-essential amino acid by NOS generates NO as well as L-citrulline. The haem-iron-dependent oxidation of L-arginine is coupled to the reductive activation of molecular oxygen and requires input of reducing equivalents shuttled from the electron donor nicotinamide dinucleotide phosphate (NADPH) to the haem through the flavins, flavin adenine dinucleotide (FAD) and flavin mononucleotide (FMN). In addition to haem, flavins and NADPH, NOS also requires the presence of tetrahydrobiopterin (BH_4), which appears to act both as allosteric effector and redox-active co-factor of the oxidation of L-arginine. Thus, NOS contains an oxygenase domain (containing the catalytic entre) and a reductase domain. The synthesis of NO from L-arginine and molecular oxygen involves the generation of N^G-hydroxy-L-arginine and water (first step) and subsequently the oxidation of N^G-hydroxy-L-arginine in the presence of molecular oxygen to form NO, L-citrulline and water. When generated, NO diffuses to adjacent cells where it activates soluble guanylyl cyclase, resulting in the formation of cyclic guanosine monophosphate (cGMP), which in turn mediates many of the effects of NO. NO is generated by many mammalian cells by at least three different isoforms of NOS. Thus, it is not surprising that NO has many biological functions in the cardiovascular, nervous and immune systems [1]. eNOS in endothelial cells and nNOS in neuronal cells are expressed constitutively, and both enzymes require an increase in intracellular calcium (Ca^{2+}) for activation. Activation of macrophages and many other cells with proinflammatory cytokines or endotoxin results in the expression of a distinct isoform of NOS (iNOS), the activity of which is functionally independent of changes in intracellular Ca^{2+} [see 2–6 for review].

1.2. Physiological Role of NO (Cardiovascular System)

Activation of eNOS by shear stress results in a continuous release of NO (active vasodilatation) which regulates blood pressure and organ blood flow. NO also reduces the adhesion of platelets and polymorphonuclear leukocytes (PMNs) to the endothelium. The latter effect of NO is, at least in part, due to the prevention by NO of the expression of the adhesion molecules P-selectin and intercellular adhesion molecule (ICAM-1) on the surface of endothelial cells. Interestingly, the enhanced expression of eNOS mRNA (e. g. following exposure to shear stress) is associated with a decrease in the transcription of the genes for E-selectin and monocyte chemoattractant protein 1 (MCP-1). In addition to preventing the adhesion of platelets to endothelial cells, NO also directly attenuates the activation of platelets. These effects of NO are associated with and/or due to prevention of (i) the expression of P-selectin (on platelets), (ii) secretion of platelet granules, (iii) intracellular calcium flux, as well as (iv) binding of glycoprotein IIb/IIIa to fibrinogen. It should be noted that both platelets and megakaryocytes are able to generate NO, as both cells contain a constitutive NOS (homologous to eNOS, but with a molecular weight of 85 kDa), and megakaryocytes also contain iNOS. NO can, in principle, also inhibit the activation of PMNs. Moreover, NO attenuates the expression of the adhesion molecules P-selectin, E-selectin and possibly vascular cell adhesion molecule (VCAM)-1 and, hence, may interfere with rolling and attachment of PMNs to the endothelium [7].

In the lung, the formation of NO by eNOS is important in maintaining a low vascular resistance. As the lung is the only organ which receives the entire cardiac output this function of endogenous NO is of utmost importance, as a significant increase in pulmonary vascular resistance leads to a dramatic rise in the workload of the right ventricle and, when excessive, to right heart failure. Hypoxia of specific areas of the lung results in vasoconstriction which serves to divert blood away from poorly oxygenated alveoli and to well oxygenated areas of the lung. In isolated perfused lungs, agents which either inhibit the formation of NO or the generation of cGMP augment the degree of hypoxic vasoconstriction. In a rabbit model of unilateral alveolar hypoxia, inhibition of NO synthesis reduces the distribution of blood flow to hypoxic alveoli resulting in a rise in arterial oxygen tension [8]. Thus, endogenous NO opposes hypoxic vasoconstriction and, hence, maintains perfusion of hypoxic lung units.

2. NO and the Pathophysiology of Septic Shock

The syndrome of shock can be defined as a progressive failure of the circulation to provide blood and oxygen to vital organs. The most common cause of shock is the contamination of blood with bacteria (bacteraemia) resulting in systemic infection and ultimately shock (septic shock). Other causes of shock include severe haemorrhage (haemorrhagic shock), trauma (traumatic shock), failure of the heart to maintain a sufficient cardiac output (cardiogenic shock), interruption of the innervation of blood vessels (neurogenic shock) and severe allergic reactions (anaphylactic shock).

In 1990, several groups independently discovered that an enhanced formation of endogenous NO contributes to (i) hypotension [9] and vascular hyporesponsiveness to vasoconstrictor agents [10, 11] in rodents with endotoxic shock, (ii) hypotension caused by cytokines and endotoxin in dogs [12, 13], (iii) the reduction in liver protein synthesis [14], and (iv) protection of liver integrity in rodents with sepsis [15]. We know today that circulatory shock is associated with an enhanced formation of NO due to the early activation of eNOS and the later induction of iNOS activity in e.g. macrophages, vascular smooth muscle, hepatocytes, cardiac myocytes etc. [16]. This overproduction of NO may contribute to circulatory failure, myocardial dysfunction, organ injury and ultimately multiple organ dysfunction syndrome (MODS; see below). The formation of NO also exerts beneficial effects in endotoxic shock including vasodilatation, prevention of platelet and leukocyte adhesion, improvement of microcirculatory blood flow and augmentation of host defence. Thus, it is not surprising that many colleagues have advocated the use of contrasting therapeutic approaches including (i) inhibition of NOS activity, (ii) enhancement of the availability of NO (NO donors, NO inhalation) or (iii) a combination of both approaches.

2.1. NO and Circulatory Failure

The circulatory failure associated with shock of various aetiologies is characterised by severe hypotension (peripheral vasodilatation), hyporeactivity of the vasculature to vasoconstrictor agents, myocardial dysfunction, maldistribution of organ blood flow and reduced tissue oxygen extraction. There is now good evidence that an enhanced formation of NO contributes to several of these pathophysiological features of septic shock. For instance, an enhanced formation of NO due to activation of eNOS (acute phase of shock) and particularly following the induction of iNOS in the vascular wall (late phase of shock) importantly contributes to the *hypotension* in animals (rat, dog, pig, sheep) and humans with septic shock [5]. Interestingly, endotoxin does not cause hypotension in mice in which the gene for iNOS has been deleted ("iNOS knockout" mice) [17]. Thus, the hypothesis [9] that an enhanced formation of endogenous NO importantly contributes to the hypotension associated with endotoxic shock, is now supported by numerous studies (in various different species from rodents to humans) using different pharmacological (e.g. prevention of iNOS expression, inhibition of iNOS activity with non-selective or iNOS-selective inhibitors, use of agents which scavenge NO etc.) or molecular biological approaches (e.g. gene-targeting of the iNOS gene). The peripheral vascular failure in animals and humans with septic shock also results in a progressive attenuation of the pressor effects afforded by noradrenaline and other vasoconstrictor agents. This phenomenon, which has also been termed *"vasoplegia"* also contributes to the therapy-refractory hypotension in septic shock. Clearly, the hyporeactivity of blood vessels obtained from animals exposed to endotoxic or haemorrhagic shock (for several hours) to catecholamines is largely, but not exclusively, due to an enhanced formation of NO secondary to the induction of iNOS. In endotoxaemia, an NO-mediated *vascular hyporeactivity* occurs in conductance, resistance as well as venous vessels [18]. Prolonged periods of septic shock also cause the development of an *endothelial dysfunction*, which is characterised by the impairment of "endothelium-dependent vasodilatation" and therefore presumably eNOS activity. The mechanism(s) of this endothelial dysfunction may include the downregulation of the expression of the eNOS gene by proinflammatory cytokines such as tumor necrosis factor (TNF)-α, endothelial cell damage due to cytotoxic effects of NO, peroxynitrite or oxygen-derived radicals, and (to a lesser extent) the inactivation of NO by oxygen radicals [5, 19].

2.2. NO and Multiple Organ Failure

The progression of shock or systemic inflammatory response syndrome (SIRS) to multiple organ dysfunction syndrome (MODS) is associated with an increase in mortality from 25–30% (in the absence of MODS) to 90–100% [see 20, 21 for review]. Although there are many investigations documenting the effects of various NOS-inhibitors on systemic or regional haemodynamics in animal models of endotoxic shock, there are few studies investigating the consequences of these interventions on the impairment of organ function associated with shock. Circulatory shock often results in a marked *defect in tissue oxygen extraction* resulting in tissue hypoxia and an increased venous oxygen concentration. As the local generation of large amounts of NO e.g. by activated macrophages, serves to kill bacteria or tumour cells as part of the host defence, it is not surprising that the generation of NO by iNOS in other cells is cytotoxic (suicide mechanism). Indeed, large amounts of NO cause an auto-inhibition of mitochondrial respiration by inhibiting several key enzymes in the mitochondrial respiratory chain (NADH-ubiquinone reductase, succinate-ubiquinone oxido-reductase) or in the Krebs' cycle (e.g. cis-acconitase) resulting in a shift in glucose metabolism from aerobic to anaerobic pathways [4, 19]. NO also causes DNA strand breakage which triggers a futile, energy-consuming repair cycle by activating the nuclear enzyme poly(ADP)ribosyltransferase (PARS). Activation of PARS results in the rapid depletion of the intracellular concentration of NAD^+ (its substrate) slowing the rate of glycolysis, electron transfer and ATP formation which ultimately results in cell death ("PARS suicide hypothesis") [22, 23]. Thus, the generation of large amounts of NO by iNOS may contribute to the defect in oxygen extraction and ultimately cell hypoxia and death by causing (i) maldistribution of regional blood flow (reduced oxygen supply), (ii) formation of a diffusion barrier for oxygen within the vascular wall (reduced oxygen transport), (iii) inhibition of the generation of ATP (reduced oxygen utilisation), and (iii) excesive and futile consumption of ATP. In concert with the severe hypotension (reduced perfusion pressure), these effects of the local overproduction of NO may importantly contribute to the organ injury and dysfunction associated with septic shock. Studies using inhibitors of NOS activity in animals with endotoxic shock have yet to convincingly demonstrate that an enhanced formation of NO by iNOS contributes to multiple organ failure. There is evidence that some inhibitors of NOS activity (e.g. those which preferentially inhibit iNOS activity) reduce the organ dysfunction, while others (e.g. relatively selective inhibitors of eNOS activity) may have no effect or even enhance the organ injury/dysfunction caused by endotoxic shock. Although selective inhibitors of iNOS activity reduce the liver dysfunction in endotoxaemia in rodents [24, 25], the degree of liver injury caused by endotoxin in mcie in which the iNOS gene was inactivated by gene targeting (iNOS knock out) is similar to the one elicited by endotoxin in wild-type mice [17]. There is little information regarding the effects of inhibitors of NOS activity on the lung dysfunction caused by endotoxin in animals. In the anaesthetised rat, endotoxaemia causes within 15 min an acute metabolic acidosis as indicated by falls in bicarbonate and base excess. This metabolic acidosis is compensated by a hyperventilation resulting in falls in arterial PO_2. Treatment of lipopolysaccharide (LPS)-treated rats with the selective iNOS inhibitor 1-amino-2-hydroxy-guanidine significantly attenuates the falls in bicarbonate and base excess as well as the secondary fall in PO_2 [25]. As the fall in PO_2 observed in this study was secondary to a metabolic acidosis rather than a direct dysfunction of the lung, this study demonstrates that endogenous NO contributes to the dysfunction of various organs (e.g. liver, pancreas) and presumably the development of a defect in tissue oxygen extraction, but does not provide direct evidence that NO from iNOS contributes to the lung dysfunction associated with endotoxic shock.

3. Modulation of NO Formation in Shock

The controversy as to whether endogenous NO has beneficial or detrimental effects in septic shock has fuelled the search for therapeutic interventions aimed at (i) reducing the formation of NO, (ii) enhancing the availability of NO or (iii) combining both approaches. In principle, there are two approaches for reducing the formation of NO in septic shock, namely inhibition of iNOS expression or inhibition of iNOS activity. The local or systemic availability of NO may be enhanced by using NO donors or NO gas inhalation either alone or in combination with NOS inhibitors. The following paragraphs discuss the effects and side effects of therapeutic approaches aimed at modulating the formation of NO in animal models of endotoxic shock.

3.1. Prevention of iNOS Expression

The list of xenobiotics which prevent the induction of iNOS activity and protein is ever growing and now includes antibodies to TNF-α, soluble TNF-α receptors, the endogenous interleukin (IL)-1 receptor antagonist, IL-4, IL-10, IL-11, IL-13, platelet activation factor (PAF)-receptor antagonists, dihydropyridine-type calcium channel antagonists, ketokonazole, glibenclamide, N-acetylserotonin (an inhibitor of the salvage pathway for the generation of BH_4), 2,4-diamino-6-hydroxy-pyrimidine (DAHP, an inhibitor of the activity of GTP cyclohydrolase and, hence, BH_4, biosynthesis), tyrosine kinase inhibitors (genistein, tryphostins, erbstatin), inhibitors of the activation of the nuclear transcription factor NFκB (rotenone, PDTC, butyrolated hydroxyanisole) or inhibitors of IκB-protease (calpain inhibitor 1); to name but a few [26]. It should, however, be pointed out that agents which prevent the expression of iNOS have to be administered prior to endotoxin to prevent induction of iNOS, circulatory failure or MODS. In contrast, once hypotension (and presumably iNOS induction) has occurred, the administration of dexamethasone (and other agents which prevent the induction of iNOS) fails to improve haemodynamics and organ function. In contrast, inhibition of the activity of NOS offers the opportunity for a late intervention in animals and patients which have developed hypotension and early signs of the onset of organ dysfunction. Nevertheless, the above interventions have helped to elucidate the signal transduction events leading to the expression of iNOS *in vitro* and *in vivo* (Fig. 1).

3.2. Non-selective, Competitive Inhibitors of NOS Activity

The discovery of L-arginine-analogues which inhibit NOS activity including N^G-methyl-L-arginine (L-NMMA) provided the first tool to explore beneficial or side effects of NOS inhibition in animals and humans with septic shock. The subsequent publication of papers describing the use of the NOS inhibitors N^G-nitro-L-arginine (L-NA) and its methyl ester (L-NAME) [27], which in contrast to L-NMMA were cheap and readily available, stimulated numerous studies aimed at evaluating the role of NO in septic shock by using L-NAME. This was somewhat unfortunate, as L-NAME is a more potent inhibitor of eNOS than iNOS activity and hence, caused many adverse effects resulting from the inhibition of eNOS activity including excessive vasoconstriction (e.g. fall in cardiac output, pulmonary hypertension, reduction in mesenteric blood flow, reduction in renal blood flow etc.) and enhanced adhesion of platelets and neutrophils to the

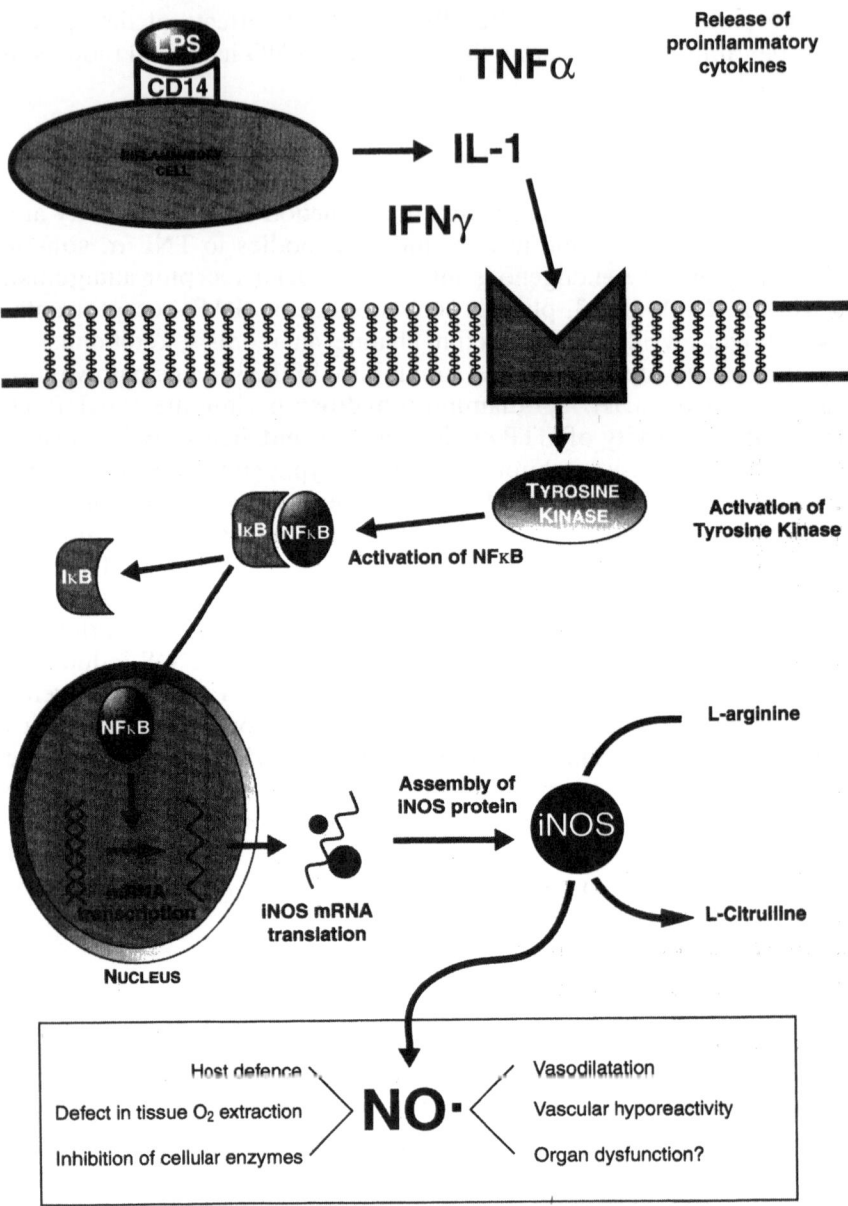

Figure 1. Schematic diagram illustrating the postulated signal transduction pathway(s) leading to the increased expression of inducible nitric oxide synthase (iNOS).

endothelium [see 19, 28]. Thus, it was not surprising that high doses of L-NAME or even L-NMMA increased mortality in mice and rabbits with endotoxic shock [29, 30]. The hypothesis that the basal relase of NO by eNOS has an important role in the regulation of regional blood flow (beneficial effects of NO), while the excessive generation of NO by iNOS contributes to some aspects of the pathophysiology of shock (harmful effects of NO), has stimulated the search for novel therapeutic approaches which maximise the benefits resulting from the inhibition of iNOS activity, while minimising the side effects arising from inhibition of eNOS activity. These therapeutic approaches include the development of selective inhibitors of iNOS activity or the combination of non-selective inhibitors of NOS activity with either NO donors (to minimise the systemic side effects arising from inhibition of eNOS activity, e.g. excessive vasoconstriction and adhesion of blood-borne cells to the endothelium) or NO gas inhalation (to minimise side effects resulting from excessive pulmonary vasoconstriction).

3.3. Relatively Selective Inhibitors of iNOS Activity

The following paragraphs highlight some aspects of the chemistry and pharmacology of NOS inhibitors which are relatively selective towards iNOS. For a more detailed and complete account of the chemistry and isoenzyme selectivity of NOS inhibitors, the interested reader is referred to a recent, excellent review of this topic [31].

Aminoguanidine was the first relatively selective inhibitor of iNOS activity discovered [32]. Although aminoguanidine is a more potent inhibitor of iNOS than eNOS activity [33–35], aminoguanidine is not a very potent inhibitor of iNOS activity. In addition, aminoguanidine is not a very specific inhibitor of NOS activity, as this guanidine has many other pharmacological properties (e.g. inhibition of histamine and polyamine metabolism, inhibition of catalase activity). Interestingly, aminoguanidine also prevents the expression of iNOS protein by a hitherto unknown mechanism [36]. Other guanidines including (in the rank order of their potency as inhibitors of iNOS activity in murine macrophages and smooth muscle cells) 1-amino-2-hydroxy-guanidine, 1-amino-2-methyl-guanidine, 1-amino-1-methyl-guanidine and 1-amino-1,2-dimethylguanidine also inhibit iNOS activity [25]. Of these, 1-amino-2-hydroxyguanidine is more potent, more selective and more soluble in aqueus solutions than aminoguanidine itself and hence, may be more suitable than the respective parent compound [25]. There is now good evidence that aminoguanidine attenuates the circulatory failure and reduces mortality caused by endotoxin in rodents. Moreover 1-amino-2-hydroxy-guanidine also reduced the liver and pancreatic dysfunction caused by endotoxin in rats [25].

S-substituted isothioureas (ITUs) are non-amino acid analogues of L-arginine and also potent inhibitors of iNOS activity with variable isoform selectivity [37–39]. The most potent isothioureas were those with only short alkyl chains on the sulphur atom and no substitutes on the nitrogen atoms. For instance, S-ethyl-ITU is a potent competitive inhibitor of all isoforms of human and murine NOS [37]. In contrast to S-ethyl-ITU, aminoethyl-ITU and S-methyl-ITU are more selective inhibitors of iNOS than of eNOS activity [39]. Aminoethyl-ITU is metabolised to mercaptoethyl-guanidine, which may represent the active principle of aminoethyl-ITU [31]. Clearly, both S-methyl-ITU as well as aminoethyl-ITU attenuate the circulatory failure caused by endotoxin even when given up to 2 h after administration of endotoxin in rats. Moreover, both isothioureas attenuate the multiple organ failure as well as the mortality caused by endotoxin in the rat [24, 38]. S-substituted ITUs and guanidines contain the amidine function, feature which they have in common with O-substituted isoureas and amidines themselves. Indeed, amidines including 2-iminopiperidine, butyramidine, 2-aminopyridine, propioamidine and (to a much lesser extent) acetamidine inhibit NOS activity. Interestingly, both 2-iminopiperidine and butyramidine were more potent inhibitors of iNOS activity than L-NMMA in murine macrophages [40].

The number of novel NOS inhibitors which differ in chemistry and selectivity towards certain isoenzymes of NOS is ever increasing and their pharmacology has recently been reviewed elsewhere [31]. It should, however, be noted that none of these agents are 100% selective inhibitors of iNOS activity and hence, may (at higher doses) cause side-effects due to inhibition of eNOS activity.

3.4. Combination of Inhibitors of NOS Activity with NO Donors

Any potential side effects of non-selective (or even iNOS-selective) NOS inhibitors may be overcome by combining these agents with NO donors which may improve regional haemodynamics and inhibit the adhesion of platelets and PMNs to the endothelium in the absence of NO synthesis by endothelial cells (due to eNOS inhibition). There is some evidence that NO donors per see may exert beneficial haemodynamic effects in animal models of endotoxic or septic shock. For instance, in a canine model of endotoxaemia the continuous infusion of low to moderate doses (1 or 2 μg/kg/min) of the NO donor 3-morpholinosydnonimine (SIN-1) caused increases in cardiac index, stroke index and left ventricular stroke work index, without causing a significant alteration in systemic or pulmonary arterial pressures. Moreover, SIN-1 increased mesenteric, but not renal blood flow. Infusion of SIN-1, however, had no effect on the increase in the plasma levels of TNF-α or lactate. In contrast, higher doses of the NO donor (4 μg/kg/min) caused reductions in blood pressure, cardiac index and stroke index. These results suggest that lower to moderate doses of the NO donor SIN-1 improve the perfusion of the mesenteric vascular bed without causing systemic haemodynamic side effects [41]. Similarly, the NO donor linsidomine (2 mg over 3 h) attenuated the fall in systemic and hepatic perfusion associated with hypodynamic, endotoxic shock in rabbits. These beneficial haemodynamic effects of the NO donor were associated with a reduction in the degree of lactic acidosis caused by endotoxaemia in this species [42, 43]. These findings support the notion that NO donors may improve regional haemodynamics without causing a further deterioration in systemic haemodynamics in animals with endotoxic shock. Pre-treatment of rabbits with a high dose of L-NMMA prior to injection of LPS augments the degree of (acute) hypotension and regional vasoconstriction as well as the mortality caused by endotoxaemia. These detrimental effects of the inhibition of NOS activity are abolished by co-administration of the NO donor S-nitroso-N-acetyl penicillamine (SNAP) [29]. These findings support the view that the detrimental effects arising from inhibition of eNOS activity can be limited by the concomitant administration of an NO donor. Further studies are necessary to elucidate the effects of the co-administration of NOS inhibitors (either non-selective or iNOS-selective) and NO donors on organ function in animal models of endotoxaemia and sepsis.

3.5. Combination of Inhibitors of NOS Activity with NO Gas Inhalation

There is now good evidence that the inhibition of the formation of NO by eNOS in the pulmonary vascular bed leads to pulmonary vasoconstriction [18, 28]. As endotoxaemia per se leads (in many species including humans) to a rise in pulmonary vascular resistance, the administration of non-selective NOS inhibitors in animals with endotoxaemia results in a further rise in pulmonary vascular resistance which (in some species such as the pig) may even lead to a fall in cardiac output due to a reduction in left ventricular filling pressures. The following paragraphs review the effects of NO gas inhalation on the alteration in pulmonary haemodynamics and gas exchange in animals with endotoxic shock. In pigs with endotoxaemia, NO inhalation (10 parts per million (ppm)) selectively attenuates the pulmonary hypertension caused by endotoxin without affecting blood pressure or cardiac output. Moreover, inhalation of NO reduces the fall in pH and arterial oxygen tension suggesting that this intervention prevents the deterioration in gas exchange caused by endotoxaemia. In this model, endotoxaemia also results in a marked activation of the sympathetic system as indicated by an increase in the plasma levels of noradrenaline and neuropeptide Y. Interestingly, this excessive activaton of the sympathetic system is also attenuated by inhalation of NO gas [44]. In pigs receiving a continuous infusion of endotoxin, intermittent inhalation of NO gas (57 ppm) prevents the initial peak rise in pulmonary artery pressure and resistance and diminishes pulmonary shunting. Most notably, inhalation of NO gas also attenuates the degree of platelet activation caused by endotoxin [45].

The severe pulmonary vasoconstriction caused by endotoxin in pigs is also associated with a decrease in right ventricular ejection fraction and an increase in right ventricular and diastolic volume. Inhalation of NO gas (40 ppm, after the onset of endotoxaemia) reduces the degree of pulmonary hypertension and significantly increases right ventricular ejection fraction [46]. Thus, inhalation of NO gas prevents or reverses the rise in pulmonary vascular resistance and the subsequent dysfunction of the right ventricle.

These beneficial effects of NO inhalation in animal models of endo-toxaemia stimulated studies which compared the effects of intravenous infusion of the NOS inhibitor L-NMMA, with that of NO gas inhalation and with that of a combination of both interventions in pigs with endo-toxaemia [47]. The infusion of endotoxin (15 pg/kg/h for 3 h) causes a pro-gressive fall in blood pressure and cardiac output and a biphasic increase in mean pulmonary artery pressure (Fig. 2) and pulmonary vascular resis-tance. In these animals, a continuous infusion of L-NMMA (0.1 mg/kg/min) significantly attenuates the fall in blood pressure, but does not affect the alteration in mean pulmonary artery pressure (Fig. 2), pulmonary vas-cular resistance or cardiac output caused by endotoxaemia. NO inhalation (50 ppm) does not affect the hypotension, but significantly blunts the biphasic rise in pulmonary artery pressure and pulmonary vascular re-sistance and delays the fall in cardiac output. Most importantly, the combi-nation of L-NMMA and NO gas inhalaton prevents the fall in blood pres-sure, significantly improves cardiac output and attenuates the biphasic rise in pulmonary artery pressure and (Fig. 2) pulmonary vascular resistance [47]. Endotoxaemia also causes a decline in PaO_2 (Fig. 3) and a rise in $PaCO_2$. Infusion of L-NMMA neither affects the fall in PaO_2 (Fig. 3) nor the rise in $PaCO_2$. In contrast, inhalation with NO gas alone as well as the combined administration of L-NMMA infusion and NO inhalation pre-vents the fall in PaO_2 (Fig. 3) and attenuates the subsequent rise in $PaCO_2$. Infusion of endotoxin for 3 h results in a mortality of 58%, which is not affected by L-NMMA (63%). In contrast, treatment of endotoxaemic pigs with either NO inhalation alone or NO inhalation plus L-NMMA abolishes the mortality caused by endotoxin. Thus, this study demonstrates that the combined treatment with NO gas inhalation and systemic administration of L-NMMA is superior to either treatment alone in preventing the endotoxin-induced alterations in gas exchange, haemodynamics and mortality in anaesthetised pigs [47]. In a similar study, Weitzberg and colleagues [48] also demonstrate that the combination of the NOS inhibitor L-NAME (50 mg/kg/h) and NO gas inhalation (50 ppm) attenuates the degree of pul-monary hypertension and improved gas exchange in pigs with endotoxic shock. Moreover L-NAME plus NO inhalation prevents the development of systemic hypotension, but impaired cardiac output and increased systemic and renal vascular resistance to supranormal levels [48]. Taken together, these studies demonstrate that NO gas inhalation may improve pulmonary and cardiac haemodynamics and attenuates the rise in pulmo-

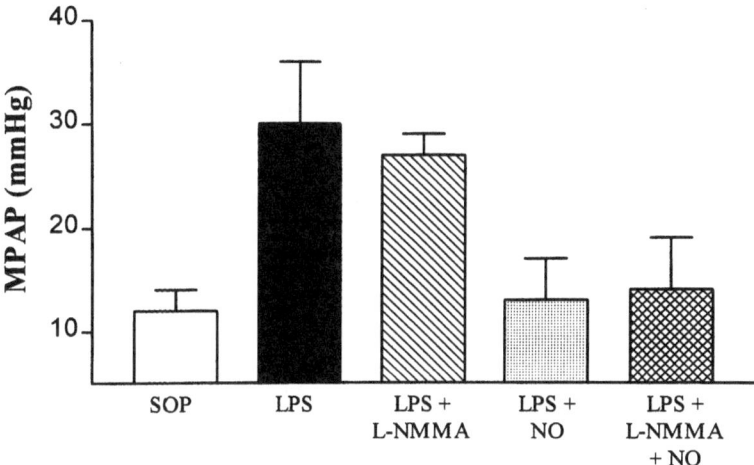

Figure 2. Effect of LPS alone nd in combination with the nitric oxide synthase inhibitor N^G-methyl-L-arginine (L-NMMA) and/or nitric oxide (NO) on mean pulmonary artery pressure (MPAP) in anaesthetised pigs. SOP; sham operated pigs.

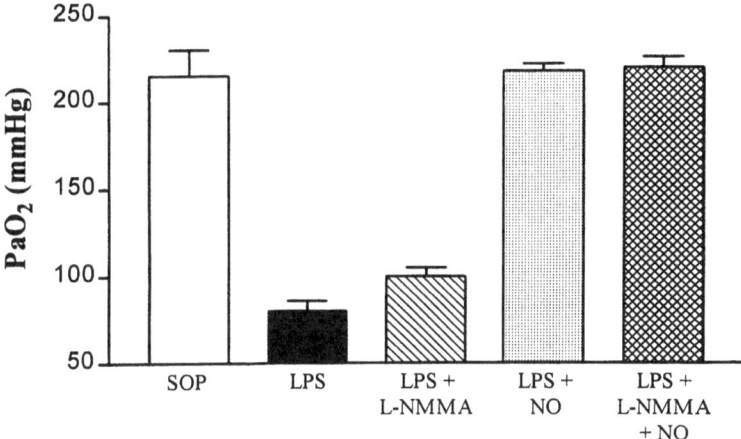

Figure 3. Effect of LPS alone and in combination with the nitric oxide synthase inhibitor N^G-methyl-L-arginine (L-NMMA) and/or nitric oxide (NO) on pulmonary artery O_2 (PaO_2) in anaesthetised pigs. SOP; sham operated pigs.

nary vascular resistance caused by inhibition of eNOS activity with non-selective inhibitors of NOS in pigs with endotoxaemia. When compared to other species, pigs are more likely to develop a rapid rise in pulmonary vascular resistance (and a subsequent dysfunction of the right heart) when exposed to infusion of endotoxin. Thus, the benefits arising from the inhalation of NO gas (either alone or in combination of NOS inhibitors) may well be greater in pigs than in other animals. Nevertheless, there is evidence that inhibition of NOS activity with L-NMMA in patients with septic shock also results in a significant rise in pulmonary vascular resistance [49]. If the ongoing multi-centre clinical trial which evaluates the effects of L-NMMA in patients with septic shock reveals that pulmonary vasoconstriction is, indeed, an important side effect of NOS inhibitors in humans, it may well be possible and useful to limit the rise in pulmonary vascular resistance caused by these agents by NO gas inhalation.

4. Concluding Remarks

Since 1990, numerous studies have documented that animal models of circulatory shock of various aetiologies are associated with an enhanced formation of NO. Similarly, patients with septic shock and IL-2 immunotherapy exhibit elevated plasma levels of nitrite/nitrate. Although the enhanced formation of NO in animals and humans with septic shock contributes to hypotension and hyporeactivity of the vasculature to vasoconstrictor agents (vasoplegia), it is still unclear whether NO (from iNOS) contributes to the organ dysfunction/failure syndrome associated with severe septic shock. The inhibition of eNOS activity in animals with endotoxic shock results in excessive vasoconstriction (e.g. increase in pulmonary vascular resistance) and augments the adhesion of platelets and neutrophils to the endothelium. This side effect of non-selective inhibitors of NOS activity may be avoided by using selective inhibitors of iNOS activity or circumvented by combining these agents with NO donors or NO inhalation therapy. It should be stressed that the many reported adverse effects of NOS inhibition are, in most studies, due to the use of large quantities of L-NAME, an agent which is a more potent inhibitor of eNOS than iNOS activity. If the results of the ongoing clincial trial evaluating the effects of L-NMMA should reveal that this NOS inhibitor causes an increase in pulmonary vascular resistance, this adverse effect may well be prevented by inhalation of NO. Although there are few studies investigating the effects of NO donors (either alone or in combination with inhibitors of NOS activity) in animal models of shock, these agents should in principle be useful to overcome the "endothelial dysfunction" associated with shock. When given together with inhibitors of NOS activity, NO donors may also limit the systemic side effects arising from inhibition of eNOS activity. The results of the multi-centre trial of L-NMMA in patients with septic shock are eagerly awaited. Obviously, the outcome of this clinical trial will importantly influence any future strategies aimed at modulating the biosynthesis of NO in shock.

5. References

1 Moncada S, Higgs A (1993) The L-arginine-nitric oxide pathway. *N Engl J Med* 329: 2202–2212
2 Nathan C (1992) Nitric oxide as a secretory product of mammalian cells. *FASEB J* 6: 3051–3064
3 Dinerman JL, Lowenstein CJ, Snyder SH (1993) Molecular mechanism of nitric oxide regulation: potential relevance to cardiovascular disease. *Circ Res* 73: 217–222
4 Morris SM, Billiar TR (1994) New insights into the regulation of inducible nitric oxide synthase. *Am J Physiol* 266: E829–839
5 Thiemermann C (1994) The role of L-arginine: nitric oxide pathway in circulatory shock. *Adv Pharmacol* 28: 45–79
6 Szabo C, Thiemermann C (1994) Role of nitric oxide in haemorrhage, traumatic and anaphylactic shock, and thermal injury. *Shock* 2: 145–155
7 Loscalzo J, Welch G (1995) Nitric oxide and its role in the cardiovascular system. *Prog Cardiovasc Dis* 38: 87–104
8 Sprague RS, Thiemermann C, Vane JR (1992) Endogenous endothelium-derived relaxing factor opposes hypoxic pulmonary vasoconstriction and supports blood flow to hypoxic alveoli in anaesthetized rabbits. *Proc Natl Acad Sci USA* 89: 8711–8715
9 Thiemermann C, Vane JR (1990) Inhibition of nitric oxide synthesis reduces the hypotention induced by bacterial lipopolysaccharide in the rat. *Eur J Pharmacol* 182: 591–595
10 Julou-Schaeffer G, Gray GA, Fleming I, Schott C, Parratt JR, Stoclet JC (1990) Loss of vascular responsiveness induced by endotoxin involves the L-arginine pathway. *Am J Physiol* 259: H1038–H1043
11 Rees DD, Celleck S, Palmer RMJ, Moncada S (1990) Dexamethasone prevents the induction of nitric oxide synthase and the associated effects on the vascular tone: an insight into endotoxic shock. *Biochem Biophys Res Commun* 173: 541–547
12 Kilboum RG, Juburan A, Gross SS, Griffith OW, Levi R, Adams J et al (1990) Reversal of endotoxin-mediated shock by N^G-monomethyl-L-arginine, an inhibitor of nitric oxide synthesis. *Biochem Biophys Res Commun* 172: 1132–1138
13 Kilbourn RG, Gross SS, Jubran A, Adams J, Griffith OW, Levi R at al (1990) N^G-methyl-L-arginine inhibits tumour necrosis factor-induced hypotension: implications for the involement of nitric oxide. *Proc Natl Acad Sci USA* 87: 62932
14 Curran RD, Ferrari FK, Kispert KH, Stadler J, Stuchr DJ, Simmons RL et al (1991) Nitric oxide and nitric oxide-generating compounds inhibit hepatocyte protein synthesis. *FASEB J* 5: 2085–2095
15 Billiar TR, Curran RD, Harbrecht BG, Stuchr DJ, Demetris AJ, Simmons RL (1990) Modulation of nitric oxide synthesis *in vivo*. N^G-monomethyl-L-arginine endotoxin-induced nitrite/nitrate biosynthesis while promoting hepatic damage. *J Leukoc Biol* 48: 565–569
16 Szabo C, Mitchell JA, Thiemermann C, Vane JR (1993) Nitric oxide-mediated hyporeactivity to noradrenaline precedes the induction of nitric oxide synthase in endotoxin shock. *Br J Pharmacol* 108: 786–792
17 MacMicking JD, Nathan C, Horn G, Chartrain N, Fletcher DS, Trumbauer M et al (1995) Altered responses to bacterial infection and endotoxic shock in mice lacking inducible nitric oxide synthase. *Cell* 82: 641–650
18 Parratt JR, Stoclet JC (1995) Vascular smooth muscle function under conditions of sepsis and endotoxaemia. In: Firik MP, Payen D (eds) Role of nitric oxide in sepsis and ARDS. Berlin: Springer, 44–61
19 Thiemermann C (1995) Inhibition of nitric oxide synthase activity in circulatory shock: Friend or Foe? In: Fink MP, Payen D (eds) Role of nitric oxide in sepsis and ARDS. Berlin: Springer, 201–216
20 Baue AE (1983) The multiple organ or systems failure syndrome. In: Schlag G, Redl H (eds). Pathophysiology of shock, sepsis and organ failure. Berlin: Springer, 1004–1018
21 Bone RC (1994) Gram-positive organism and sepsis. *Arch Intem Med* 154: 26–34
22 Schraufstatter L, Hinshaw D, Hyslop P, Spragg R, Cochrane C (1986) Oxidant injury of cells. DNA strand breaks activate polyadenosine diphosphate ribose polymerase and lend to depletion of nicotinamide adenine dinucleotide. *J Clin Invest* 77: 1312–1319

23 Zingarelli B, O'Conner M, Wong H, Salzman AL, Szabo C (1996) Peroxynitrite-mediated DNA breakage activates polyadenosine diphosphate ribosyl sythetase and causes cellular energy depletion in macrophages stimulated with bacterial lipopolysaccharide. *J Immunol* 156: 350–358

24 Thiemermann C, Ruetten H, Wu CC, Vane JR (1995) The multiple organ dysfunction syndrome caused by endotoxin in the rat: Attenuation of liver dysfunction by inhibitors of nitric oxide synthase. *Br J Pharmacol* 116: 2845–2851

25 Ruetten H, Southan GJ, Abate A, Thiemermann C (1996) Attenuation of the multiple organ dysfunction caused by endotoxin by 1-amino-2-hydroxy-guanidine, a potent inhibitor of inducible nitric oxide synthase. *Br J Pharmacol* 118: 261–270

26 Szabo C, Thiemermann C (1995) Regulation of the expression of the inducible isoform of nitric oxide synthase. *Adv Pharmacol* 34: 113–154

27 Moore PK, Al-Swayeh OH, Chong NWS, Evans RA, Gibson A (1990) L-N-nitro-arginine, a novel, L-arginine reversible inhibitor of endothelium-dependent vasodilatation *in vitro*. *Br J Pharmacol* 99: 408–412

28 Cobb JP, Danner RL (1996) Nitric oxide and septic shock. *JAMA* 275: 1192–1196

29 Wright CE, Rees DD, Moncada S (1991) Protective and pathological roles of nitric oxide in endotoxic shock. *Cardiovasc Res* 26: 48–57

30 Park JH, Chang SH, Lee KM, Shin SH (1996) Protective effect of nitric oxide in an endotoxin-induced septic shock. *Am J Surg* 171: 340–345

31 Southan GJ, Szabo C (1996) Selective pharmacological inhibition of distinct nitric oxide synthase isoforms. *Biochem Pharmacol* 51: 383–394

32 Corbett JA, Tilton RG, Chang K, Hasan KS, Ido Y, Wang JL, Sweetland MA, Lancaster JR, Williamson JR, McDaniel ML (1992) Aminoguanidine, a novel inhibitor of nitric oxide formation, prevents diabetic vascular dysfunction. *Diabetes* 41: 552–558

33 Misko TP, Moore WM, Kasten TP, Nickols DA, Corbett JA, Tilton RG et al (1993) Selective inhibition of the inducible nitric oxide synthase by aminoguanidine. *Eur J Pharmacol* 233: 119–125

34 Wu CC, Chen SJ, Szabo C, Thiemermann C, Vane JR (1995) Aminoguanidine attenuates the delayed circulatory failure and improves survival in rodent models of endotoxic shock. *Br J Pharmacol* 114: 1666–1672

35 Wu CC, Ruetten H, Thiemermann C (1996) Comparison of the effects of aminoguanidine and N^G-nitro-L-arginine methyl esteron the multiple organ dysfunction caused by endotoxaemia in the rat. *Eur J Pharmacol* 300: 99–104

36 Garvey PE, Oplinger JA, Tanoury GJ, Sherman PA, Fowler M, Marshall S et al (1994) Potent and selective inhibition of human nitric oxide syntheses. Inhibition by non-amino acid isothioureas. *J Biol Chem* 269: 26669–26676

37 Szabo C, Southan G, Thiemermann C (1994) Beneficial effects and improved survival in rodent models of septic shock with S-methyl-isothiourea sulfate, a novel, potent and selective inhibitor of inducible nitric oxide synthase. *Proc Natl Acad Sci USA* 91: 12472–12476

38 Sontham G, Szabo C, Thiemermann C (1995) Isothioureas: potent inhibitors of nitric oxide syntheses with variable isoform selectivity. *Br J Pharmacol* 114: 510–516

39 Sontham GJ, Szabo C (1996) Selective pharmacological inhibition of distinct nitric oxide synthase isoforms. *Biochem Pharmacol* 51: 383–394

40 Southan GJ, Szabo C, O'Conner MP, Salzman AC, Thiemermann C (1996) Amidines are potent inhibitors of constitutive and inducible nitric oxide syntheses: Preferential inhibition of the inducible isoform. *Eur J Pharmacol* 291: 311–318

41 Zhang H, Rogiers P, Friedman G, Prelser JC, Spapen H, Buurman WA, Vincent JL (1996) Effects of nitric oxide donor SIN-1 on oxygen availability and regional blood flow during endotoxic shock. Arch Surg 11: 767–774

42 Pastor CM, Payen DM (1994) Effect of modifying nitric oxide pathway on liver circulation in a rabbit endotoxin shock model. *Shock* 2: 196–202

43 Pastor CM, Losser MR, Payen D (1995) Nitric oxide donor prevents hepatic and systemic perfusion decrease induced by endotoxin in anesthetized rabbits. *Hepatology* 22: 1547–1553

44 Weitzberg E, Rudehill A, Lundberg JM (1993) Nitric oxide inhaltion attenuates pulmonary hypertension and improves gas exchange in endotoxic shock. *Eur J Pharmacol* 233: 85–94

45 Dalim P, Blomquist S, Martensson L, Thorne J, Zoucas E (1994) Circulatory and ventilatory effects of intermittent nitric oxide inhalation during porcine endotoxaemia. *J Trauma* 37: 769–777
46 Offner PJ, Ogura H, Jordan BS, Pruitt BA, Cioffi WG (1995) Effects of inhaled nitric oxide on right ventricular function in endotoxin shock. *J Trauma* 39: 179–185
47 Klemm P, Thiemermann C, Winklmaler G, Martorana PA, Henning R (1995) Effects of nitric oxide synthase inhibition combined with nitric oxide inhalation in a porcine model of endotoxic shock. *Br J Pharmacol* 114: 363–368
48 Weitzberg E, Rudehill A, Modin A, Lundberg JM (1995) Effect of combined nitric oxide inhalation and N^G-nitro-L-arginine infusion in procine endotoxin shock. *Crit Care Med* 23: 909–918
49 Petros A, Lamb G, Leone A, Moncada S, Bennett D, Vallance P (1994) Effects of a nitric oxide synthase inhibitor in humans with septic shock. *Cardiovasc Res* 28: 34–39

Subject index

α-adrenergic agonist 189

β_2-agonist, inhaled long-acting 178
β_2-agonist, inhaled short-acting 178

5-HT 103

acetylcholine 130, 140, 141
acute respiratory distress syndrome (ARDS) 25, 28–30, 204
adenosine monophosphate (AMP) 99
adenosine 175
ADP-ribosylation 145
adult respiratory distress syndrome 176
airway 41, 151, 167
airway disease 204
airway disease, chronic 176
airway disease, pathophysiology of 167
airway edema 136
airway eosinophilia 155
airway epithelial cell 152
airway epithelium 111
airway hyperresponsiveness 115, 134
airway inflammation 113, 128, 133, 134, 136, 152, 167, 178
airway inflammation, measuring of 178
airway neuron, intrinsic 147
airway obstruction 136, 138
airway resistance (Rperiph), peripheral 140
airway response, constrictor of 131
airway response, neural dilator of 131
airway responsiveness 142, 173
airway smooth muscle 41, 152, 140
airway, lower 152
airway, microvascular leak of 147
airway, upper 152
allergen 118
allergen challenge 112, 155, 173
aminoguanidine 115, 178, 217
angiotensin II (A-II) 99, 103
antibiotics 177
antigen 134, 136
antiserum, immunohistochemistry of 72
antiserum, postembedding immunohisto-chemistry of 73
antiserum, preembedding immunohisto-chemistry of 73
apocynin 115
apoptosis 31, 32
arachidonic acid 115
arginine vasopressin (AVP) 99

L-arginine 105, 170, 178, 189
arteries, leakage of 194
asthma 42, 112, 142, 143, 152, 167, 173, 174
asthma, bronchial 152
ATP 96, 103

beating, ciliary 171, 177
biopsy, bronchial 173, 178
blood flow 141
bradykinin (BK) 99, 128
breath-holding 173
bronchial circulation 194
bronchial smooth muscle 136, 137, 140, 144
bronchialveolar lavage (BAL) 172, 178
bronchiectasis 81, 167
bronchiolitis, obliterative 171
bronchitis, chronic 176
bronchoconstriction 129, 131, 141, 142, 154
bronchoconstriction, capsaicin-induced 133
bronchoconstriction, histamine-induced 135, 139, 140
bronchoconstriction, methacholine-induced 138, 141
bronchoconstriction, modulation of 130
bronchoconstrictor, response of 136
bronchodilation, neural 74, 128
bronchodilator 128, 133, 140, 142, 143, 145, 146
bronchoscopy, fibreoptic 172

calcium homeostasis 12
cancer 82
capsaicin 131, 133
catecholamine 103
cell/pathogen killing, NO-mediated 14
chemiluminescence 168
chemokine 155
chronic obstructive pulmonary disease (COPD) 141, 176
cilia 191
ciliary activity, defect of 177
circulatory failure 212
circulatory shock 209
CO_2 141
constrictor, neural 130
contraction, adrenergic 91, 92
contraction, hypoxic 103, 104
contraction, modulation of adrenergic neural 91
cyclic guanosine monophosphate (cGMP) 55, 97, 139, 144, 145

cyclic guanosine monophosphate (cGMP) kinase, cytosolic 11
cyclooxygenase 102, 117
cystic fibrosis (CF) 81, 171, 176, 191
cytokine, proinflammatory 171, 177

disease, nasal 177
dose-response effect 179
dynamic respiratory compliance (Cdyn) 136, 137, 138
dysfunction, endothelial 213

electrical field stimulation (EFS) 42
electrochemical probe, NO-sensitive 134
endothelial cell 80
endothelial cell, bronchial 167
endothelial cell, vascular 147
endothelin 128
endotoxin 173
eosinophil 178
eosinophil, apoptosis of 156
eosinophil, migration of 153, 157
epithelial cell 167, 171
epithelial cell, bronchial 147
epithelial cell, murine 171
epithelium 129, 130
epithelium, tracheal 130
ethanol 171
exercise, physical 173,189

forced expired volume in one second (FEV1) 178

ganglium, parasympathetic 76
glucocorticoid 173, 189
glucocorticoid prednisolone, oral 177
glucocorticoid therapy 167
glutathione 188
Griess reagent method 129
guanylyl cyclase 10, 145, 146
guanylyl cyclase, soluble 55 72

haemoglobin 145
haemorrhagic shock 211
histamine 103, 130, 131, 133, 135, 136, 139, 140, 141, 144, 145, 173
histamine, responsiveness of 130, 131
host defence 190
human 141, 146
hybridisation, in situ 73
hyperaemia 172
hyperoxia 26
hyperresponsiveness, bronchial 135, 136
hypertension, systemic 176

hyperventilation 170, 173, 190
hypocapnia 140, 141
hypotension 212
hypoxia 104
hypoxia, chronic 105
hypoxic pulmonary vasoconstriction (HPV) 102, 103

infection 176
infection, respiratory viral 119
inflammation 42
inflammation, chronic 81
inflammation, neutrophilic 176
inflammatory cell 152
innervation 73
innervation, non-adrenergic non-cholinergic (NANC) 42
iron-heme center 145
ischaemia reperfusion injury 26, 27, 28

Kartagener's syndrome 177, 191

leukotriene 117
leukotriene B4 (LTB4) 100
leukotriene C4 133
leukotriene D4 (LTD4) 144, 145
lipopolysaccharide, inhalation of 176
lipoxygenase 117
lung 51, 152
lung disease, interstitial 176
lung injury 28, 29
lung resistance (Rlung) 131, 137, 138, 141

macrophage 167
macrophage, alveolar 158
mast cell 157, 175
measurement, nasal 185
metastasis 82
methacholine 133, 138, 139, 142, 143, 144, 145, 173
methemglobinemia 138
mucosa, nasal 178

nasopharynx 168
necrosis 31
neonate 203
nerve 41
nerve, cholinergic 93
nerve, parasympathetic 97, 167
nerve, sympathetic 90, 97
neuropeptide Y (NPY) 99
neurotransmission, nitrergic 57
neurotransmitter, excitatory non-adrenergic non-cholinergic (eNANC) 95

neurotransmitter, inhibitory non-adrenergic non-cholinergic (iNANC) 95, 97
NG-monomethyl-L-arginine (L-NMMA) 178, 215
NG-nitro-L-arginine methyl ester (L-NAME) 178, 215
nitric oxide (NO) 41, 94, 95, 97, 99, 100, 151, 167
nitric oxide (NO), as a bronchodilator neurotransmitter 173
nitric oxide (NO), as a vasodilator 172
nitric oxide (NO), bacterial 188
nitric oxide (NO), biosynthesis of 9
nitric oxide (NO), endogenous 91
nitric oxide (NO), exhaled 112, 154, 175
nitric oxide (NO), exogenous 137
nitric oxide (NO), expired 133, 136
nitric oxide (NO), expired levels of 136
nitric oxide (NO), inhaled 137–143, 146, 210
nitric oxide (NO), inhibitor of 10
nitric oxide (NO), level in mixed expired gas 133, 147
nitric oxide (NO), nasal 172
nitric oxide (NO), non-enzymatic 188
nitric oxide (NO), production of 104, 105, 134-136
nitric oxide (NO), pulmonary production of 133
nitric oxide (NO), release of 97, 101
nitric oxide (NO)-related compounds 137, 143
nitric oxide synthase (NOS) 51, 105, 167, 209
nitric oxide synthase (NOS) activity, inhibitor of 215
nitric oxide synthase (NOS), inhibitors of 173, 175
nitric oxide synthase (NOS), neuronal isoform of 78
nitric oxide synthase (NOS), subcellular location of 78
nitric oxide synthase (NOS), ultrastructural studies of 78
nitric oxide synthase (NOS), constitutive 111
nitric oxide synthase, endothelial (eNOS) 6, 79, 105, 167
nitric oxide synthase, inducible (iNOS) gene expression of 154
nitric oxide synthase, inducible (iNOS) mRNA, expression of 175
nitric oxide synthase, inducible (iNOS) 7, 78, 111, 167, 185, 189
nitric oxide synthase, neuronal (nNOS) 5, 73, 97, 167
nitrite 172
nitroglycerin 143
nitroprusside 143, 144

nitrosylation 145
nitrothiol 172
nitrotyrosine 114
nuclear factor B (NF-B) 177
nucleus, vagal 93

ONOO⁻ 24, 29–31, 113
organ dysfunction 212
oropharynx 188
ovalbumin 113, 136
oxidative damage 31
oxygen delivery 141
oxygenation 194
oxygenation, arterial 141

peptide, atrial natriuretic (ANP) 99
peptide, calcitonin gene-related (CGRP) 96, 99
peroxidation, lipid 23, 28, 29
peroxynitrite 13, 113
plasma, extravasation of 75
platelet-activating factor (PAF) 103
polypeptide, vasoactive intestinal (VIP) 96, 99, 128
post synaptic density protein (PSD), 93 78
post synaptic density protein (PSD), 95 78
primate 188
prostaglandin D2 99, 103
prostaglandin E1 99
prostaglandin E2 99, 103, 117
prostaglandin F2a 99, 103
prostaglandin I2 99
protein, expression of 105
pulmonary artery 76
pulmonary circulation 89, 171, 194
pulmonary hemodynamics 141
pulmonary hemodynamics, vascular 146
pulmonary hypertension 82, 173, 176, 194
pulmonary hypertension, hypoxic 105
pulmonary hypertension, persistent 203
pulmonary hypertension, primary (PPH) 205
pulmonary vascular pressure 141
pulmonary vascular resistance 141

reactive nitrogen species (RNS) 22, 24, 26, 29–32
reactive nitrogen species (RNS), as second messenger 31
reactive oxygen species (ROS) 22, 26, 27, 29–32
reactive oxygen species (ROS), as second messenger 31
receptor, muscarinic 94
reflex 92, 94
regulation, cholinergic 93

regulation, humoral 99, 100
relaxation, iNANC 97
relaxing factor, endothelial-derived (EDRF)
    4
relaxing factor, epithelium-derived 115
respiratory resistance (Rresp) 131, 136
respiratory tract 152
respiratory tract, infection of the lower 173
respiratory tract, infections of the upper
    170
respiratory tract, upper 168
response, adrenergic 91
response, cholinergic 94
responsiveness, bronchial enhanced 133
responsiveness, bronchial 130, 133, 143
rhinitis, allergic 193

salbutamol 173
sclerosis, systemic 176
shunt fraction 141
signal transduction 31
sinuses, paranasal 172, 187
sinusitis 192
smoking 173
smoking, acute and chronic effects of 171
smooth muscle, relaxation of 42, 74
S-nitrosothiol (RSNO) 137, 144, 145
S-NO-cysteine 144
S-NO-glutathione 144
S-NO-thiol 146
soft palate 170
specific lung conductance (sGaw) 141, 142
sputum, induced 178
Staphylococcus aureus 177
steroid, inhaled 173
substance P (SP) 96, 133

sulfhydryl group 145
superoxide dismutase (SOD) 13
superoxide 113

T lymphocyte 157
techniques, immunohistochemical 72
Th2 cytokine 157
thiol group, nitrosylation of 12
thromboxane A2 (Tx A2) 100
tidal breathing 170
tissue oxygen extraction, defect of 213
tomography, computerised 175
tomography, high-resolution computed
    139
tumor 82

vagal reflex 140
vagal stimulation 93, 130
vascular hyporeactivity 213
vascular smooth muscle 141, 144
vascular tone, pulmonary 90, 98, 99, 106
vascular tone, regulation of 90
vasoactive intestinal peptide (VIP) 45
vasoconstrictor 100
vasodilatation, cholinergic 93
vasodilatation, iNANC-mediated pulmonary
    98
vasodilator, response of 94
vein, pulmonary 77
ventilation-perfusion (V/Q) 141, 146, 172
virus infection 170
virus, parainfluenza type 3 119, 133

xanthine oxidase (XOD) 24, 27, 28